RELIGION, HEALTH AND SUFFERING

RELIGION, HEALTH AND SUFFERING

Edited by

JOHN R. HINNELLS AND ROY PORTER

Routledge
Taylor & Francis Group
LONDON AND NEW YORK

First published in 1999 by
Kegan Paul International

This edition first published in 2011 by
Routledge
2 Park Square, Milton Park, Abingdon, Oxon, OX14 4RN

Simultaneously published in the USA and Canada
by Routledge
711 Third Avenue, New York, NY 10017

Routledge is an imprint of the Taylor & Francis Group, an informa business

First issued in paperback 2016

British Library Cataloguing in Publication Data
A catalogue record for this book is available from the British Library

ISBN13: 978-0-7103-0611-1 (hbk)
ISBN13: 978-1-138-99722-6 (pbk)

Publisher's Note
The publisher has gone to great lengths to ensure the quality of this reprint but points out that some imperfections in the original copies may be apparent. The publisher has made every effort to contact original copyright holders and would welcome correspondence from those they have been unable to trace.

The Editors
wish to dedicate their work
in this workshop and volume
to

MR KEVIN HARDINGE M.CH.ORTH, FRCS
CONSULTANT ORTHOPAEDIC SURGEON
AT WRIGHTINGTON HOSPITAL

as a mark of great respect for his skill and care
in keeping John Hinnells
'on the road' for a quarter of a century.

ACKNOWLEDGEMENTS

The editors wish to thank the Wellcome Trust and SOAS for their generous financial assistance in supporting the conference on this theme, held at the Wellcome Institute in September 1996, which has formed the basis of this book. Thanks as always to Frieda Houser for her organisational skills, without which neither the conference nor the book could have happened. Tony Jeffery proved an excellent copy-editor, Roger Knowles has formatted the typescripts with extraordinary efficiency and Jean Runciman has contributed the excellent index. Our thanks to all.

CONTENTS

INTRODUCTION

The interaction between religion and medicine is universal throughout recorded history. They meet at the great turning points of life: at birth, at moments of acute suffering and at death. Not only are priest and doctor often needed at the same time and place, the two roles have also been combined in ancient and modern societies. Indeed, the separation of the roles in Western society may be seen as a consequence of modern secularising trends. In the medieval and pre-modern West, the Church was the main source of aid for those who were ill. Even in the twentieth century, Christian medical missions, Buddhist monks, Shamans, diviners, all combine the role of religious and medical practitioner. In most religions and cultures, the position of the healer has been seen not simply as socially respectable, but also as religiously important.

However, relations between healers and religious leaders have not always been good. In modern Western society established churches, both Catholic and Evangelical, have objected, indeed obstructed, some surgical procedures such as abortion. Similarly in the nineteenth century, many Christians objected to the medical alleviation of pain in childbirth because of the passage in Genesis (3:16) where God punishes Eve for eating of the fruit of the tree of knowledge and says: 'I will greatly multiply your pain in child-bearing; in pain shall you bring forth children.' It should also be said that many religious leaders in religions the world over, have inflicted suffering and torture in order to obtain converts or punish heretics. Religions have not always been the caring forces their adherents sometimes emphasise!

But whether healers and religions have worked in harmony or been in conflict, what cannot be doubted is their frequent and substantive interaction. It is, therefore, remarkable how few books have been written on the subject,[1] and explains why the editors chose to organise the International Workshop which lies behind this volume. One of the distinctive features of this project is that it brought together scholars of religion, historians of medicine, anthropologists and medical practitioners.

Patients approach suffering with a whole range of presuppositions about the nature of suffering, its cause, consequence and treatment. A holistic medical approach cannot ignore the patient's emotional or cultural 'baggage'. Whether the health care worker shares the patient's religious views is irrelevant. If such views affect the patient's physical or psychological condition, they should form an important part of the care programme. Western medical treatment, not least the Cartesian mind/body dichotomy, and conventional psychiatric practice of talking out traumatic experiences, can be wholly inappropriate in some cultures, as Honwana shows so vividly in her chapter on post-war Mozambique in this volume. The treatment in the West of patients from non-Western societies requires sensitivity to their cultural and religious background, as Cohen illustrates in his chapter.[2]

There is also a range of theological questions relating to religion, health and suffering. Monotheistic religions have particular problems with the explanation of suffering. If God is all loving and all powerful, why do the righteous and the innocent (e.g. babies) suffer? Religions which teach rebirth have an obvious explanation, namely that one is suffering as a consequence of sins committed in a previous life. But in that case why should one seek a medical cure, if it is an effect which has to be lived through? If suffering is a form of divine punishment, is it religiously right to seek to cure it? Most religions believe in miracles, but they too present theological problems. Why does God, or the gods, answer the prayers of some, and not of others? It is patently clear that it is not always the virtuous or the religious who experience miraculous cures. The belief in a just and powerful God is difficult to maintain in the face of life experiences.

Religions have offered many explanations of why the innocent suffer. Plagues have often been attributed to God's wrath against sinners in Judaism, Christianity and Islam, how else can one explain the experiences of the godly or the innocent in such afflictions? (see the chapters by Solomon, Melling, Conrad and Sachedina). In the 1990s some Christian fundamentalists attributed problems of BSE to divine punishment. The idea that suffering is a punishment is common in many cultures, not least in the Western world. Suffering is seen as 'the wages of sin', both in popular television programmes (see the chapter by Julia Leslie) and of formal theologies (see, in addition to the chapters just listed, that of Singh). Disabled people in all societies are commonly made to feel inferior. A short time in a wheelchair will soon disabuse anyone of the idea that there is no prejudice against the disabled, and people with lengthy illnesses all too quickly are seen as burdens, as though their condition is something for which they are responsible. These frequent prejudices may be explicable without recourse to religious teachings, but certainly religious teachings have legitimated or reinforced them. It would, for example, be naive to depict Christianity as being a religion which only teaches loving care of the sick. Perhaps the clearest link between suffering and sin is in the New Testament, where Jesus cures the sick by forgiving their sins. Although the Church did aid plague victims, the first step was to call for repentance (see Wear's chapter). A consequence of linking sin and suffering is not only that some people see the sick as being at fault, patients themselves have felt a sense of guilt. Perhaps the only religion to formulate a doctrine which depicts suffering as wholly evil and separate from the will of God is Zoroastrianism (see the chapter by Hinnells).

Religions are rarely internally logically self consistent. There are many and diverse explanations of suffering in all the religions. In Christianity, as in some secular Western views, suffering is said to be good for you. It is seen as character building (usually an explanation offered by the healthy!); as an opportunity to share in the passion of Jesus. Self-inflicted suffering is a part of various religions, for example, flagellation, asceticism and mortification of the flesh are part of Islamic practice, notably in Shi'ism, and Christianity. Similarly in various forms of Indian religions, conquering the body is seen as a necessary step on the path to liberation. Overcoming suffering is sometimes, therefore, seen as a religious opportunity, to demonstrate the mastery of the spirit over the flesh. Suffering on earth may be seen as the anticipation of post mortem punishments, and thereby obviating the need for them in the hereafter. As Conrad notes, plague victims were placed alongside martyrs in some Islamic teaching. Although Hinduism traditionally explains suffering as due to the effect of *karma*, action in a previous life, as Leslie comments, many Hindus do not wish to acknowledge personal 'fault' for their suffering and so explain their own suffering as due to the curse of another person. Although others may explain suffering as due to the fault of an individual, that individual rarely accepts such an explanation for themselves.

Just as religions may cause suffering through missionary endeavours, so they may do also at a personal level, for example by causing huge guilt complexes through damming what others would see as natural instincts and activities (e.g. masturbation or homosexuality). But they sometimes also provide the cure, through confession or sacrificial offerings. Religious activities can, whether the religion be seen as 'true' or 'false', be therapeutic. The point made by Singh concerning the positive effects of Sikh prayers on stress-related illnesses, might be made for other religions also through prayer, worship and meditation (see the chapter by Rawcliffe). Intercession in prayer, hoping for a miracle, can give hope where nothing else helps. Religious ceremonies can provide a catharsis for grief, when words fail.

Religion often overlaps with what are sometimes (though not always helpfully) referred to as folk traditions and remedies. In the ancient Mediterranean world, temple and secular medicine were not rigidly separated (Horden, King and Wear). Similarly in other cultures, ancient and modern, traditional healing medicine embraces a world view and understanding of human nature which is shared by the religions of the respective regions, for example some of the underlying ideas behind herbal medicine or the Taoist teachings on managing one's bodily energies (Bray), or the concepts underlying acupuncture and the principles behind Ayurvedic medicine (Wujastyk).[3] Although emerging from a different world view many of these practices are attracting growing interest in Western society (Saks).

Academics frequently debate at length on what is meant by the term 'religion'. This book takes an inclusivist view and does not draw a tight boundary between religion and culture. Religion is far more than a mere set of beliefs, or an optional way of life. It is also a conditioning, a powerful expression of identity, the embodiment of a received tradition of world views, of personal understanding, of values, priorities, hopes and fears. It is for that reason that chapters are included both on formal Buddhist doctrines (Skorupski) and an anthropological perspective on Tibetan medicine (Samuel), on classical Hindu literature (Leslie) and on more 'popular' Indian tradition (Wujastyk), and why there are chapters on traditional (Bray) and 'alternative' medicines (Saks), alongside others on formal Christian, Jewish, Islamic, Sikh, etc. theologies. Within other individual chapters authors have discussed both 'official' and 'popular' teaching and customs, and point out some of the practical implications for health care workers of the beliefs and practices of the religions.

If 'religion' is a debated term, 'magic' is even more so. Writers have often made attempts to distinguish between a religious prayer as being a request to the divine which may or may not be successful, and magic which is thought of as an automatic process. This is grossly over simplistic. Religious people believe in the power of prayer, people who practice magic are well aware that it does not always work. All too often 'magic' is other people's prayers. Consequently, this book includes what some call magic, just as it includes establishment religion. What is, perhaps, striking, is that although the religions differ between and within themselves on doctrines, there is a remarkable degree of similarity between the 'folk traditions' or magical practices. Not only in the use of herbs, diviners, amulets, astrology but also with the belief in the evil eye. It is necessary for all to be included in this book because however the Western trained health care worker may view folk traditions, religious people the world over rarely separate official theology and traditional practice. Commonly religions incorporate the folk traditions into their belief systems and formal practices. In Western multi-religious societies, health care workers should realise that patients will commonly resort to traditional practices alongside conventional medicine, be those practices prayers in church or temple, the lighting of votive candles, the invocation of ancestors, herbal remedies, the wearing of amulets, Christian or non Christian, and the driving out of malign spiritual forces. The more serious the condition, the more likely a patient is to take out a 'comprehensive' religious insurance policy. Indeed it is precisely at such times that many people become more rather than less religious. Religious assumptions and sensitivities are inevitably at their most acute at the time of death and bereavement.[4] Any health care worker who is not sensitive to the patient and the family's religious needs and values cannot be said to be caring for the whole person (see in particular the chapter by Cohen). There are also different patterns of illness, as well as different attitudes to various illnesses among the sick of various communities.[5]

If the terms religion and magic require comment, so too does 'suffering' (see especially the chapter by Porter). Pain, physical disability and disease are far from being the only experiences of suffering. In one sense all suffering is in the mind – does an unconscious person feel pain? Buddhist teachings (see the paper by Skorupski) emphasise that the basic cause of suffering is not pain, but craving, the desire to be other than what we are. Suffering can be said to be culturally conditioned.[6] As Solomon comments, being childless is in some traditions an especially acute form of suffering. If religions have theological problems with physical suffering, many have yet greater difficulties with psychiatric illness.[7] The problems again vary between and within religions and cultures. People claiming to be divine may in some ages or places be accepted as such, others be considered insane.[8] What is for one person a serious psychiatric illness, may for another be spirit possession. If the patient believes in the latter, does the medical care have to accept that and practice accordingly? Does a diviner need to be consulted alongside any treatment with medication? But more than that what is 'normal' behaviour in one society, may be deviant in another. Rack relates how a Pakistani woman in Bradford was thought by her relatives to be mad because she behaved coquettishly towards the men folk, whereas the psychiatrist they took her to thought she was behaving normally.[9] Most societies, not least Western, find psychiatric illness difficult to accept. The depressed are commonly told to 'snap out of it' – the very thing they cannot do. Illnesses may be described as 'psychosomatic' and therefore in a sense not 'real'. Asian religions and cultures struggle perhaps even more with the notion of psychiatric illness, and so patients and family may be yet more reluctant to 'admit' to it.[10] A physical explanation, with placebo treatment alongside any other, may result in a readier acceptance of the condition. In all medicine, but especially in psychiatric care, ignoring a patients 'cultural baggage' must almost inevitably result in loss of effective treatment for anything but the most straightforward problems such as a broken leg. But as Littlewood demonstrates so clearly in his chapter in this book, even in Britain's officially highly acclaimed health care system, in practice, the care for those with a psychiatric illness is negligible. This often affects particular classes and groups, notably those inner city populations, which is where many Black and Asian families live. There is also a strong sense among many of Britain's minority groups that racial bias is evident in the staffing (especially regarding promotion), in research priorities and not least in the stereotyping of patients by health care workers,[11] again an issue which medical staff should be alert to.

Despite the size of the workshop and the book, there remain many related issues still to be addressed. Three obvious ones are attitudes to the body, to sexuality and to death and bereavement – issues which may be addressed in future workshops. The editors are grateful to their respective institutions for the financial and material support given to this project, and to the contributors for their co-operation. We both hope that the future collaboration will be as much fun as this one has been.

NOTES

1. Two books which consider the attitudes of various religions to suffering are: J. Bowker, *Problems of Suffering in Religions of the World* (Cambridge: Cambridge University Press, 1970); L. E. Sullivan (ed.), *Healing and Restoring, Health and Medicine in the World's Religious Traditions* (New York, London: Macmillan Press, 1989). On a related theme there is also Jane M. Law (ed.) *Religious Reflections on the Human Body* (Bloomington: Indiana University Press, 1995).
2. See also J.H.S. Fuller and P.D. Toon, *Medical Practice in a Multicultural Society* (Oxford: Heinemann, 1988) and C. Helman, *Culture, Health and Illness* (Bristol: Wright-PSG, 1984, repr. 1986); Waqar I.U. Ahmad, *'Race' and Health in Contemporary Britain* (Buckingham: Open University Press, 1993 repr. 1994).
3. The standard work on Ayurvedic medicine is J. Filliozat, *Classical Doctrine of Indian Medicine,* trans by Dev Raj Chanana (Delhi: Munshiram Mancharlal, 1964). See also C. Leslie (ed.), *Asian Medical Systems: a comparative study* (Berkeley: University of California Press, 1976).
4. See D.P. Irish, K.F. Lundquist and V.J. Nelsen (eds.), *Ethnic Variations in Dying, Death and Grief: Diversity in Universality* (Washington: Taylor and Francis, 1993); G. Howarth and P. C. Jupp (eds.), *Contemporary Issues in the Sociology of Death, Dying and Disposal* (New York: St. Martins Press; Basingstoke: Macmillan, 1996); D.W. Moller, *Confronting Death: Values, Institutions & Human Mortality* (New York/Oxford: Oxford University Press, 1996).
5. R. Littlewood and M. Lipsedge, *Aliens and Alienists: Ethnic Minorities and Psychiatry* (London: Routledge, 3rd ed. 1997), especially ch. 12.
6. See Helman, *Culture Health and Illness*, ch. 6.
7. See P. Rack, *Race, Culture, and Mental Disorder* (London: Tavistock Publications, 1982); S. Fernando, *Mental Health in a Multi-ethnic Society: A Multidisciplinary Handbook* (London: Routledge, 1995); and the review of recent writings and developments in the 3rd edition of Littlewood and Lipsedge, *Aliens and Alienists: Ethnic Minorities and Psychiatry.*
8. See Helman, *Culture, Health and Illness*, ch. 9.
9. Rack, *Race, Culture, And Mental Disorder*, 97f.
10. Littlewood and Lipsedge, *Aliens an Alienists*, ch. 12.

11. See especially, W.I.U. Ahmad, *Race and Health in Contemporary Britain* (Buckingham: Open University Press, 1993).

I

HEALTH AND SUFFERING IN ZOROASTRIANISM

John R. Hinnells

Introduction

Zoroastrianism is the religion started in Iran by the prophet Zoroaster in approximately 1,200 BCE. It is, therefore, one of the earliest of the prophetic religions. For over a thousand years, from the founding of the Persian empire in the sixth century BCE until the rise of Islam in the seventh century CE, it was the official religion of the world's largest empires of those eras. When Islam conquered Iran, the Zoroastrians were increasingly oppressed and forced to retreat into the secure obscurity of remote desert settlements, mainly near Yazd and Kerman, where a few thousand survive to the present day.[1] During the regime of the last Shah many Zoroastrians flourished, but with the founding of the Islamic Republic by the Ayatollah Khomeini in 1979 they assumed a lower public profile, and a number (mostly, but not only, well-to-do people from Tehran) migrated to the West, mainly to California and British Columbia and some to Europe.

But the more numerous Zoroastrians are the Parsis in India. When life under Islam became severe in the ninth century, a small band of Zoroastrians set out from the province of Pars and settled on the North West coast of India and were known as the people from Pars, or Parsis. Under British rule they flourished as middlemen in trade, pursued Western education in proportionately large numbers and thereby became leaders in various professions and in politics. Their educated Bombay leaders became very Westernised.[2] From the eighteenth, but especially in the nineteenth and twentieth centuries, they travelled around the world for trade and for study, establishing small communities in Hong Kong, East Africa, America and Australia. Their oldest and largest settlement outside India is in London.[3] This paper will consider the Zoroastrian teachings on health and suffering under four headings: (a) the theology of the classical literature; (b) the ancient folklore out of which much theology grew, but which survives in some popular practices; (c) modern beliefs and practices both in the old countries and in the dispersion; (d) a conclusion on the implications for health care workers caring for Zoroastrians.

(A) Traditional Zoroastrian Theology

This section is based primarily on texts written down around the ninth century in the Middle Persian (or Pahlavi) language to support the faithful in the face of Islamic persecution.[4] Some of the texts are summaries and translations of the ancient Avestan scriptures in a language now little understood; other texts are expositions of the faith in the light of contemporary experiences. Much of the theology expounded here is, therefore, an expression of earlier thought, some going back to the time of the prophet, and is based on an even older cosmology. The logical point at which to begin the exposition is with the concept of creation.[5]

Fundamentally, Zoroastrians believe that if good in the world makes you believe in God, Ohrmazd, then the reality of evil, exemplified in the suffering of the innocent, logically leads to a belief in a devil, Ahriman.[6] There appear to have been several ancient Iranian creation myths.[7] In what emerged as the classical Zoroastrian doctrine of creation, God and the 'devil', Ohrmazd and Ahriman, existed independently of each other from the beginning. Ohrmazd dwells on high in endless light, perfect but not all powerful because of the existence of Ahriman who dwells below in deepest darkness. Due to his inveterate ignorance, Ahriman was unaware of Ohrmazd's existence, but Ohrmazd in his omniscience knew of Ahriman and created the world as a trap in which to ensnare and destroy evil.[8] First the world was created in *mēnōg* form, that is invisible and intangible. After three thousand years Ohrmazd then created the *mēnōg* world in *gētīg*, that is visible, tangible form. The material world is not, therefore, the opposite of the spiritual, as it is in many religions, but rather the embodiment of the spiritual. The world of *mēnōg* and *gētīg* is commonly referred to in Zoroastrianism as 'the Good Creation'. In its original state the world was perfect. Humanity, the plant and animal creations were without need, at peace, deathless. But on seeing this Good Creation, Ahriman, typical of his destructive instincts, attacked the world inflicting suffering, misery, disease and death. In Zoroastrian thought the whole of existence reflects the ultimate cosmic battle between good and evil: opposed to light there is dark; to the heavenly beings there are the demonic forces; to life there is death; to divinely created health there is demonically caused suffering; to beauty there is ugliness; to beneficent, holy animals like the dog or cow, there are evil creatures (*khrafstras*) characterised by their destructive instincts, such as snakes, lizards and scorpions, though the most common image of death is the polluting fly. And so the Good Creation was subject to evil assault. The face of the earth was seething with noxious creatures, the sacred creation of the fire was afflicted by smoke; plants withered and died, and the archetypal creature and person were assaulted with pain, suffering and ultimately death. The natural human condition, therefore, is a state of perfection, health and immortality. Pain, fever, ill health and mortality are unnatural conditions. Disease and infection are the works of Ahriman.[9]

The history of the world is the story of the battle between the forces of good and evil. Humanity is thought of as Ohrmazd's chief weapon or helper (*hamkār*). Zoroastrians believe that if people follow the ideals of the Good Religion, as revealed through Zoroaster, then ultimately good will triumph over evil. They look forward not to the end of the world, for that would be the end of Ohrmazd's Creation, but to its renovation (*frašegird*). There will, at the end of history, be a final cosmic battle as the forces of good and evil pair off in combat. In its death throes, evil will unleash one last assault on the world so that all social values will be overthrown, the young will not respect their elders, nor the students their teachers; the chaos will be cosmic also, the sun and moon will not give their light. But good will triumph. A saviour will come and raise the dead, for if death were the end of life then Ahriman's destruction of the divinely created body would represent his victory. When everyone dies they face a judgement before the divine scales. If the good thoughts, words and deeds outweigh the evil then the soul is guided across the bridge of judgement by a beautiful maiden, the manifestation of the person's conscience, to the house of light and song, heaven. If the evil outweigh the good then the soul is led trembling by an ugly old hag, the manifestation of the soul's conscience, across the bridge from where it falls into hell, a place of darkness, foul stench, bad food and punishment. The rewards and punishments are made to fit the crime, or the virtue, for the purpose of hell is corrective. This first judgement after death is clearly one of the *mēnōg* dimension of a person, for its *gētīg* body can be seen to remain on earth after death. The purpose of the resurrection is, in part, to enable the judgement of the *gētīg*, and body and soul return to heaven and hell, as appropriate. But once rewarded or punished and after passing the trial of molten metal, the purified person dwells in heaven, which is literally the best of both worlds, of the *mēnōg* and the *gētīg*. The second reason for the resurrection is that the whole human being, body and soul, can dwell with Ohrmazd. With evil defeated, Ohrmazd is now not only all good and omniscient, but also all powerful. Suffering, misery, disease and death are eradicated.

The myth expresses key ideas for the traditional Zoroastrian understanding of the body and of suffering. The material world is not opposed to the spiritual but its expression. Because the spiritual and material worlds are so interrelated, health necessarily involves the good state of both aspects of human life. The *gētīg* world is the divine creation, consequently evil cannot assume *gētīg* form. It can only dwell like a parasite within the *gētīg* body, or work through the form of noxious creatures. In one sense, therefore, evil does not really exist for it can exist only in the unseen *mēnōg* Whereas in some religions, the human being is a spiritual entity trapped in the body in an evil, alien material world, in Zoroastrianism the opposite is the case. To use Western terms, the devil is an evil spiritual force trapped in what is for it the alien environment of a good material world.[10]

How does this understanding of human nature demand that one should live? The basic duty is summed in a Pahlavi text, the *Dēnkard*:

> It is possible to put Ahriman out of the world in this manner, namely every person, for their own part, chases him out of their body, for the dwelling of Ahriman in the world is in people's bodies. When he will have no dwelling in people's bodies, he will be annihilated from the whole world, – for as long as there is in this world dwelling even in a single person a small demon, Ahriman is in the world. [Instead] The heavenly forces should be made to inhabit that place which if they inhabit, they are made to inhabit the whole of this world, and the heavenly forces, too, when they made rulers over people's bodies, they are rulers over the whole world.[11]

The demons which are to be ejected include Violence, Fury, Greed, Wrath, Sloth, and the essence of all evil, the Lie. But while people are caught up in this conflict, they are assaulted by such evils as pain, suffering and death.

The concept of pollution is important for an understanding of Zoroastrian attitudes to health and medicine. Any dead object is the scene where evil is powerfully present. The greatest focus of such evil pollution is the corpse of a holy person, for that is evil's greatest triumph. As soon as death occurs, the demon Nasu, described as a hideous, mottled fly, comes from the north, the home of the demons. If Nasu is strengthened she multiplies diseases, distress and destruction.[12] But anything which is dead, or decaying matter, is also polluting, whether that is dirt or rotting matter. Similarly, anything leaving the body such as excreta, nail clippings or cut hair, is dead matter. Even blood, which while it is in the body is life sustaining, is dead and therefore polluting when out of the body. The obvious example of this is menstruation. In Zoroastrianism, the religious roles are the same for men and women. Both wear the same symbols of the religion, the sacred shirt and cord, or *sudrē* and *kustī*; both have the same obligations of prayer; both have the same responsibilities in temple worship and the funeral rites are the same. But women have a particular role. As human life is the Good Creation of Ohrmazd, so the womb may be seen as the special locus for the daily conflict of good and evil. Just as the evil Ahriman attacked life at the beginning of creation, so he does in the womb. The monthly flow of blood, and the death often associated with childbirth in antiquity, was seen by Zoroastrians as the renewed assaults of evil. During her periods, therefore, and shortly after giving birth, a woman is the hapless victim as evil seeks to attack. The woman is, at these times, impure. There is no implication of sinfulness, but there is a strong sense of evil forces lurking waiting to attack, and so her movements, social and religious contacts, are restricted. It is because of this monthly pollution that women cannot be priests in Zoroastrianism.

These beliefs concerning the nature of pollution and death determine funeral practices. Since the dead body is the locus of evil it cannot be buried in the sacred earth for that would result in the pollution of the holy, similarly it cannot be disposed of at sea because the waters are sacred; nor can it be cremated because that would pollute the sacred element of fire. Instead, the traditional Zoroastrian funeral involves exposing the corpse in a *daxma*, or

'Tower of Silence' as the British called them, where the flesh is consumed by vultures (believed to have been created by Ohrmazd for the purpose of saving the creations from such pollution). The bones are powdered by the heat of the sun and disposed of in a central pit. Many modern Parsis argue that such a practice is hygienic, economic with land, natural (for as humans eat meat in life so in death we feed the birds), and expressive of the fundamental democracy of the religion for all, rich and poor, male and female, are treated alike.

But menstruation and death are not the only occasions when evil forces lurk. In order to protect humanity from evil's assaults which cause such suffering and death, Ohrmazd sent 9,999 medicinal herbs to counter the same number of diseases which Ahriman let loose on earth.

> One ought to be diligent and eager to know each medicinal plant and drug, for by knowing medicinal plants and drugs one may abolish ailments and diseases in the world against which there is no (other) stratagem. Besides, Ohrmazd the lord created a medicine for each ailment and disease which Ahriman brought into the world.[13]

Chief among the medicinal plants is Haoma (the Iranian form of the Indo-Iranian Soma) who is said to enfeeble the demons, fiends, wizards and witches. The plant Haoma is crushed in an ancient and central Zoroastrian liturgy, the *Yasna*, and represents,the heavenly priest who protects people from evil and gives divine inspiration.[14] Similarly Ohrmazd sent his holy word in the prophet's teaching and the holy prayers which, when recited in purity and faith, can protect people from the powers of evil. For those affected by pollution, for example corpse bearers, or for people seeking real purity, such as practising priests, there are a number of purificatory rites ranging from a bath and associated prayers, to a nine day purification ceremony.[15] An important means of purification is the use of cow's urine (*gōmēz*) especially in its consecrated form (*nīrang*). Cow's urine has a high ammonia content, and what can disinfect physically is thought by both Hindus and Zoroastrians to be able to cleanse spiritually when sipped. Some Parsis argue that the consecration process removes all harmful bacteria and that this is an aid sent by God to help people cleanse themselves spiritually.[16] Above all, if people expel the demons from within and give a home to the heavenly forces they receive protection. How people have faced up to the suffering inflicted upon them will count in their favour at the final judgement:

> When a man stands in the religion of the gods, the gods notice the pain endured by him in the world . . . and they carry and keep for him in the Reckoning of the Spirits, the discomfort, hunger, thirst, worry and disease which affect him.[17]

But in this present state of existence where good and evil are mixed together, and Ohrmazd is not omnipotent, evil remains free to attack.

Various Zoroastrian texts offer different analyses of human nature, the most common being that each person consists of five parts: body, soul, consciousness, heavenly self (or *fravaši*) and the ideal form.[18] Evil seeks to destroy people by dividing the human self so that internal disharmony undermines the person. Zoroastrians believe that it is important that body and soul are in harmony, with the health of one depending on the health of the other. If the body is not kept healthy, then the divine forces will not dwell within it.

> It is necessary to keep one's body in joy and to hold one's hand from doing harm. For a man whose body is in joy Wahman [one of the most powerful of the holy forces] dwells in his body, and when Wahman dwells in the body it is difficult to commit sins . . . a man who desires to be wise . . . should always keep his body under guard so that demons do not become victorious and ruling over his body. [19]

Any activity which develops one aspect of human nature to the detriment of the other is harmful. For example, both fasting and asceticism are wrong because they exalt the *mēnōg* over the *gētīg*, equally gluttony and debauchery are wrong because they exalt the *gētīg* over *mēnōg*. A central principle of Zoroastrian ethics is to follow the middle path. They deployed Aristotle's notion of the Golden Mean to express what is a fundamental Zoroastrian idea. Sin is defined as excess or deficiency, and virtue is seen as the middle point between contrasting vices. Ill health due to excess or deficiency in a way of life that is freely chosen is, therefore, sinful.[20] Inevitably in such a thought frame, the physicians who ease externally afflicted suffering are seen as performing a holy role. So in Sasanian times (third to seventh century CE) the priests were often doctors and the priest of the holy word is said to be the greatest healer in the ancient (pre-Christian) hymn, *Yašt* III.6. Some of the ancient religious heroes, notably Thraetaona, and the ideal king Yima (or Jamshid) brought healing for the people.[21] The latest Zoroastrian High Priest in Britain, Dastur Sohrab H. Kutar[22] exemplified this ancient link in the modern world, for he was also a medical doctor. He has been the only priest outside Iran and the Indian sub-continent to be formally recognised by the senior authorities in the old country as a high priest. Before his installation as a dastur there was debate about whether his work as a doctor necessarily involved him in having to deal with impurity (corpses, blood, urine samples, etc.) that however holy a person he may be (and none doubted that), was he not necessarily polluted? The decision was that being a doctor was a holy profession and could be combined with the highest priestly standing. A number of priests in India also engage in healing work through the teaching of special personal prayers or mantras.

(B) Ancient Iranian Folklore Regarding Health and Suffering

Having discussed traditional Zoroastrian doctrines on the subject it will be helpful to turn backwards, chronologically, to the bedrock of traditions from which we may assume Zoroastrian theologians developed their doctrines, apart that is from Zoroaster's prophetic inspiration. There was in ancient Iran a widespread belief in the demons of sickness and death controlled by witches or wizards, *pairikās* and *yātus*[23] They are referred to in many ancient Zoroastrian texts, sometimes negatively, as for example in the Pahlavi text the *Greater Bundahišn* V. 1 where the sorcerer's spell is seen as the evil counterpart of the holy prayer of Zoroastrians. But there are other passages where these are evidently seen simply as part of the unseen, yet real, world. In particular, there was in Iran, as in many societies, a belief in the evil eye.[24] This belief appears also in some of the secular epic literature, a genre often more indicative of 'popular' religion than the 'official' theological texts. So in the Parthian romance dating from the early years of the Common Era, there are references to a mother breathing on a beautiful daughter's face so that the evil eye may not harm her,[25] or the heroine's nurse utters a charm so that she is not harmed by the evil eye.[26] The same text also illustrates the point that witchcraft, spells and incantations were not necessarily thought of as harmful, or what we would call 'Black Magic', for the same nurse is described in several passages as using incantations to aid her charge's love life and to inspire the (semi) hero Vis to love the beautiful Ramin.[27] A similar contrast in the image of *pairikās*, translated above as witches, has been noted by Bivar[28] who suggests that in the epic literature the term 'fairy' – i.e. not a malevolent being – may be more appropriate at least in some contexts. Here, as commonly in academic studies, there is no translation without interpretation and the use of terms such as 'witches and wizards' conditions the Western reader's perception of the subject. In some of the official Zoroastrian literature, there may be such connotations but even here the concept of the holy mantra, the sacred prayer, and its use by many followers of the religion, may not in practice have been too far removed from what is translated as the spells and incantations of popular religion. Countless amulets have been discovered by archaeologists from ancient times in which some of the figures from Zoroastrian texts and Iranian folklore are invoked against the itch, hot fever and the humours.[29] Zoroastrianism, like other religions, absorbed, reinterpreted and used ancient demonic folklore. However witches, spells and the evil eye were depicted in such 'official' texts as the *Bundahišn*. It is also clear from more secular literature, and from archaeological excavations, that at the popular level such people and forces were seen as powerful, effective and not necessarily harmful. In ancient Iran, as elsewhere, many people, not least the majority underclass, felt themselves helpless in the face of unseen threatening forces which assaulted them fiercely, frequently and unpredictably in health, safety and general misfortune. It was, therefore, only natural to seek the aid of protective powerful forces. What Zoroastrian theologians did was to incorporate these common fears, beliefs and practices, into a coherent theological understanding of good and evil, one which resulted in a unique answer to the problem of suffering, of the religious duty of bodily care and healing.

(C) Some modern Zoroastrian Attitudes to Health and Suffering

Just as Christianity has changed from, say, the teaching of the medieval theologian, St Thomas Aquinas, down to the twentieth century, so too has Zoroastrianism. The initial point to emphasise is the diversity of modern Zoroastrian teaching. The first division is between the beliefs and practices of Iranian Zoroastrians and the

Parsis in India. The former have generally kept within the metaphoric walls of their own community, because of the hostility they have faced from Muslim authorities. As a result Iranian Zoroastrians, especially in the rural areas, have been subject to less external influence.[30] In so far as they have been influenced by the external religious environment, they have reaffirmed those aspects of the religion most in accord with Islam, the respect for the holy book, the access of non Zoroastrians to worship, the relative unimportance of what Parsis see as the external badges of the faith, the *sudre* and *kustī*, the (at least theoretical) possibility of conversion – theoretical because in practice Muslims did not convert, for such apostasy warranted execution. But it is an idea which Iranian Zoroastrians have carried with them into the diaspora. Parsis, especially from cosmopolitan Bombay where they have acquired significant levels of Western education and have not felt threatened by Hindus, have been more open to both Westernising and Hinduizing trends. This may be seen in the Protestantising of their attitudes to prayer, and also, especially since Indian Independence, in the acquisition of beliefs in rebirth, *karma* and the respect for the pure priesthood. Another contrast has already been implied, namely between rural and urban Zoroastrians. There are ways in which Bombay and Tehran Zoroastrians have more in common than either of them have with their rural counterparts. Partly because of my speciality, but also because they have produced more available literature, the following account focuses mainly on the Bombay (and Karachi) Parsis. Before considering their teaching it is necessary to give what might be described as a 'post-modernist' excursus. Scholars commonly have a perception of what the 'real' form of a religion is, what constitutes 'true Christianity' or 'the real Zoroastrianism', etc., which is commonly identified as the ancient faith. I would argue that a religion is what it has become; that a religion is what its members think and do when they believe that they are functioning as Zoroastrians, Christians, etc. Religions necessarily change if they are to be meaningful in different times and settings. It should not, therefore, occasion any surprise to find that the living form of Zoroastrianism, be that in Bombay, Tehran, or any Western city, appears different from the classical form outlined above.

The Liberal Protestants who influenced Western educated Parsis at the end of the nineteenth and early twentieth centuries provoked Zoroastrians to turn away from their traditional mythology, including the concept of Ahriman as an independent evil force, as a devil. They challenged them instead to look for an abstract philosophical faith, to demythologise their beliefs, and taught them to attach little, or minimal, importance to complex priestly rituals and the purity laws. Once the concept of Ahriman was demythologised as being simply an evil inclination within a person then the linchpin of traditional Zoroastrian teachings on suffering and death was undermined.[31] The purity laws were no longer seen (by the Western educated) as the prevention of pollution caused by Ahriman, but rather in terms of medical hygiene.[32] Some early twentieth-century Parsi writers used the Christian notion of suffering as a test imposed by God, referred to death as Ohrmazd calling people back to himself, and explained the death of children by saying that they were so good that they could not live on earth but had returned to their heavenly abode. Hell is interpreted by such writers, not as a mythical place, but as a state of mind.[33]

Such accounts have not resonated with younger Parsis who have been brought up in Hindu India. Many of them believe in rebirth and therefore see earthly suffering as the consequence of their actions in a previous life, as their *karma*. My impression, based on several years of visiting Bombay, is that Parsis are not alone among the non-Indian religions in incorporating such ideas into their daily life, be they Christian or even some Muslims. Similarly the notions of the divine incarnation, the Hindu teaching on the *avatār*, has affected how some Parsis see Zoroaster. Some Parsis use Hindu accounts of the material world as *māyā* (illusion) or the Hindu ideas of *Puruṣa* and *Prakṛiti* to explain their ideas on the material and spiritual worlds, and a number refer to yoga as a spiritual discipline leading to enlightenment.[34]

Many educated early twentieth-century Parsis, like many educated contemporary Hindus, reacted against the Protestantising, the rationalising, of their beliefs, by turning to the occult teachings of Theosophy. A number of Parsis were involved in the Theosophical Society while its headquarters were in Bombay (1879–1907). Theosophists taught that Western academics read ancient texts literally, and missed their mystical or occult significance. Theosophical belief was a mixture of Jewish kabbalah, Buddhist, Sufi and Hindu teachings. The founders, Madame Blavatsky and Col. Olcott, claimed to have received their inspiration from secret Tibetan masters. The appeal was, therefore, that it was a mystical movement, with Western connections, but which incorporated Asian teachings and reaffirmed hallowed ancient practices. This early Parsi involvement in Theosophy had longer term impact for a number of Theosophical ideas were internalised within the Zoroastrian community in a new Parsi religious movement founded by Behramshah Shroff (1858–1927) called Ilm-i Khshnoom 'the path of spiritual satisfaction'. Essentially it teaches rebirth and that, through a succession of disciplined lives, the soul progresses up the spiritual ladder, or along a path of spiritual unfoldment, until it is ready for birth as a Zoroastrian. The true Zoroastrian is in his/her last life before ultimate liberation. Each person has their own 'aura', or spiritual force field, which like the body, is strengthened by the traditional prayers and the purity laws.[35] The religious path involves the soul unfolding itself from the lower levels of physical matter to develop its latent higher spiritual powers. It can, therefore, be a more ascetic tradition than the classical position outlined above. One part of this process is becoming vegetarian, otherwise one swallows dead matter, which is against the moral order.

But it would be wrong to give an account of living Zoroastrianism among the Parsis as though it was all far removed from the ancient faith. Influential at the end of the twentieth century is a Parsi teacher, Khojeste Mistree, who studied under Mary Boyce in London. She inspired this mystically inclined lay man with a deep respect for the ancient tradition, including the Pahlavi teachings outlined in Part A of this chapter. In the 1970s Mistree began a teaching mission among Bombay Parsis and then to Zoroastrian communities around the world. He expounds the broad teachings outlined above in his book. At one point he states:

> The great strength of Zoroastrian doctrine lies in the fact that the agency which perpetrates excess or deficiency by way of poverty, chaos, disease and eventually death, is not that which is ordained by God but that which is perpetrated by the antagonistic spirit of evil.
>
> To conclude then, death, the negation of life, is the maleficient action of a hostile evil spirit who is fundamentally antagonistic to the inherent goodness of God. Therefore in Zoroastrian doctrine, God cannot be held responsible for death nor can He be deemed to be the creator or perpetrator of evil in the world.[36]

And later he writes:

> . . . the inequalities reflected through poverty, despair, misery, pain, suffering, disease are not due to a previous life punishment [i.e. not through rebirth], but exist as a result of the constant battle between the antagonistic forces in this life.[37]

The classical teaching outlined earlier is therefore reasserted vigorously by one of the most active (but also controversial) religious teachers among the Parsis. An attempt to popularise some of Mistree's teachings has been made in the form of a novel by his friend and former student, Tina Mehta,[38] whose daughter had earlier, produced a book reflecting Mistree's teaching on Zoroastrianism for young Parsis.[39] The ancient traditions have, therefore, been revived and are part of the living and the popular religion. The problem with the modern literature discussed above, is that it is the work of the literary religious 'activist'. What of the beliefs and practices of the ordinary Zoroastrian? Ultimately this can be understood only by extended periods of fieldwork. My own research in Bombay since the early 1970s suggests that a reasonable representation of the daily beliefs and practices of the majority of ordinary Zoroastrians is depicted in what is the fairly new genre of Parsi literature, the (English) novel. Eighteen novels (or collections of short stories) have been written by Parsis since 1968.[40] These, I suggest, can be a good insight not only into the 'soul' of the author, but sometimes also into the soul of the community from which they emerge. In the case of the Parsi novels it is important to exercise some caution. Just as there is no better source of anti-Jewish jokes than the Jewish community, so also the typical Parsi humour, and the novels, do 'send up' the Parsis. The apparent self-mocking has to be allowed for. Not all Parsis have quite such a bawdy sense of humour, as big a nose nor such large appetites for food and alcohol, as the novels suggest. On the whole, however, it seems to me that their pictures of religious belief and practice have some foundation in the contemporary community.

The first point to make is the Parsi involvement in Western medicine. To my knowledge this microscopic community of approximately 120,000 persons world wide, has helped fund forty-three hospitals,[41] and the first Indians to study medicine in the West were Parsis in the 1860s.[42] A medical career is particularly respected in Parsi society both because it is consistent with traditional

Zoroastrian values, and because it gives respectability in contemporary society. Both within Parsi novels, and in real Bombay life, Parsis commonly search diligently for Parsi practitioners of Western medicine not just out of tribal loyalty, but also because they believe them to be better, and as a result of the Parsi purity laws, they are commonly seen as more careful about hygiene.

But few Parsis in the novels, or in my experience, are ready to put all their trust in Western medicine. Many accept traditional Indian medicine, not least the views on the healing potential of what are categorised as hot and cold foods (not in terms of cooked and uncooked, but in terms of their perceived effect on the body). But beyond that, devotion towards Indian miracle working holy men; the recital of curative, personal holy mantras; visits to medicine men who dispense secret powder recipes, the consumption of herbs with healing powers and magical talismans;[43] the 'God forbid' gesture[44] to ward off the harmful powers of the evil eye,[45] and the offering of prayers to the gods of other religions, and astrology,[46] are common throughout both the novels and the Indian community. One quotation from a Parsi novel may illustrate this point. The loveable rascal hero, Faridun, or Freddy, is becoming increasingly desperate about his interfering mother-in-law and seeks supernatural aid to remove her and goes to a Muslim fakir.

> The fakir was not a phoney, Freddy decided, recollecting the enigmatic display of vials, powders and parchment. Surely the man had been in communion with spirits, unsavoury ones no doubt, when Freddy looked into the backroom hesitatingly from the threshold. He [Freddy] never had doubted black magic and witchcraft. Of course, he would take the precaution of counter-balancing any risk to his relationship with God with extra prayer and alms-giving.[47]

Sidhwa explains these beliefs in magic, ghosts, witches and the evil eye as due to Hindu influence on the Parsi,[48] but as noted above, much of this is found in the earlier sacred and secular literature. In Zoroastrianism, as in many traditions, the influence of folklore practices are as long lasting as the official teaching, if not more so. For those who believe in astrology, either the writers of ancient texts or members of the modern communities, their suffering is part of their fate. Historians of religion, and health care professionals alike, need to consider both popular customs and formal teachings, for it is often the customs not the learned texts which dominate at life-threatening, or anxious, moments. Whether or not historians or doctors believe in astrology, magic, witchcraft and the evil eye, if the Zoroastrian case is anything to go by, the religious patient may do so.

(D) Conclusion: Implications for Health Care Workers

The most convenient way to consider the implications of sections A–C is under the headings of the main life cycle events.[49]

In childbirth, the family may want to observe certain purity laws and ceremonies. There are no rites equivalent to baptism if the child's life is in danger, though a priest is necessary immediately if death occurs, or if that of the mother is under threat. Parsis commonly practice contraception, but barrenness would be seen by a traditional Zoroastrian as an evil curse. Impotency on the part of either partner is, however, in Parsi marriage and divorce law, a ground for the annulment of the marriage.[50] Intercourse in the later stages of pregnancy is said in the classical literature to be a sin, and the pregnant mother should avoid any pollution. Among Westernised Parsis, childbirth practices have few distinctive features, though if the birth is to occur at home, it would be traditional to invite a priest to bless the room where delivery is expected to take place, and to keep an oil lamp lit in the room after the birth. Traditionally, after the birth the woman remains at home for forty days, and the bedding used should be destroyed, but this is not common in the diaspora.

If surgery is required, there are no restrictions on blood transfusion as there are with Jehovah's Witnesses, although there have been several calls in recent times (mostly in Bombay) for the establishment of a Parsi blood bank, because of the belief that religion is part of the very person, in the blood or genes. There are no doctrinal arguments against *in vitro* fertilisation, though in India at least there would be priestly objection to the insemination of a Parsi woman with non-Parsi semen.

Although contraception is common among Zoroastrians, in theory the purpose of sex is the procreation of children so that homosexuality is traditionally seen as theologically sinful and referred to as the 'unnatural sin'. Masturbation is doctrinally wrong because of the waste of semen. In practice, homosexuality is becoming more acceptable among the young, but Kanga's novel shows what community pressures remain.[51] Because of the typical

Bombay Parsi quest for education and career advancement, among women as well as men, the average age at marriage is quite old (around 28 for women) which restricts the period of fertility.[52] There have been studies, though few published, suggesting that Parsis are prone to certain cancers rather than others. Breast cancer seems to be particularly common amongst Parsi women. It is feared that marriage within the family (between first cousins especially) is resulting in certain medical problems, from infertility to high levels of insanity. These suggestions are part of common discourse, but as yet with little hard medical evidence. Parsi women have, however, been found to be particularly prone to G6PD enzyme deficiency, making them highly susceptible to certain drugs, and prone to jaundice among the new-born and possibly causing severe haemolytic crisis in adults.[53]

The taking of human life is perhaps the greatest sin a person can commit, for it is ending what God created. Suicide and euthanasia are, therefore, doctrinally wrong. In India, a suicide would (where the facilities exist) be exposed in a separate Tower of Silence, because the sin is so serious. The easing of pain, and the restoration of health, is, conversely, working in support of the divine creation and therefore not merely a humane but a holy act. Abortions are rare, but I have known of them, more among the younger people in the West. Where the object is to save the mother's life there is no serious objection. In theological thought at least, abortion for social reasons would be considered the taking of life. But in view of the Westernised nature of the community, in India as well as in the diaspora, Western attitudes are strong. Probably all patients who have abortions need counselling, but this may be especially true of the religious Zoroastrian for it is not really consistent with traditional values.

Death and funerals are the time when the greatest sensitivity is required. A priest should be summoned, if possible, before death so that the repentance prayer (*Patēt*) may be offered. He would advise on appropriate religious procedures with the corpse. It is not common in the diaspora to follow all the practices such as bringing a dog into the presence of the corpse. But the family will want to gather and pray, and may want a Zoroastrian of the same sex to wash the body with *gōmēz* (though in general, Zoroastrians are closer to Western, than to Muslim, ideas on gender relations between patients and health carers). Traditionally the body should not be laid with the head facing north, for that was considered to be the region of the demons.[54] The bereaved will want to dress the body in the traditional *sudre* and *kustī* and to hold the funeral as soon as possible after death (though not after dark). Western funeral undertakers do not usually have the resources to observe all the practices (for example the body should be laid on a non-porous surface, e.g. a stone slab, so that the infection or pollution may not spread). Permission to leave a small burning oil lamp (*divo*) near the deceased, to represent the protecting presence of the divine, will give comfort. The place where the body was lain should normally be cleansed with *gōmēz*. Some Zoroastrians wish to have the body returned to India for the traditional disposal in the Tower of Silence, but few can afford this. The most common form of funeral is cremation, and burial of the ashes in a Zoroastrian cemetery. Some Parsi religious teachers prefer burial to cremation, because of the pollution of the sacred flame, and that form of funeral is more common among Iranian Zoroastrians. But other Parsi religious teachers believe that where exposure in a Tower of Silence is not possible then cremation is preferable as it involves pollution for moments rather than the years taken by decomposition. People need to rationalise what is fundamentally alien to their tradition. Many modem Parsis argue that it is not a pure flame which burns the corpse in a crematorium, but intense heat generated by electricity and therefore modern crematoria are not as doctrinally wrong as the form of cremation traditional in India. Whether this logic convinces the outsider is irrelevant. The important ceremonies for the soul have to be conducted in a ritually pure temple, i.e. in the old country. Having stayed with Zoroastrian families at times of bereavement, my subjective impression is that because the families find it impossible to carry out the rites which they have been conditioned from infancy to believe are important for the spiritual care of the deceased, a sense of guilt (however unjustified) may compound the natural grief. The family is expected to observe some social restrictions while praying for the deceased, but excessive mourning is considered harmful to the living, and unhelpful to the deceased. So although there are monthly and annual ceremonies for the deceased, there is rarely an extensive display of grief. The *fravašis* (heavenly selves) of the deceased are invoked at important festivals, but this is said to be so that they may share in the joy of the living, not with what a Westerner may consider a morbid intent. The annual rite of *muktād* (a Parsi term, *Fravardīgān* among Iranian Zoroastrians), when the dead are remembered, is a time when particular care is taken to observe the purity laws and non-Zoroastrians are not welcomed at such rites because they do not observe the purity laws. This exclusion may even be imposed where the spouse is non-Zoroastrian.

The ancient classical tradition, exemplified in the myths, and the popular practices, remain strong even among the Westernised, educated Zoroastrians of the diaspora. If a doctor is to treat the whole Zoroastrian person, some sensitivity towards their religious and cultural conditioning is important.

NOTES

1. The best single volume on Zoroastrianism from its earliest times to the present day is M. Boyce, *Zoroastrians: their religious beliefs and practices,* (London: Routledge and Kegan Paul, 1979, revised repr. 1988).
2. On the Parsis in British India see E. Kulke, *The Parsees in India: A Minority as Agent of Social Change* (Munich: Weltforum Verlag, 1974).
3. On the modern Zoroastrian diaspora see R. Writer, *Contemporary Zoroastrians: an Unstructured Nation.* (Lanham: University Press of America, 1994); J.R. Hinnells, 'The Modern Zoroastrian diaspora' in J. Brown and R. Foot (eds.), *Migration the Asian experience* (London and New York: Macmillan, 1994) 56–82; Hinnells, *Zoroastrians in Britain* (Oxford: Clarendon Press, 1996).
4. On this body of literature see M. Boyce, 'Middle Persian Literature', in B. Spuler (ed.), *Iranistik Literatur* in *Handbuch der Orientalistik.* IV, 2, 1, (Leiden: E.J. Brill, 1968) and Boyce, *Zoroastrians: their religious beliefs and Practices,* for the general history.
5. For a compendium of translations see M. Boyce, *Textual Sources for the Study of Zoroastrianism.* (Manchester: Manchester University Press, 1984, repr. Chicago: Chicago University Press, 1990). For a fuller exposition of the theology see R.C. Zaehner, *The Teachings of the Magi* (London: Allen and Unwin, 1956); Zaehner, *The Dawn and Twilight of Zoroastrianism* (London: Weidenfeld and Nicolson, 1961) chs. 12–15). For the mythology see Hinnells, *Persian Mythology* (London: Hamlyn Books, 1973, 2nd edition, London: Newnes Books, 1985) and on the notions of *mēnōg* and *gētīg* see S. Shaked, *From Zoroastrian Iran to Islam.* (Aldershot and Vermont: Variorum, 1995) chs. 2 and 3. On medicine in ancient Iran see J. Hampel, *Medizin der Zoroastrier im vorislamischen Iran* (Husum: Abhandlungen zur Geschichte der Medizin und der Naturwissenschaften 45, 1982). The three main Pahlavi texts to expound the creation, with some variations (see S. Shaked, *Dualism in Transformation* (London: School of Oriental and African Studies, 1995), are the *Greater Bundahišn*, especially, chs. 1–6 see B.T. Anklesaria, *Zand-Ākāsīh, Iranian or Greater Bundahišn* (Bombay: Rahnumae Mazdayasnan Sabha, 1956), *Zātspram*, ch. 1 see R.C. Zaehner, *Zurvan: a*

Zoroastrian Dilemma (Oxford: Clarendon Press, 1955) 339–43; *Dēnkard III* (J. de Menasce, *Le Troisieme Livre du Denkart* (Paris: Librairie C. Klincksieck, 1973). On the literature in Pahlavi see Boyce 'Middle Persian Literature.' There are inevitably important cosmological and cosmogonic details in numerous other texts, some indicating doctrinal variations see A.V. Williams, *The Pahlavi Rivāyat Accompanying the Dādestān ī Dēnīg* (Copenhagen: Royal Danish Academy of Sciences and Letters, 1990) Part II, 72–76. For the eschatology see B.T. Anklesaria, *Zand-ī Vohman Yasn* (Bombay: private publication, 1957). Note: there is no standard form of transliteration of Avestan or Middle Persian words. In this chapter the transliteration used is that of the author being referred to. This occasionally results in inconsistency, for example in this footnote the titles of the books by Shaked's *Dēnkard* and de Menasce *Dēnkart*. This may occur in some of the words used in the text. The intention behind the adopted practice is to avoid confusing any reader who wishes to pursue a reference. The text uses the transliteration of the book referred to in the associated footnote.

6. See Zaehner, *Teachings of the Magi*, ch. 4.
7. A. Christensen, *Les Types du Premier Homme et du Premier Roi dans l'Histoire Legendaire des Iraniens* (Stockholm: Kungl. Boktryckeriet & P.A. Norstedt & Soner, 1917). The extent to which a single 'orthodox' Zoroastrian system of myth and doctrine emerged prior to the Islamic era is currently a matter of debate, see Shaked *Dualisms in Transformation,* and the review of that book by M. Boyce: 'On the orthodoxy of Sasanian Zoroastrianism', *Bulletin of the School of Oriental and African Studies,* lix (1996), part 1, 11–28.
8. Translation in Zaehner, *Teachings of the Magi*, 49–51.
9. See the Avestan text, the *Vendidād* 20:3 and 9f. Unfortunately the only complete translation of this text remains the dated one by J. Darmesteter, vol. IV in the *Sacred Books of the East* (ed. F. Max Muller, Oxford: Oxford University Press, 1880 and repr. Delhi: Motilal Banarsidas, 1965).
10. Shaked, *Dualisms in Transformation*, chs. 2&3.
11. VI. 264f, S. Shaked, *Wisdom of the Sasanian Sages*, (Boulder, Colorado: Westview Press, 1979),103f.
12. *Vendidād* 9.47f; 5, 27–32; 7.9f.
13. *Dēnkard* VI. 308, Shaked, *Wisdom of the Sasanian Sages*, 123.
14. See M. Boyce, 'Haoma, priest of the sacrifice' in M. Boyce and I. Gershevitch (eds.), *W.B. Henning Memorial Volume*, (London: Lund Humphries, 1970) 62–80.
15. On these purification ceremonies see J.J. Modi, *The Religious Ceremonies and Customs of the Parsees*. (Bombay: 1922: J. Karani & Sons, 2nd ed. 1937, repr. Bombay and New York, 1980).
16. The late High Priest in London, Dastur Dr S.H. Kutar, himself a medical doctor, sent a sample of *nīrang* for analysis at the London School of Hygiene and Tropical Medicine which reported that no harmful bacteria were found. He published the report in the May issue of the popular Parsi journal, *Parsiana*. Bombay, 1969.
17. *Dēnkard* VI. 106. Shaked, *Wisdom of the Sasanian Sages*, p. 43.

18. A classic study of this material is H.W. Bailey *The Zoroastrian Problems of the Ninth Century Books.* (Oxford: Clarendon Press, 1943, 2nd ed. 1971) ch. 3. See also Zaehner, *The Dawn and Twilight of Zoroastrianism*, 269ff and Shaked, *Dualisms in Transformation*, 134–45.
19. *Dēnkard* VI. 193 & 250, Shaked, *Wisdom of the Sasanian Sages*, 75 & 99.
20. Zaehner, *The Dawn and Twilight of Zoroastrianism*, 270–86.
21. See the scriptural text *Vendidād* 20 for the former and the great epic composed, largely from ancient sources, the *Shāh Nāma*, for the second see, R. Levi, *The Epic of the Kings, Shāh Nāma*, (London: Routledge and Kegan Paul, 1967) 11 and related in Hinnells, *Persian Mythology*, 33–40.
22. Died 1984, see Hinnells, *Zoroastrians in Britain*, 141f.
23. L.H. Gray, 1930, *The Foundations of the Iranian Religions*, (Bombay: K.R. Cama Oriental Institute, 1930) 195–7.
24. See B.N. Dhabhar, B.N., 1963, *Translation of the Zand-i Khūrtak Avistāk*, (Bombay: K.R. Cama Oriental Institute, 1963) 114, 142f, 193f, 196 and *Greater Bundahišn* V.i in Anklesaria, *Zand-Ākāsīh*.
25. O. Wardrop, *Visramiani* (London: Royal Asiatic Society, 1966) para 13.
26. Wardrop, para 62.
27. Wardrop, paras 80, 97, 100, and 269.
28. 'A Persian Fairyland' in H.W. Bailey, A.D.H. Bivar, J. Duchesne-Guillemin, and J.R. Hinnells, (eds.) *Papers in Honour of Mary Boyce.* (*Acta Iranica*. vols. 24 and 25, Leiden: E.J. Brill, 1985) 25–42.
29. A.D.H. Bivar, *Catalogue of the Western Asiatic Seals in the British Museum. Stamp seals: II The Sasanian Dynasty*, (London: The British Museum, 1969) and see *Vendidād* 20.
30. See especially M. Boyce, *A Persian Stronghold of Zoroastrianism*, (Oxford: Clarendon Press, 1977, repr. Lanham: University Press of America, 1989), and on the more urbanised Tehran Zoroastrians, see J.K. Amighi, *The Zoroastrians of Iran: Conversion. Assimilation, or Persistence*, (New York: AMS Press, 1990).
31. See for example the writings of the New York educated Karachi High Priest, M.N. Dhalla, *Homage Unto Ahura Mazda*, (Karachi: Private publication, 1942 and numerous Indian reprints) and Hinnells 'Modern Zoroastrian Philosophy' in B. Carr and I. Mahalingam (eds.), *Companion Encyclopaedia of Asian Philosophy*, (London: Routledge, 1997) 64–92.
32. See, for example, the writings of the scholar priest Sir J.J. Modi, notably his *A Catechism of the Zoroastrian Religion.* (Bombay: Parsi Punchayet, 1911, repr. 1962) and his *Religious Ceremonies and Customs of the Parsees.* (Bombay, Karani & Sons, 1937 repr. New York, 1980).
33. Notably Dhalla, *Hommage unto Ahura Mazda.*
34. I.J.S.Taraporewala, *The Religion of Zarathushtra* (Bombay: B.I. Taraporewala, 1926, revised ed. 1965); F.A. Bode, *Sharing the Joy of Learning* (Bombay: P.N. Mehta Education Trust, 1978).
35. P.S . Masani, *Zoroastrianism. Ancient and Modern.* (Bombay: private publication, 1917) 84. On Theosophical and Khshnoomic teaching, see further Hinnells, 'Modern Zoroastrian Philosophy.'
36. K.P. Mistree, *Zoroastrianism: an ethnic perspective.* (Bombay: Private publication, 1982) 50.

37. Op. cit. p. 54.
38. T. Mehta, *The Zarathushtrian Saga*. (Calcutta: Writers Workshop, 1995).
39. A. Mehta, *The Story of Our Religion*, (Bombay: Zoroastrian Studies, 1976).
40. See Hinnells, 'Novel Religion: the Reflection of Zoroastrianism in Modern Parsi Secular Literature,' in A. Sharma (ed.), *The Sum of Our Choices: Essays in Honour of Eric J. Sharpe*. (Atlanta: Scholars Press, 1996) 384–407. In the eighteen months since that article was written, three more English language Parsi novels have appeared, reinforcing the point made there that it is a growing genre. They are: Mehta, *Zarathushtrian Saga*, 1995; R. Mistry, *A Fine Balance* (Toronto and London, Faber and Faber, 1995); A. Vakil, *Beach Boy* (London: Hamish Hamilton, 1997). I take this opportunity to thank Dr Michael Stausberg for his help in my work on these novels. The rush to meet a deadline meant that I failed to acknowledge his help as I should have done and for this I apologise. I am indebted to him for his characteristically helpful comments on this paper.
41. Hinnells, 'The flowering of Zoroastrian Benevolence: Parsi charity in the nineteenth and twentieth centuries' in Bailey *et al., Studies in Honour of Prof. Mary Boyce*, 261–326.
42. Hinnells, *Zoroastrians in Britain*, 82–3.
43. F. Kanga, *Trying to Grow*. (London: Bloomsbury Publishing, 1990) 3; B. Desai, B., *The Memory of Elephants*. (London: Andre Deutsch, 1988) 280.
44. B. Sidhwa, *The Crow Eaters* (Delhi, Sangam Books, 1978) 28, 34, 43f; R. Mistry, *Such a Long Journey* (London: Faber and Faber, 1991) 63ff; 96, 109; B. Desai, *Memory of Elephants*, 232f; Kanga, *Trying to Grow*, 28; Mehta, *Zarathushtrian Saga*, 306.
45. R. Mistry, *Tales from Firozsha Baag*, (Markham, Ontario: Penguin Books, 1987) 53; *Such a Long Journey*, 1:121; T. Mehta, *Zarathushtrian Saga*, 29, 103, 251; B. Sidhwa, *An American Brat* (Minneapolis: Milkweed Productions 1993) 194, 303. Milkweed have also published American editions of Sidhwa's other novels.
46. Mistry, *Such a Long Journey*, 149f; Sidhwa, *An American Brat*, 24, 46f. 162; Sidhwa, *Crow Eaters*, 34. 157; B.K. Karanjia, *More of an Indian*. (Bombay: Sindhu Publications, 1970) 23. For astrology in the ancient tradition see among many instances the *Greater Bundahišn V A*. Anklesaria, *Zand-Ākāsīh*, 59–65. For astrology etc. in the epic tradition see Wardrop's *Visramiani*. paras 15, 280, 318, 346, 390, 434, 441, 449. It occurs too often in the *Shāh Nāma* to be detailed, but see Levi *Epic of the Kings*. Intro. at p. xxv. Astrology appears in the epic on pp. 2 and 66; *pīris* or fairies p. 6; wizardry, pp. 15, 24; spells and incantations pp. 47, 88 to give but a small sample.
47. Sidhwa, *Crow Eaters*, 28.
48. Op. cit. 145f.
49. I am grateful to Ervad Rustom Bhedwar, the most active of London's Zoroastrian priests, for his comments, especially on this section. Of course responsibility for errors remains my own. Details of the traditional ceremonies mentioned here can be found in Modi's *Religious Ceremonies and Customs of the Parsees*, though some small details are

incorrect as this scholar of priestly lineage did not actually function as a priest.

50. M. Shabbir and S.C. Manchanda, *Parsi Law in India*. (the fifth edition, amended in the light of the 1988 Act) (Allahabad: The Book Company, 1991) 30–5.
51. Kanga, *Trying to Grow*.
52. M. Karkal, *Survey of Bombay Parsi Population–1982*. (Bombay: Parsi Punchayet, 1983).
53. Reported in the Bombay magazine, *Parsiana*, July–August, 1996, p. 186 – though in conversation some Parsi doctors have suggested to me that this is a general problem among the Indian population, and not a specifically Parsi characteristic. Thus far the only published specialist study of Parsi genetics is J.V. Undevia, *Population Genetics of the Parsis* (Miami, 1973). But that is clearly dated and there is scope for important original research here.
54. There is a common problem faced by expositers – how much of the detailed historical origins to relate? I know of no living Zoroastrian who thinks that the north is the home of demons. This manner of laying out the dead has simply become 'the proper thing to do'. One might compare the role of bridesmaids in Western Christianity. The original intention was to dress up young girls to look like the bride in order to confuse the demons of barrenness, attract them to themselves and so preserve the fertility of the bride. Few brides or bridesmaids know this, but maintain the custom as the nice and proper thing to do. Customs often last longer than doctrines. 'Doing the right thing' at key moments in life matters to people in all cultures, even if the people involved do not know the historical or religious origins of the practice.

THE IMPLICATIONS OF THE PHYSICAL BODY: HEALTH, SUFFERING AND *KARMA* IN HINDU THOUGHT

Julia Leslie

1. Introduction

How does Hinduism explain suffering? Since 'Hinduism' is an elastic term denoting a bulging compendium of religions, there can be no simple answer. This chapter will range across the classic statements of the Sanskritic textual tradition, including both soteriological and narrative material, and end with some of the shifting positions of contemporary belief and practice. I take the term 'suffering' to include everything from the status of the individual at birth (such as matters relating to caste and gender) to personal misfortune (such as poverty and bereavement) and specific physical problems (such as disability and disease).[1] In the process, I shall outline Hindu beliefs regarding the doctrine of *karma* and explore some of the implications of this doctrine for our understanding of the physical body.

But in case anyone thinks this material is too far removed from Western culture, I shall begin with *Casualty*, the popular hospital drama shown regularly on British television. The word 'casualty' derives from the Latin *casualitas*, meaning 'chance' or 'accident'. In recent years, however, this drama series has been suggesting the reverse. As Steven Poole puts it in an article in *The Independent*, 'disease and injury, these days, are never accidents but rather the wages of sin'. He provides three examples:

> A construction worker, who spends his family's housekeeping money on gambling, is listening to a race on the radio one day in his JCB. His horse loses, and in despair he accidentally crushes a colleague with a big chunk of concrete. An alcoholic advertising executive takes his girlfriend out on a massive drinking binge; the next day she vomits blood and is admitted

> to Holby [hospital] for detoxification. He, of course, vows to give up the liquor for good. Or again, a single father is alone with his young daughter at home one day when he suffers a cardiac arrest. His former wife comes to visit him in hospital, and when her toy-boy turns up she decides to dump him. See: such are the penalties of gambling, drink and home-wrecking.

The unambiguous and essentially religious message is that wrongdoing causes suffering, including physical problems. That is why *Casualty's* 'victims of gory mishap' are usually found confessing their sins, often to Charlie, the 'twinkly, caring head nurse'. For it seems that patients come to this hospital not to be cured or sewn up but to learn moral lessons. But there is an obvious catch. The message might be reassuring to the healthy – in the sense that it provides an explanation – but the additional burden of moral guilt is surely unbearable for the sick.[2]

If we take this idea of causation and moral responsibility into the context of Hindu thought in general, extending the time frame into past and future lives, we have a rough version of the doctrine of *karma* and rebirth.[3]

2. *Karma* and Rebirth

I shall merely note in passing that there is a major scholarly debate concerning the origins of this complex of ideas. According to some historians of Indian religion, the seeds of *karma* and rebirth can be found in the earliest extant form of Hinduism, the four Vedas (*c.* 1200 BC onwards), and in the later liturgical treatises referred to as the Brāhmaṇas.[4] According to others, these 'seeds' do not constitute convincing evidence of the existence of a *karma* theory prior to the speculative and essentially soteriological dialogues recorded in the Upaniṣads (the oldest of which may be as early as the eighth century BC). According to this view, the origins of the doctrine must therefore be sought outside the corpus and culture of the early Aryans and their Vedic tradition: perhaps among the early Dravidians, possibly including the Harappan Civilisation;[5] or among the heterodox sects, such as the Jains, the Buddhists and the Ājīvikas;[6] or among ancient tribal sources.[7] Some scholars reject the historical approach altogether in favour of a discussion of the three textual corpora – Vedas, Brāhmaṇas, Upaniṣads – not as three chronological stages but as three different aspects of the same question: that is, according to the schools of ritual practice in the Vedas, of theory in the Brāhmaṇas, and of mystical interpretation in the Upaniṣads.[8]

Whichever position one takes in this debate, a glance at the earliest of the four Vedas, the *Ṛgveda*, reveals a number of themes relevant to our discussion. First, the word *karma* (or *karman*) denotes the sacrificial act that upholds and ultimately controls the universe. For many scholars, the Vedic belief in correct ritual practice foreshadows the later *karma* doctrine for it encapsulates the belief that actions can produce effects in the often distant future 'without the ordinary process . . . of visible agents of . . . cause and effect'.[9] More generally, a person's behaviour (usually defined in terms of sacrifices to the gods, or giving sacrificial gifts to the priests, or heroism in battle) is seen to affect their future existence. The rewards for correct action include prosperity, long life, and health for oneself, one's offspring and one's cattle in this life, and the transition after death to the blissful 'region of the pious'.[10] The implication is that incorrect action (similarly defined) will bring the perpetrator none of these things. A further implication, raised but barely stressed, is that those who suffer have done something to incur that suffering. Thus a man plagued with dropsy – stumbling and trembling 'like a puffed up goatskin' – cannot remember committing any offence to warrant such a punishment: he begs the god Varuṇa to have mercy on him in his ignorance of his own evident wrong-doing.[11]

With regard to the mystery of what happens after death, we may note that in the *Ṛgveda* the notion of 'immortality' (*amṛta*) implies the full extension of life to one hundred years without excluding death: death is an accepted part of human existence. There are references to death in the next world too, even for the gods. But the location of this next world is vague and inconsistent: the abode of Yama, the god of death, is one possibility; a gesture towards metempsychosis is another.[12]

The *Śatapatha Brāhmaṇa* provides what is probably the earliest textual reference to the possibility of existing without the physical body. In an intriguing passage, Death complains to the gods that, due to the power of the sacrifice, human beings are now able to become immortal and escape his clutches. The gods make him a promise. From this moment on, no one will become immortal in the physical body. When 'as a result of knowledge or sacred action' a person is about to become immortal, he will do so only after he has separated himself from his body, that is, after Death has taken that body as his share. The reference to 'knowledge or sacred action' is then explained as the building of the fire altar for the sacrifice. The passage continues that those who understand this and perform the sacrifice will come to life again in the next world: eternal life in heaven (*svargaloka*). But these individuals are in the minority. Most people fall into the categoy of those who do not understand and who do not perform the sacrifice: they will come to life in the gloomy 'world of the fathers' (*pitṛloka*) where they will become 'the food of Death' again and again.[13]

The *Bṛhadāraṇyaka Upaniṣad* presents us with the first explicit account of the doctrine of *karma* and rebirth. The idea that human life might be extinguished altogether is not discussed: life continues, either in the bliss of 'immortality' or in another temporal existence that will culminate in another death. Since by dying in this world one reaches the next world, it seems logical that dying in that world should bring us back to this one. Instead of recurrent death (*punarmṛtyu*), therefore, we now find recurrent birth: *punarāvṛttiḥ*, literally 'revolving again'.

An early form of the Upaniṣadic doctrine proves to be an elaboration of the Brāhmaṇic distinction between 'the way of the gods' and 'the way of the fathers'. The vivid symbolism of the sacrifice permeates the whole passage. Man is likened to a sacrificial fire: 'in that very fire gods offer food, and from that offering springs semen'.[14] Sex is also a sacrifice, and woman the sacrificial fire:

> Her firewood is the vulva; her smoke is the pubic hair; her flame is the vagina; when one penetrates her, that is her embers; and her sparks are the climax. In that very fire gods offer semen, and from that offering springs a man.
>
> He remains alive for as long as he lives, and when he finally dies, they offer him in the [cremation] fire. . . . In that very fire gods offer man, and from that offering springs a [new] man of brilliant colour.
>
> The people who know this, and the people there in the wilderness who venerate truth as faith – they pass into the flame [of the cremation fire], from the flame into the day, from the day into the fortnight of the waxing moon, from the fortnight of the waxing moon into the six months when the sun moves north, from these months into the world of the gods, from the world

> of the gods into the sun, from the sun to the region of lightning. A person consisting of mind comes to the regions of lightning and leads him to the worlds of *brahman*. These exalted people . . . do not return.
>
> [But] the people who win heavenly worlds . . . by offering sacrifices, by giving gifts, and by performing austerities – they pass into the smoke [of the cremation fire], from the smoke into the night, from the night into the fortnight of the waning moon, from the fortnight of the waning moon into the six months when the sun moves south, from these months into the world of the fathers, from the world of the fathers into the moon. Reaching the moon they become food . . . [and] the gods feed on them . . . When that ends, they pass into this very sky, from the sky into the wind, from the wind into the rain, from the rain into the earth. Reaching the earth, they become food. They are again offered in the fire of man [the fire of digestion] and then take birth in the fire of a woman [the fire of sexual intercourse]. Rising up once again to the heavenly worlds, they circle around in the same way.
>
> Those who do not know these two paths, however, become worms, insects, or snakes.[15]

There is a significant change of emphasis here. The Brāhmaṇas stress the importance of the sacrifice to enable one to reach the heavenly worlds. The Upaniṣads keep the symbolism of the sacrifice but subordinate ritual to esoteric knowledge. They tell us how the laws of *karma* and rebirth take effect in human life.

For example, there are several earnest discussions between a teacher named Yājñavalkya and his student (one Jāratkārava Ārtabhāga) regarding the process of dying. The following conveys something of this teacher-pupil discourse:

> 'Yājñavalkya,' Ārtabhāga said again, 'tell me – when a man dies, do his breaths depart from him, or do they not?' 'They do not,' replied Yājñavalkya. 'They accumulate within this very body, causing it to swell up and to become bloated. So a dead man lies bloated.
> . . . 'Yājñavalkya,' Ārtabhāga said again, 'tell me – when a man has died, and his speech disappears into fire, his breath into the wind, his sight into the sun, his mind into the moon, his

> hearing into the quarters, his physical body into the earth, his self (*ātman*) into space, the hair of his body into plants, the hair of his head into trees, and his blood and semen into water – what then happens to that person?' Yājñavalkya replied: 'My friend, we cannot talk about this in public. Take my hand, Ārtabhāga; let's go and discuss this in private.'
>
> So they left and talked about it. And what did they talk about? – they talked about nothing but action [*karma*]. And what did they praise? – they praised nothing but action. Yājñavalkya told him: 'A man turns into something good by good action and into something bad by bad action.'
>
> Thereupon Jāratkārava Ārtabhāga fell silent.[16]

The furtive behaviour suggests that the doctrine of *karma* was at that time still a closely guarded secret, a truly esoteric doctrine.

In another conversation, Yājñavalkya is more overtly informative. This time, he describes how at the point of death the transmigrating soul withdraws from the physical body:

> Now, as this self (*ātman*) grows steadily weaker and begins to lose consciousness, these vital functions (*prāṇa*) throng around him. Taking into himself these particles of light, he descends back into the heart. When the person connected with sight turns back, the man loses his ability to perceive visible forms. So people say: 'He's sinking; he can't see!' – 'He's sinking; he can't smell!' – 'He's sinking; he can't taste!' – 'He's sinking; he can't speak!' – 'He's sinking; he can't hear!' – 'He's sinking; he can't think!' – 'He's sinking; he can't feel a touch!' – 'He's sinking; he can't perceive!' Then the top of his heart lights up, and with that light the self exits through the eye or the head or some other part of the body . . .
>
> It is like this. As a caterpillar, when it comes to the tip of a blade of grass, reaches out to a new foothold and draws itself onto it, so the self (*ātman*), after it has knocked down this body and rendered it unconscious, reaches out to a new foothold and draws itself onto it.

Yājñavalkya reaches his conclusion:

> What a man turns out to be [in his next life] depends on how he acts [in this one] . . . If his actions are good, he will turn into

> something good. If his actions are bad, he will turn into something bad.[17]

Another slant on the doctrine is produced by the role of desire. A person is impelled by desire, resolves to act in accordance with that desire, and then turns out in the next life in accordance with the resulting action. This idea feeds into an important thread in Indian religious thought: the issue of whether it is action or desire that fuels the karmic cycle of births; hence the notion – found most famously in the *Bhagavadgītā* – that salvation (*mokṣa*, 'release') derives not from ceasing to act but from ceasing to desire.[18]

With these two variations, then, we have the classic doctrine of *karma* and rebirth, first explicitly met with in the Upaniṣads. But what scholars refer to as a 'theory' of *karma* is a self-evident fact for most, if not all, Hindus.[19] It solves several major problems at once. The fear of death is resolved by the widespread expectation that one will survive and be reborn into another household. The existence and apparent injustice of suffering is resolved by an all-inclusive (if ultimately uncomfortable) theory of causality, of cosmic justice: there are no innocent victims. The desire to avoid suffering and rebirth altogether is met by the complementary doctrine of *mokṣa*, salvation defined as permanent release from the cycle of birth and death.

But the psychological consequence of this stress on moral responsibility – the burden of moral guilt that I mentioned in the context of the unfortunate patients in *Casualty* – remains unresolved.

3. The Problem of Moral Responsibility

The fact is that soteriological texts like the Upaniṣads do not adequately convey the emotional context of suffering. For this we must turn to the narrative tradition. In the context of classical texts, this means the two great Sanskrit epics: the *Mahābhārata* and the *Rāmāyaṇa*.[20] The core of each of these works can be dated to about the fifth or fourth century BC; however, while the world reflected there is earlier still, the reworking of both texts probably continued until about the fourth century AD.[21] My point here is that the epic narrative – told and retold in every vernacular down the ages – allows the human response to suffering to be articulated far more clearly than is possible in any soteriological text. I shall briefly draw attention to two examples taken from the Sanskrit *Rāmāyaṇa*: the suffering experienced by, Rāma's parents – King Daśaratha and Queen Kausalyā – at the start of the epic, and their rationalisation of that suffering in terms of *karma*. Daśaratha explains his misfortune in terms of *karma* incurred in his youth; Kausalyā explains hers in terms of *karma* incurred in a previous life. In both cases, current suffering neatly fits the remembered or imagined crime.

The story is well known. Daśaratha's favourite wife and Rāma's stepmother is a beautiful and spirited lady named Kaikeyī. In the past, she saved her husband's life twice on the battlefield and as a reward was granted two wishes. Now, when Rāma is about to be consecrated as Daśaratha's heir, Kaikeyī demands the fulfilment of those wishes: her own son, Bharata, must become king, and Rāma must go into exile for fourteen years. When Daśaratha hears her demands, his distress is overwhelming. He is 'shaken and unnerved, like a stag at the sight of a tigress', then sinks to the floor in a stupor, 'his heart crushed by grief'.[22] Regaining his senses, he begs Kaikeyī to reconsider:

> 'The greatest joy I know is seeing my first-born son. If I cannot see Rāma, I shall lose my mind.
>
> . . . I beg you! Must I get down and bow my head to your feet?'
>
> His heart in the grip of a woman who knew no bounds, the guardian of the earth began helplessly to cry, and as the queen extended her feet he tried in vain to touch them, and collapsed like a man on the point of death.[23]

When he comes to, Daśaratha begs again: 'Please, I am an old man, my life is nearly over.' He laments 'frantically and piteously, his eyes reddened and dimmed by tears', and again he falls unconscious to the floor.[24] Daśaratha's collapse destroys what is left of his life. Shortly before he dies of a broken heart, however, this violent grief revives a memory 'of something evil he once did'.[25] Long ago, while hunting in the forest, he killed a young ascetic by mistake. The young man's blind father cursed Daśaratha: 'Just as I now sorrow over my son's calmity, so you, too . . . shall end your days grieving for a son.'[26] The moral of the story is clear. As Daśaratha himself puts it, 'Whatever a person does, be it good or evil . . . he receives in like measure, the direct result of the deeds he has done himself.'[27]

I shall consider the suffering of Rāma's mother, Kausalyā, even more briefly. When she hears that her beloved son is to be exiled to the forest, her distress too is heart-rending. Vālmīki describes her as 'tortured by such unhappiness as she had never known before'.[28] To Rāma, she says:

> What will it be like when you are gone, my child? Surely nothing is left me but to die.
>
> . . . My heart must be made of iron that it does not split and shatter upon the ground, and my body too, under this crushing sorrow.[29]

Only later is she able to find a rational answer for her pain. 'I guess,' she says to her husband,

> . . . yes, it must no doubt be that once upon time, when calves were thirsting to drink, I ruthlessly hacked off the udders of the cows, their mothers.
>
> And so now . . . I who love my child so have been made childless by Kaikeyī as brutally as a lion might do to a cow with a young calf.'[30]

Later still, Rāma makes a similar imaginative guess to justify his mother's pain: 'It must be that in some past life women were separated from their sons by my mother's doing . . . and so this has happened to her.'[31] The karmic connection made, even as tenuously as it is in this case, and it seems we are expected not to dwell on the situation any further. Fault and guilt are theirs alone. But this is little consolation to Daśaratha and Kausalyā: for them as for us, the bitter pill of karmic explanation is easier to distribute than to swallow.

The anthropologist, David Pocock, puts it another way. 'Rebirth,' he suggests, 'is primarily for other people.' In the context of his own fieldwork among Gujarati peasants, he explains:

> It is when they speak of others, when they are looking for some wider theory to explain the misfortune . . . of others, that they have recourse to the theory of re-birth . . . The belief in some kind of eternal salvation relates to the future whereas the belief in re-birth relates to the past.[32]

The textual tradition betrays a similar tendency to use the *karma* doctrine as a means of explaining away the misfortunes of others. Even soteriological advice, which is clearly dispensed with an eye to the future, also explains the present in terms of the past. For example, the Upaniṣads teach us to avoid future rebirth by being 'mindful' and 'pure'; consequently, the fact that one has been born at all means that previously one was neither mindful nor pure.[33] All those who are to be reborn will demonstrate their spiritual status in the circumstances of their birth: those who have been good will enter the womb of a high-caste Brahmin, Kṣatriya or Vaiśya woman, while those of 'stinking conduct' will enter the 'stinking womb' of an Untouchable woman or a female animal.[34] While this teaching serves as a memorable warning to those looking to the future, for the lucky ones it also provides a reassuring explanation of the present. Birth as a male or a female on this continuum of births demonstrates a further hierarchical arrangement of good (i.e. male) and bad (i.e. female) – or good and not so good, or bad and even worse – with similar occasion for admonition and self-congratulation. Then there are the long lists of future penalties for wrong-doing that are to be found in the prescriptive texts known as the Dharmaśāstras, the earliest and most famous of which is the *Manusmṛti* (*c.* second century AD).[35] For example, a man who steals gold will have 'mangled fingernails' in his next life; a man who drinks alcohol will have discoloured teeth; a priest-killer will suffer from consumption; and a man who 'violates his guru's marriage-bed' will have a skin disease.[36] These penalties and many more like them are surely recorded in order to enlist good behaviour in the future, but they can also be used most effectively to justify the current misfortune or ill health of others.

In the context of the textual tradition, then, the *karma* doctrine seems to be fundamental to Indian thought. This is not to say that there is one consistent version of *karma* throughout the texts. A range of ideas is in evidence: group *karma*, the transference of karmic debt from one individual to another, the issue of the cycle of rebirths versus a cosmology of heavens and hells, the balancing of merits against demerits in the interpretation of karmic consequences, the railing against 'fate' (*daiva*), the power of the ascetic's curse or the anger of the gods when set against the *karma* of the individual, and the changing implications of devotional religion with its reliance on the grace of god to side-step even the consequences of *karma*.[37] Yet, beneath this variety of explanations lies the catch-all doctrine of *karma*, its scope so far-reaching that it seems it can never wholly be denied.[38]

The major shortcoming of the doctrine is that it does not tackle fully the resulting psychological burden of moral guilt, the burden no doubt experienced by the patients in *Casualty* when it is implied that they have only themselves to blame. The variety of responses to suffering revealed by contemporary accounts reveals that the situation is rather more complex than the texts often seem to allow. Before examining some of these accounts, however, I shall briefly explore the link between the inner self and the outer physical body.

4. The Self and the Body

By the self, I mean both the individual 'soul' or *ātman* and the wider complex of personality that in Indian religions is the result of the accumulated *karma* of many births. Both one's mental (including spiritual) state and one's physical body are defined by *karma*, and the latter reflects the former. This is, of course, a familiar idea: one's inherent nature (*svabhāva*) is the result of the merits and demerits of past lives, and one's physical birth and material circumstances are made to match. Thus the high-caste Kṣatriya is born with both a king's body and a regal nature. The low-caste Śūdra is born with a labourer's body and a servant's nature. When a person is born, he or she is (or at least should be) all of a piece. While there are mythological examples of mismatches between inherent nature and birth-and-circumstance packages, these merely serve to underline the traditional expectations of Indian religious thought.[39] The Śūdra's nature embedded in a royal body is unthinkable. The reverse, a Kṣatriya's nature in what is apparently a Śūdra body is the temporary but tragic fate of Karṇa: abandoned by his unmarried mother, Kuntī, he has the instincts and physical shape of the Kṣatriya but the social circumstances of his Śūdra foster-parents. Such a mismatch can only lead to tragedy.[40] Tragedy also befalls Ekalavya, the tribal boy who threatens to surpass the Pāṇḍavas in fighting skills. Their weapons' teacher, Droṇa, demands Ekalavya's thumb as his sacrificial fee: the mutilation makes a mockery of the boy's martial aspirations. Here the mismatch is resolved by cutting the errant body down to size.[41]

Physical appearance

Let us now focus on one part of what I have called the 'birth-and-circumstance package': a person's physical appearance. It is a commonplace in classical Sanskrit literature that a good man can be recognised by his good looks. To continue with my epic example, Rāma's beauty is well known, his physical form a perfect reflection of the perfection within:

> He was extremely handsome and his face had the lovely glow of moonlight. With his beauty and nobility he ravished both the sight and hearts of men.[42]

This explicit link between inner and outer perfection explains why texts like the *Manusmṛti* advise the king to select as his minister a man who is 'goodlooking' (*vapuṣman*).[43] Similarly, medical texts such as the *Suśruta Saṃhitā* recommend that, for his own safety, the king should choose a 'nice-looking man' (*priyadarśana*) as his personal physician.[44] The implication is clear: a man's good looks reflect the moral integrity within. A further implication is that an ugly man cannot be trusted.

Is this equally true in the case of women? The answer is as one might expect of a literature renowned for its ambivalence towards women: a woman's beauty may indeed reflect her inner goodness, as it does for the great heroines of the culture such as Sītā and Sāvitrī, but it may also be a trap set to ensnare the unwary. To continue my examples from the *Rāmāyaṇa*, Kaikeyī, Rāma's manipulative stepmother, is described as entrancingly beautiful but this seems merely to demonstrate that Daśaratha is not to blame: he is under the spell of a beauty which cannot be trusted.[45] A woman's lack of beauty is less problematic. External ugliness is always a warning of inner evil; hence the many epic examples of hideous demonesses. A particularly illuminating example is provided by Rāma's encounter with the demoness Śūrpanakhā, a *rākṣasī* or female *rākṣasa*.[46] In Vālmīki's Sanskrit version, the physical contrast between the two is striking:

> Rāma was handsome, the *rākṣasa* woman was ugly, he was shapely and slim of waist, she misshapen and potbellied; his eyes were large, hers were beady, his hair was jet black, and hers the color of copper; he always said just the right thing and in a sweet voice, her words were sinister and her voice struck

> terror; he was young, attractive, and well mannered, she ill mannered, repellent, an old hag.[47]

Interestingly while the Sanskrit *Rāmāyaṇa* clearly portrays Śūrpanakhā as hideous, the sixteenth-century Hindi *Rāmcaritmānas* by Tulsīdās describes her as beautiful; more significantly, both are equated with female iniquity.[48]

Disability

If we narrow our focus even more, the implications of a disabled body become clear. A person who is in some way disabled or deformed is assumed to have a distorted or immoral personality. That the physical deformity is the result of sins in past lives goes without saying. As the *Manusmṛti* puts it, 'because of the particular effects of their past actions, men who are despised by good people are born idiotic, mute, blind, deaf, and deformed'.[49] What is not always so clearly articulated is that it is the distorted inherent nature that gives rise to physical deformity, and not the other way around. The defective personality causes the defective body. In this context, it makes no sense to treat a disabled person as if their physical form has no bearing on their inner state; it is precisely that distorted inner state (the result of sins in past lives) that has given rise to, and is expressed in, the deformity.

My epic example is provided by Kaikeyī's servant in the *Rāmāyaṇa*. Mantharā is described as *kubjā*, a term usually translated 'hunchback',[50] and she is often depicted as an old woman with a pronounced curvature of the spine.[51] This portrayal suggests the conflation of two separate possibilities: a deformity from birth, and the spinal curvature produced by increasing age. According to at least one traditional interpretation, however, the term *kubja* more properly indicates a form of dwarfism, often accompanied by a curved or deformed spine;[52] in this case, a *kubja* need not be elderly but Mantharā probably was. This detail aside, Mantharā's disability is pronounced and conspicuous.[53]

As the story of Rāma's enforced exile proceeds, the blame for the upheaval of the kingdom shifts from the beautiful but duplicitous Kaikeyī to her ugly, crippled servant. Mantharā becomes the target of both verbal and physical abuse.[54] The justification is implicit: her physical body betrays her guilt. For the physical body is not simply a reward or punishment for the accumulated effect of past merits and demerits; it precisely manifests the condition of the mind and nature within. The female body demonstrates that Mantharā has attained a less advanced spiritual state than her male counterpart; the disabled body by definition contains a defective personality.

Heads and bodies

There is an interesting and typically Indian conundrum here. If the head represents a person's mind and inner nature, and the body the physical effect of *karma*, then what would be the result of a switching of heads and bodies?[55] This question was recently explored by Girish Karnad in his Kannaḍa-language play, *Hayavadana* ('The Man with the Horse's Head').[56] The play is based on a modern short story by Thomas Mann[57] which in turn was inspired by an ancient collection of Sanskrit tales, *Vetālapañcaviṃśatī* ('The Twenty-Five Tales of the Vampire'), embedded in Somadeva's *Kathāsaritsāgara* ('Oceans of Streams of Story').[58] Karnad's twentieth-century retelling of the story stresses the different physiques and personalities of two friends: Devadatta, poet and 'man of intellect', is contrasted with Kapila, wrestler and 'man of the body'. At the climax of the drama, in a deserted temple, each man in turn decapitates himself. When Devadatta's distraught wife, Padmini, is commanded by the Goddess to replace the heads so that the two men can be brought back to life, she becomes confused. By mistake, she attaches the decapitated heads to the wrong bodies. Faced with the choice of two composite men, she elects to stay with Devadatta's head on Kapila's body, on the grounds that the head is the thinking part of the individual and thus the real person. The athletic body on her educated husband is an admitted bonus, but temporary: by the end of the play the two bodies have transformed themselves so that they perfectly match the heads (and, by implication, the natures) to which they are now attached.[59]

This story obviously belongs in the realm of folklore. But the implication for real human beings is unavoidable: our physical form reflects our inner nature which in turn is the result of the accumulation of *karma* in past lives. So what does this mean in the context of physical health?

Disease

The message of the vast body of religious law (*dharmaśāstra*) is unambiguous: physical problems are the result of bad *karma*. 'He who does X will be reborn with affliction Y.'[60] Sometimes it is suggested that the behaviour of one person will have a karmic effect on another, an idea often applied to women. Thus a wife's good behaviour can ensure a better future for her husband, wiping out the effects of his own bad *karma*.[61] Similarly, the prohibitions directed at the menstruating or pregnant woman are reinforced by threats of defects accruing to the unborn child. For example, if she uses collyrium, her child will be blind; if she combs her hair, he will be bald; if she massages her body with oil, he will have a skin disease; and so on.[62] There are plenty of epic examples of this kind of transference from mother to child. In the *Mahābhārata*, for example, Dhṛtarāṣṭra is born blind because his young mother closed her eyes at the sight of the hideous old man sent to impregnate her according to the rules of levirate, while his stepbrother, Pāṇḍu, is born with an unnaturally pale skin because his mother turned pale with shock.[63] While the blame is placed squarely on the two mothers, however, the fact that Dhṛtarāṣṭra's blindness disqualifies him from kingship demonstrates that his disability identifies him (and not his mother) as inherently defective.

One way or another, then, karmic explanations place the burden of moral responsibility for physical affliction on the sufferer's own past actions. Indeed there is a type of literature, a 'set piece', that deals solely with such explanations: these passages on the 'ripening of *karma*' (*karmavipāka*) explain the precise consequences of every possible sin, using *karma* 'as a club with which to beat the listener into a suitably contrite frame of mind'.[64] But if all illness is the inescapable consequence of sin, what can be the role of the medical practitioner? How does one reconcile the implied determinism of the *karma* doctrine and a medical system that presupposes at least the possibility of a cure?

Mitchell Weiss, writing on *karma* in medical texts, discusses this problem at length.[65] As he points out, the impasse of karmic determinism versus the human need to act is addressed in a variety of religious and narrative texts as well as in the medical literature. The basic principle is the same: diseases do not afflict the person whose thoughts, words and deeds are as they should be. None the less, a healthy lifestyle and the use of appropriate medicines can overcome or ameliorate a medical condition whether it is the result of bad *karma* or of a curse, a spell, or divine or demonic anger. Only the effects of very bad *karma* cannot be averted.[66] The general conclusion is as one might expect: a disease may be cured by consulting this doctor or taking that remedy, but if it persists then the patient's bad *karma* is simply – and demonstrably – too strong.

5. Contemporary Explanations

Contemporary explanations of human suffering and ill health are, if anything, even less tidy than those provided by the textual tradition.[67] For example, in her study of a community in Himachal Pradesh, Ursula Sharma found that the choice of explanation for misfortune was largely derived from the desire to evade personal responsibility. Thus a man explained his severe rheumatism as the result of unknown *karma* from past lives; since the offence was both unknown and in the remote past, he evidently felt no need for remorse. By contrast, his neighbours preferred to blame him, attributing his ill health to the fact that he had felled a sacred pipal tree the previous year. In another case, a Brahmin woman with a skin disease that medication would not cure allowed two possible explanations: the practice of sorcery by her sister-in-law, or the anger of the goddess on account of her failure to fulfil a vow made earlier that year. Sharma notes that the woman both took ritual precautions against the possibility of divine anger and stopped eating at her sister's house; but she clearly preferred the explanation of sorcery since it placed all responsibility outside herself.[68]

A similar preference is suggested by a nineteenth-century account of the first outbreak of cholera in British India. According to Sleeman's report, the villagers blamed the outbreak squarely on the British, that is, outside their stricken community, apparently without any reference to their own karmic guilt. Their interpretation of events ran as follows. In 1817, in order to provide beef for the troops of Lord Hastings, a cow had been slaughtered in a sacred grove despite the remonstrations of the resident priest; as a result, cholera attacked the camp and from there spread throughout India.[69] It is tempting to think that the *karma* doctrine was given no explanatory power in this case. However, a comparison with another well-known example of a community disaster, the fire of Karimpur described by Susan Wadley and Bruce Derr, suggests otherwise.[70] The general opinion in Karimpur village was that the fire was caused by the sins of the Brahmin leaders; yet alongside this view was the widely held belief that all those who suffered or died in the fire had in some way incurred blame. Some sins were obvious to all (gambling, lechery, drunkenness . . .); others, not in evidence in this life, were surmised by reference to previous lives; while notorious sinners who had escaped the fire were deemed to have earned invisible merit that effectively counterbalanced their sins. If we relate this explanatory paradigm to the outbreak of cholera reported by Sleeman, we would expect to find similar kinds of karmic explanations for the suffering or deaths of specific individuals. But we must remember Pocock's remark about *karma* being for other people. As so many anthropologists have pointed out, and as the textual tradition repeatedly demonstrates, it is the unscathed commentator who is so free with explanations of karmic blame.[71] Those involved are far more likely to merge overarching karmic explanations with (or subordinate them entirely to) more specific (and, preferably, external) causes.[72]

In some ways, this subordination of *karma* is the mark of an individual's ability to tell his or her own story. Hence perhaps A K. Ramanujan's declaration that, in the folktales that he spent much of his adult life collecting, 'there is no *karma*'. Unlike in the great epics 'where the chain of cause and consequence is unrelenting', traditional storytellers seem to operate within a more personal theory of action. Through the process of telling, the story becomes the teller's own, no longer one more action in the karmic chain.[73] In the context of religious teaching, however, the doctrine of *karma* seems inescapable. As Narayan puts it, 'the average person is seen to be bound up in a tangle of relationships bred from past karma, generating new karma as he or she bumbles along'. People are linked by their *karma*, dependent on each other for the resolution of their karmic burdens. Even the saint or *guru* is implicated in this karmic 'tangle'. Like a washerman whose job it is to handle dirty clothes, the *guru* may become contaminated by the sins of his flock. Hence the ill health of many saintly individuals, whose only sin (or weakness?) seems to be the tendency to absorb (in the form of physical ailments) the sins of others. But the case of the enlightened individual is different in one crucial respect: while the physical body works though the karmic residue of past lives (hence the weakness, the vulnerability to others' pain), no new *karma* is created. At the death of the physical body, with no further impulse towards a new body, release (*mokṣa*) is theirs.[74]

Conclusions

I conclude that there are many problems with the notion of *karma* as a universal explanation for suffering and ill health. I have mentioned only some of them. However, both in the textual tradition and in contemporary accounts, the doctrine of *karma* remains as a kind of metaphysical safety net. As Sharma puts it, 'whilst the karma principle need not be the theory which the villager turns to first of all in his search for a meaning for the misfortune he suffers, it is generally the last which he will abandon.'[75] That the doctrine of *karma* appeals more to the physically and socially healthy (the higher castes, the wealthy, men, the able, and the well) than to the sick (the lower castes, the poor, women, the disabled, and the ill) is as obvious to the commentator on Indian society and culture as it must be to followers of the hospital drama, *Casualty*.

NOTES

1. For a more comprehensive analysis of Indian notions of suffering as it is expressed in the ancient and modern texts, see Kapil N. Tiwari (ed.), *Suffering: Indian Perspectives* (Delhi: Motilal Banarsidass, 1986).
2. Steven Poole, 'Help, Doctor! I've Got a Dose of Moral Sickness', *The Independent* (Saturday 24 February 1996), 17.
3. For varying accounts of the chief features of the doctrine of *karma* and rebirth, see Julius Lipner, *Hindus: Their Religious Beliefs and Practices* (London/New York: Routledge, 1994), 230 ff.; Wendy Doniger O'Flaherty, 'Introduction', in Wendy Doniger O'Flaherty (ed.), *Karma and Rebirth in Classical Indian Traditions* (Berkeley: University of California Press, 1980, Delhi reprint 1983), ix–xxv; Richard Gombrich, 'On Pain of Retribution', *Times Literary Supplement* (4 September), 995–6. For a philosophical as opposed to a text-historical approach, see Bruce R. Reichenbach, *The Law of Karma: A Philosophical Study* (Honolulu: University of Hawaii Press, 1990).
4. E.g. Surendranath Dasgupta, *A History of Indian Philosophy* (Cambridge: Cambridge University Press, 1922, reprint 1969), i, 22, 53–4; W. Doniger O'Flaherty, 'Karma and Rebirth in the Vedas and Purāṇas', in O'Flaherty (ed.), *Karma and Rebirth in Classical Indian Traditions*, 3–37.
5. George L. Hart, III, 'The Theory of Reincarnation among the Tamils', in O'Flaherty (ed.), *Karma and Rebirth in Classical Indian Traditions*, 116–33.
6. James P. Macdermott, 'Karma and Rebirth in Early Buddhism', in O'Flaherty (ed.), *Karma and Rebirth in Classical Indian Traditions*, 165–92; Padmanabh S. Jaini, 'Karma and the Problem of Rebirth in Jainism', in O'Flaherty (ed.), *Karma and Rebirth in Classical Indian Traditions*, 217–38. For an account of the Ājīvikas, see A.L. Basham, *History and Doctrines of the Ājīvikas: A Vanished Indian Religion* (London: Luzac & Co., 1951).
7. Gananath Obeyesekere, 'The Rebirth Eschatology and its Transformations: A Contribution to the Sociology of Early Buddhism', in O'Flaherty (ed.), *Karma and Rebirth in Classical Indian Traditions*, 137–64.

8. E.g. Sylvain Lévi, 'La transmigration des âmes dans les croyances hindoues', in *Mémorial Sylvain Lévi* (Paris: Paul Hartmann, 1937), 25 ff. For a useful summary of the chronological approach to the history of Indian religions, with particular reference to these early texts, see J.L. Brockington, *The Sacred Thread: Hinduism in its Continuity and Diversity* (Edinburgh: Edinburgh University Press, second edition 1996), 7–29.
9. Dasgupta, *History of Indian Philosophy*, i, 71–2.
10. E.g. *Ṛgveda* 10.16.4; 10.17.4. Translations of the hymns of the *Ṛgveda* are taken from Wendy Doniger O'Flaherty, *The Rigveda: An Anthology* (Harmondsworth: Penguin, 1981); see also Ralph T.H. Griffiths, *Hymns of the Rigveda* (1889; second revised edition, Delhi: Motilal Banarsidass, 1976).
11. *Ṛgveda* 7.89.
12. E.g. *Ṛgveda* 10.16, 10.15.
13. *Śatapatha Brāhmaṇa* 10.4.3.9–10. For an English translation, see J. Eggeling, *The Śatapatha Brāhmaṇa according to the Text of the Mādhyandina School*, Sacred Books of the East vol. 44 (Oxford: Clarendon Press, 1882–1900, Delhi reprint 1972–8).
14. *Bṛhādaraṇyaka Upaniṣad* 6.2.12.
15. *Bṛhādaraṇyaka Upaniṣad* 6.2.13–16. Translations from the Upaniṣads are taken from Patrick Olivelle, *The Upaniṣads* (Oxford: Oxford University Press, 1995), with my own additions in square brackets.
16. *Bṛhādaraṇyaka Upaniṣad* 3.2.11, 13.
17. *Bṛhādaraṇyaka Upaniṣad* 4.4.1–2, 5.
18. *Bhagavadgītā* 3.37 ff. For English translations, see R.C. Zaehner, *The Bhagavad-gītā* (Oxford: Oxford University Press, 1969) and Franklin Edgerton, The *Bhagavad Gītā*, Harvard Oriental Series 48–9 (Cambridge, Mass.: Harvard University Press, 1972).
19. It is possible to be a Hindu without believing in *karma* and the cycle of rebirths, of course, and to believe in them without being a Hindu (Brockington, *The Sacred Thread*, 5).
20. For scholarly but incomplete English translations of these two texts, see J.A.B. van Buitenen *et al.*, *The Mahābhārata* (Chicago and London: University of Chicago Press, 1973–) and Robert P. Goldman (gen. ed.), *The Rāmāyaṇa of Vālmīki: An Epic of Ancient India* (Princeton, New Jersey: Princeton University Press, 1986–); for earlier but complete translations, see Kisari Mohan Ganguli, *The Mahabharata* (Delhi: Munshiram Manoharlal, 1970) and Hari Prasad Shastri, *The Ramayana of Valmiki* (London: Shanti Sadan, 1962–76).
21. Brockington, *The Sacred Thread*, 54.
22. *Rāmāyaṇa* 2.10.30–1. English translations are taken from Sheldon I. Pollock, *The Rāmāyaṇa of Vālmīki: An Epic of Ancient India, Vol, 2: Ayodhyākāṇḍa*, general editor: R.P. Goldman (Princeton, New Jersey: Princeton University Press, 1986).
23. *Rāmāyaṇa* 2.10.38–41.
24. *Rāmāyaṇa* 2.11.12–15.
25. *Rāmāyaṇa* 2.55.21.
26. *Rāmāyaṇa* 2.58.46.
27. *Rāmāyaṇa* 2.57.4.

28. *Rāmāyaṇa* 2.17.19.
29. *Rāmāyaṇa* 2.17.24, 30.
30. *Rāmāyaṇa* 2.38.16–17.
31. *Rāmāyaṇa* 2.47.19.
32. David F. Pocock, *Mind, Body and Wealth: A Study of Belief and Practice in an Indian Village* (Oxford: Blackwell, 1973), 37–9.
33. *Kaṭha Upaniṣad* 3.7. Cf. *Bṛhadāraṇyaka Upaniṣad* 6.2.16, *Chāndogya Upaniṣad* 5.10.5–6.
34. *Chāndogya Upaniṣad* 5.10.7.
35. Brockington, *The Sacred Thread*, 92–4. For an English translation, see Wendy Doniger with Brian K. Smith, *The Laws of Manu* (Harmondsworth: Penguin, 1991).
36. *Manusmṛti* 11.49.
37. For many of these issues, see Reichenbach, *The Law of Karma*; for *karma* and cosmology, see Richard F. Gombrich, 'Ancient Indian Cosmology', in Carmen Blacker and Michael Loewe (eds), *Ancient Cosmologies* (London: Allen and Unwin, 1975), 121; for a discussion of fatalism in the epics, see Pollock, *The Rāmāyaṇa of Vālmīki*, vol. 2, 33–5 and Bruce Long, 'The Concepts of Human Action and Rebirth in the *Mahābhārata*', in O'Flaherty (ed.), *Karma and Rebirth in Classical Indian Traditions*, 38–60; for the link between *karma* and the common motif of the curse, see Robert P. Goldman, 'Karma, Guilt, and Buried Memories: public fantasy and private reality in traditional India', *Journal of the American Oriental Society* 105.3 (1985), 413–25; for *karma* and the grace of God, see Hart, 'The Theory of Reincarnation among the Tamils', in O'Flaherty (ed.), *Karma and Rebirth in Classical Indian Traditions*, 116–33; for a discussion of how the notion of *karma* resolves the problem of misfortune at the 'cognitive' but not the 'affective' level, see Richard F. Gombrich, *Precept and Practice: Traditional Buddhism in the Rural Highlands of Ceylon* (Oxford: Clarendon Press, 1971), 150 ff.
38. Hence Zaehner's conclusion that the *karma* doctrine is 'one of the presuppositions of post-Vedic Hinduism which are rarely, if ever, disputed'; R.C. Zaehner, *Hinduism* (Oxford: Oxford University Press, 1966), 4–5; but cf. Brockington, *The Sacred Thread*, 5.
39. For a discussion of the concept of inherent nature with particular reference to women and kings, see I. Julia Leslie, *The Perfect Wife: The Orthodox Hindu Woman according to the Strīdharmapaddhati of Tryambakayajvan* (Delhi: Oxford University Press, 1989), 246–72.
40. The contrast between Karṇa's regal appearance and his presumed lowly origins is highlighted in *Mahābhārata* 1.126.1–1.127.30. For a brief but insightful discussion of Karṇa's impossible situation, see Iravati Karve, *Yuganta: The End of an Epoch* (1974; Bombay: Disha Books, 1990), 106–22.
41. *Mahābhārata* 1.123.10–35. Ekalavya belongs to the Niṣāda tribe, regarded as 'aboriginal' and therefore extremely low caste. For a modern rendering of this episode, see Jean-Claude Carrière, *The Mahabharata: A Play Based upon the Indian Epic*, translated from the French by Peter Brook (London: Methuen, 1985), 30–2.

42. *Rāmāyaṇa* 2.3.12.
43. *Manusmṛti* 7.64. The commentators provide a series of synonyms: *surūpa, sundara, priyadarśana*; see V.N. Mandlik (ed.), *Mānava-Dharma-Śāstra [Institutes of Manu] with the Commentaries of Medhātithi, Sarvajñanārāyana, Kullūka, Rāghavānanda, Nandana and Rāmachandra; and a Supplement of the Commentary of Govindarāja* (Bombay, 1886). These commentaries have not been translated into English.
44. *Suśruta Saṃhitā: Kalpasthāna* 1.8. For an English translation, see Dominik Wujastyk, *The Roots of Āyurveda: Selections from Sanskrit Medical Writings* (Delhi: Penguin, 1998), p. 173. The composition of the *Suśruta Saṃhitā* is usually placed in the early centuries BC.
45. For a description of the power of Kaikeyī's beauty and her use of that power to manipulate her husband, see *Rāmāyaṇa* 2.9.17 ff.; for a description of Daśaratha as being unable to free himself from Kaikeyī's 'snare', see *Rāmāyaṇa* 2.12.8, 2.72.4 etc.
46. *Rāmāyaṇa* 3.16–17.
47. *Rāmāyaṇa* 3.16.8–10.
48. For an English translation of the Hindi passage, see R.C. Prasad, *Tulasidasa's Shriramacharitamanasa: The Holy Lake of the Acts of Rama* (Delhi: Motilal Banarsidass, 1990), 399–400. For a comprehensive discussion of the various versions of the episode, see Kathleen M. Erndl, 'The Mutilation of Śūrpanakhā', in Paula Richmond (ed.), *Many Rāmāyaṇas: The Diversity of a Narrative Tradition in South Asia* (Berkeley: University of California Press, 1991), 67–88.
49. *Manusmṛti* 11.53.
50. *Rāmāyaṇa* 2.7.6 ff., 2.9.28 ff., etc.
51. See, for example, the hugely popular comic book retellings of the epic story: Anant Pai (ed.) *Ramayana*, Arnar Chitra Katha series (Bombay: India Book House, 1988),15–16, and *Ramayana* (Delhi: Dreamland Publications, 1993), 8–9.
52. K.T. Pandurangi, personal communication (Bangalore, 1995).
53. For a survey of current research and historical data on disability in Hinduism, Buddhism and Islam, see M. Miles, 'Disability in an Eastern Religious Context: historical perspectives', *Disability & Society*, 10.1 (1995), 49–69; for a discussion of disability aimed at American therapists, see M. Miles, 'Some Influences of Religions on Attitudes towards Disabilities' (forthcoming). Other relevant work by M. Miles includes: 'Responses to Mental Retardation in South Asia: a 3,000-year review', in G. Woodill and R. Hanes (eds), *The History of Disabilities: International Perspectives* (New York and London: Garland, forthcoming); 'Goitre, Cretinism and Iodine in South Asia: historical perspectives on a continuing scourge', *Medical History* (in press); and 'References to Physical and Mental Disabilities in the Mahabharata (in English Translation)', *Asia-Pacific Journal of Disability and Rehabilitation* 8/2 (1997), Supplement: 1–7.
54. *Rāmāyaṇa* 2.72.5–25.
55. In traditional Indian medicine (*āyurveda*), of course, the heart (*hṛdaya*) is the seat of thought and identity (*cetanā*), not the head. In fact, the brain seems not to have been recognised as an organ at all, and was certainly not the seat of thought.

56. Girish Karnad, *Hayavadana* (Dharwar: Manohara Grantha Mala, 1971). For an English translation, see Girish Karnad, *Hayavadana* (Delhi: Oxford University Press, 1975).
57. For an English translation, see Thomas Mann, 'The Transposed Heads', in *Mario and the Magician and Other Stories*, tr. by H.T. Lowe-Porter (1940; London: Penguin, 1975),158–235.
58. For the classic English translation of the *Kathāsaritsāgara*, see N.M. Penzer (ed.), *The Ocean of Story: Being C. H. Tawney's Translation of Somadeva's Kathā Sarit Sāgara (Or Oceans of Streams of Story)*, 10 vols. (London: Chas. J. Sawyer Ltd., 1924–8). Volume 6 contains Somadeva's version of the *Vetālapañcaviṃśati*, with the key episode on pages 204–8.
59. Interestingly, the play's sub-plot of the man with the horse's head subverts this traditional meaning. The horse head thinks and speaks like a man: this composite creature has a human mind and body, but the physical head of a horse. By the end of the play, the human elements have all disappeared: mind and body have transformed themselves into those of a complete horse.
60. I am simplifying here. For a more detailed account of the various versions of the *karma* theory embedded in the Dharmaśāstras, see Ludo Rocher, 'Karma and Rebirth in the Dharmaśāstras', in O'Flaherty, *Karma and Rebirth in Classical Indian Traditions*, 61–89, and Ariel Glucklich, 'Karma and Pollution in Hindu Dharma: distinguishing law from nature', *Contributions to Indian Sociology* (n.s.) 18,1 (1984), 25–43.
61. A particularly striking example is the idea that the wife who dies on her husband's pyre can rescue him even from the gates of hell: 'Just as the snake-catcher drags the snake from its hole by force, even so the virtuous wife (*satī*) snatches her husband from the demons of hell and takes him up to heaven' (Leslie, *The Perfect Wife*, 294).
62. See Julia Leslie, 'Some Traditional Indian Views on Menstruation and Female Sexuality', in Roy Porter and Mikuláš Teich (eds), *Sexual Knowledge and Sexual Science: The History of Attitudes to Sexuality* (Cambridge: Cambridge University Press, 1994), 73.
63. *Mahābhārata* 1.99.28–1.100.30.
64. O'Flaherty, 'Karma and Rebirth in the Vedas and Purāṇas', 14–15.
65. Mitchell G. Weiss, '*Caraka Saṃhitā* on the Doctrine of Karma', in O'Flaherty (ed.), *Karma and Rebirth in Classical Indian Traditions*, 90–115.
66. Weiss, '*Caraka Saṃhitā* on the Doctrine of Karma', 92–6.
67. For a comprehensive summary of popular attitudes towards misfortune, see C.J. Fuller, *The Camphor Flame: Popular Hinduism and Society in India* (Princeton: Princeton University Press, 1992), 224–52. Fuller underlines an important point (p. 248): 'All these popular ideas about *karma* . . . actually have close analogues in the textual tradition. The common assumption in anthropological literature that popular thinking deviates from *the* textual theory of *karma* – mistakenly identified with the radically individualistic Brahmanical version – is incorrect. Rather, a range of similar ideas about *karma* exist in both popular and textual Hinduism.'

68. Ursula M. Sharma, 'Theodicy and the Doctrine of Karma', *Contributions to Indian Sociology* (n.s.) 4 (1973), 1–21.
69. W.H. Sleeman, *Rambles and Recollections of an Indian Official* (1844), revised by Vincent A. Smith (Karachi: Oxford University Press, 1915), 162–3.
70. Susan S. Wadley and Bruce W. Derr, 'Eating Sins in Karimpur', *Contributions to Indian Sociology* (n.s.) 23 (1989), 131–48.
71. E.g. Fuller, *The Camphor Flame*, 248–9; Lawrence A. Babb, 'Destiny and Responsibility: karma in popular Hinduism', in Charles F. Keyes and E. Valentine Daniel (eds), *Karma: An Anthropological Inquiry* (Berkeley: University of California Press, 1983), 168; Gananath Obeyesekere, 'Theodicy, Sin and Salvation in a Sociology of Buddhism', in E.R. Leach (ed.), *Dialectic in Practical Religion* (Cambridge: Cambridge University Press, 1968), 21.
72. Fuller, *The Camphor Flame*, 249.
73. A.K. Ramanujan, 'Telling Tales', *Daedalus: Journal of the American Academy of Arts and Sciences* (Fall 1989), issue entitled 'Another India' (Proceedings of the American Academy of Arts and Sciences 118/4), 247–8.
74. Kirin Narayan, *Storytellers, Saints, and Scoundrels: Folk Narrative in Hindu Religious Teaching* (Philadelphia: University of Pennsylvania Press, 1989),172–3.
75. Sharma, 'Theodicy and the Doctrine of Karma', 358.

SUFFERING AND SANCTIFICATION IN CHRISTIANITY

David J. Melling

In the plague-ridden city, is faith a prophylactic against disease?

In the year 252 CE plague infested Carthage. Cyprian, bishop of the city, describes its horrors with graphic precision: 'This trial, that now the bowels, relaxed into a constant flux, discharge the bodily strength; that a fire originated in the marrow ferments into wounds of the fauces; that the intestines are shaken with a continual vomiting; that the eyes are on fire with the injected blood; that in some cases the feet or some parts of the limbs are taken off by the contagion of diseased putrefaction; that from the weakness arising by the maiming and loss of the body, either the gait is enfeebled, or the hearing is obstructed, or the sight darkened; . . .'[1]

The Christian community of Carthage was evidently greatly disturbed by the plague. '. . . it disturbs some', Cyprian notes,[2] 'that the power of this Disease attacks our people equally with the heathens . . . It disturbs some that this mortality is common to us with others; and yet what is there in this world which is not common to us with others, so long as this flesh of ours still remains, according to the law of our first birth, common to us with them? . . . Thus, when the earth is barren with an unproductive harvest, famine makes no distinction; thus, when with the invasion of an enemy any city is taken, captivity at once desolates all; and when the serene clouds withhold the rain, the drought is alike to all; and when the jagged rocks rend the ship, the shipwreck is common without exception to all that sail in her; and the disease of the eyes, and the attack of fevers, and the feebleness of all the limbs is common to us with others, so long as this common flesh of ours is borne by us in the world.'

Cyprian's answer: suffering as a 'proof of faith'

Cyprian himself saw the plague as 'profitable as a proof of faith.'[3] For Cyprian, faith is no defense against illness and misfortune.[4] Far from it; 'if the Christian know and keep fast under what condition and what law he has believed, he will be aware that he must suffer more than others in the world, since he must struggle more with the attacks of the devil. Holy Scripture teaches and forewarns, saying, . . . 'In pain endure, and in thy humility have patience; for gold and silver is tried in the fire, but acceptable men in the furnace of humiliation.'[5] Suffering, Cyprian is arguing, is not only common to all humanity, it has, for the Christian, a special role in the spiritual life. His image of the precious metals tried in the furnace suggests two functions; suffering is a means of spiritual purification and purgation, and it is a means whereby believers are put to the test.

Cyprian writes from a plague-ridden city, confronting the plague and his community's response to the plague. He writes as a pastor, a theologian and as a spiritual teacher trying to make sense of the suffering his community is enduring, offering not promises of miraculous healing or selective preservation, but rather an interpretation of the sickness as a challenge to virtue and a testing ground of faith.

Why do we suffer?

At a popular level, and in preaching and apologetics, Christians have not infrequently spoken of specific misfortunes as a punishment for sin. In some cases it is clear that a direct link can be made between a disordered and vicious style of life and a range of unpleasant consequences, from friendlessness to dyspepsia which are a direct or indirect result of the particular repertoire of vices an individual has chosen to practice. Indeed, an explanation of how it has come about that a specific sickness is afflicting a particular person in terms of a disordered and self-indulgent lifestyle may be offered by a medical adviser as readily as by a spiritual counsellor. There remains, however, a significant difference between seeing suffering as a consequence of disordered living and seeing suffering as a punishment inflicted by God.

While preachers often presented plagues and epidemics as visitations of the wrath of God on contemporary wickedness, Christian theology has normally rejected any attempt to account for the existence of suffering *as such* in terms of collective punishment. The vivid picture of the sufferings of the righteous Job in the Book of Job had already dealt a powerful blow to any such theory. Nor can such an approach account for the suffering of animals. Indeed, particularly amongst philosophical theologians of the modern period, the existence of suffering has been very widely seen as providing the most serious problem for Christian theodicy, that of reconciling the claim the God is omniscient, omnipotent and all-loving with the existence in the created world of unnecessary suffering.

Equally, however, Christian tradition, especially as it responded to the challenge of Gnostic and Manichean thought, has been resolutely hostile to any thoroughgoing dualism which would attribute the existence of suffering to the creative action of an Anti-God.

This leaves open a variety of theological approaches to the general explanation of the existence of suffering. The existence of suffering can be interpreted as an inevitable consequence of the process of development and transformation of the created world, or as providing a necessary field for moral and spiritual growth and development. Alternatively, the existence of suffering can be interpreted as a consequence of the existence of free created agents. Such accounts see suffering as a consequence of the intrusion of evil disorder into the created world by the primordial fall, either the fall of the Dawn-bearer, Lucifer and the other rebel angels, or the fall of Adam[6] and Eve, the first-created parents of the human race.

Cyprian, however, faced with the misery and doubts of his plague-ridden community, focuses not on the question of the origin of suffering, but on the significance of suffering to the Christian spiritual life. He points not to the question of the cause or origin of suffering *as such* but of why God has inflicted *this* particular suffering on me, and what response I am called to make to it.

The Venerable Bede (d.c.735), commenting on the story of Jesus' curing the paralytic in the second chapter of the Gospel of Mark, says: 'We are told, too, that many bodily sicknesses arise from sins, and so it is, perhaps, that sins are first forgiven so that once the causes of the sickness are removed, health may be restored. People suffer bodily afflictions for five reasons: to increase their merits, as Job and the Martyrs; to preserve their humility, as Paul by Satan's messenger; or in order that they should perceive and correct their sins, as Miriam, the sister of Moses, and this paralytic; for the glory of God, as the man born blind and Lazarus; or as the start of the pains of damnation, as Herod and Antiochus.'[7]

Bede's list of five reasons for suffering offers four which locate the reason for the person's suffering in the spiritual state of the person himself.

Like Job and the martyrs a person may suffer as a means of increasing merit. This as it is stated, Protestant theology would generally find unacceptable, given the Reformation rejection of the doctrine of merit. What Bede is pointing to, however, is that suffering offered Job the opportunity to practise the virtue of patience and offered the martyrs the opportunity to practise long-suffering, constancy, hopefulness, trust and fidelity. In other words, Job and martyrs flourish spiritually by their response to the sufferings inflicted on them.

The second function of suffering in a person's spiritual life which Bede identifies is that of preserving humility. This too is a case of suffering offering the occasion for the practice of virtue. It is more. He is thinking of cases where a person suffers a sickness, disability or deformity which both serves as an obstacle to any deluded heroic perception of oneself, and at the same time promotes an awareness of one's weakness, fragility and transience.

The third of the personal reasons Bede offers is drawn from the specific Gospel text on which he is commenting. Jesus tells the paralytic that his sins are forgiven, and then, to show those standing by that he has the power to forgive sins, he tells the man to take up his bed and walk, curing him. Interestingly, Bede does not assimilate this case to that of the man born blind, whose disability he sees as given 'for the glory of God', but sees the paralysis the man in the story suffers from as inflicted on him to help him perceive his sin. The implication of Bede's account is that Jesus, when he tells the man that his sins are forgiven, is responding to the real, though silent, request the man is making. The subsequent cure testifies to Jesus's power to forgive sin by removing a disability which has now served its spiritual purpose.

Bede's fourth personal reason is more disturbing. He interprets the hideous suffering of Herod, his living flesh consumed by worms, and the similar fate that befell Antiochus Epiphanes[8] (d.163 BCE) as a first taste of the torments of Hell. Christianity has normally offered a vision of human life as ultimately directed to one of two ends, eternal bliss in unity with God and the saints and angels or eternal misery, alienated utterly from God in Hell. The undying worm, like the unquenchable fire, is part of the image of Gehenna Jesus uses in Mark 9. 48 and from which later Christian images of the Hell of damnation are derived. In the original text, Gehenna is the rubbish tip in the vale of Hinnom where the garbage of Jerusalem was burned. Bede clearly sees Herod and Antiochus as examples of human beings who have attained the state of damnation even before death; the reverse, presumably, of the greatest saints.

The fifth reason for 'bodily affliction' that Bede offers is not rooted in the spiritual state or need of the person who suffers. Some afflictions, he says are 'for the glory of God'. The gospel story of Jesus's cure of the man born blind begins with the disciples asking 'Rabbi, who sinned, this man or his parents, that he was born blind?'[9] Jesus rejects both explanations, thereby leading Christian tradition to reject any theology that sees disability or sickness as always or necessarily a punishment or even a result brought about by wrongdoing. In the case of the man born blind and of his friend Lazarus who is raised from the dead, and presumably in other cases, the condition of the person is not to be explained as a result of that person's conduct or of any other person's conduct: it is for the glory of God. The importance of this answer is precisely that it does not offer an easily assimilated explanation of disability or sickness; rather it puts firmly aside the notion that anyone who suffers must have sinned or someone else's sin must have caused their suffering, and points instead to the mystery of the Divine will.

Bede's comments on the story of the paralytic move us from seeking any single cause of suffering, to seeing suffering in terms of the spiritual life of the person who suffers and in terms of the mystery of the will of God. If we ask what range of significances suffering can have in the spiritual life of an individual, Christian theology offers many possible answers: as, for example, a reminder of the transience of life; as an opportunity for self-discovery; as a reminder of solidarity with the whole human race in its fragility; as a reminder of solidarity with all living, sentient things; as a training ground in virtue; as a means of putting virtue to the test; as an opportunity for spiritual and moral growth in the face of adversity; as an opportunity for sacrificial self-offering; even as a way of sharing in the salvific sufferings of Christ and as a way of experiencing the Divine Energies and of deification. Not all Christians would agree with every item on this list, and some would, no doubt, have others to add. The list could be summarised as claiming that suffering can be interpreted as an opportunity for learning and development, as a vehicle for insight, as a mode of ascetic discipline, as an opportunity for growth and transformation, as a means of sacrificial action, and as a means of the sufferer's participating in the divine life and the salvific work of Christ.

Voluntary Suffering

The Christian proclamation of the suffering Saviour and the importance of the passion and death of Jesus to Christian faith offer a focus for theological thinking on suffering. Traditional Christianity affirms strongly that Jesus *voluntarily* accepted suffering and death. He is not merely a passive victim: he chooses the path of suffering. He offers the model of suffering voluntarily endured, though as the incarnate Word of God he is perfect and sinless, so that there is nothing in his own life that needs purgation or expiation by suffering.

A vigorous image of the willing suffering of Christ is offered, for example, in the Anglo-Saxon poem, the 'Dream of the Rood'. The Cross itself speaks to the poet in a vision:

'. . . Mankind's Lord I saw
hasten in mighty resolve to mount me. . . .
The young hero ungirded himself, He, God Almighty!
Strong and steadfast he mounted the gallows.'[10]

The spiritual writings of the early Christian centuries are rich with affirmations of the value of suffering voluntarily endured. Indeed self-inflicted suffering in the form of fasting, sleep-fasting, wearing chains and hair-shirts and even self-flagellation have often been part of the ascetic practice of devout Christians in the unreformed churches. Though the Reformation cast grave doubt on the value of such ascetic practices, even in the Anglican tradition we see the picture of Dr Johnson (1709–84) doing penance standing in the rain. The main focus of Christian spiritual writers has not, however, been on the value of self-inflicted suffering, but rather on the value of the voluntary acceptance of suffering.

'A person definitely wants to be healed if he does not put up any resistance to the healing remedies: These are the pains and hurts brought on by many different circumstances. The one who resists does not know what is being worked out here nor what advantage he would draw from it when he leaves this world.'[11] says Maximus the Confessor. Suffering, he is saying, can be medicinal, exercising a function of moral and spiritual katharsis. 'Suffering cleanses the soul infected with the filth of sensual pleasure and detaches it completely from material things by showing it the penalty incurred as a result of its affection for them. This is why God in His justice allows the devil to afflict men with torments.'[12]

Maximus's contempt for 'sensual pleasure' is not something peculiarly Christian; it derives directly from the values of Platonic, Stoic and Cynic philosophy, all of which exercised a significant influence on the development of Christian thought,[13] Platonism in furnishing a technical vocabulary for spiritual psychology, Stoicism and Cynicism in shaping Christian ethics. Maximus's emphasis on suffering as leading to detachment and on the didactic role of suffering is of particular interest, especially since he seems to see the devil as a causal agent in human suffering. Perhaps his thought is that pain and misery caused by a lifestyle based on an excessive attachment to material things can provide us with the means of escape from that attachment once we perceive the causal link between obsessive attachment and the pain, sickness and misery it causes. The devil's role is as tempter, leading us into attachment and the vices that flow from it, he afflicts us, co-operatively, since we also inflict ourselves, with the miserable consequences that then ensue. But, Maximus argues, the devil's victory is also his defeat, if we allow our sufferings to teach us detachment.

The end to which the purifying action of divine justice is directed is not simply retribution, but the radical transformation of human life and consciousness. 'God made us so that we might become, "partakers of the divine nature"[14] and sharers in His eternity, and so that we might come to be like Him through deification by grace. It is through deification that all things are reconstituted and achieve their permanence; and it is for its sake that what is not is brought into being and given existence.'[15]

Positive affirmations of the spiritual value of suffering voluntarily accepted are not restricted to the earlier centuries of Christianity. In 1984 Pope John Paul II issued an Apostolic Letter, '*Salvifici Doloris*,'[16] which argues powerfully and at length for a positive Christian understanding of suffering. He presents suffering as something which is 'particularly essential'[17] to human nature,[18] something, that is, which is a fundamental aspect of our being human. Not, however, simply as aspect of what as a matter of fact is involved in being human, for the Pope suffering 'seems to belong to man's transcendence: it is one of those points in which man is in a certain sense "destined" to go beyond himself, . . .'[19]

Theological address to suffering becomes possible when the vocabulary becomes available to distinguish the mere fact of being affected by evil from the actual experience of evil. 'In the vocabulary of the Old Testament,' the Pope writes, 'suffering and evil are identified with each other. In fact, that vocabulary did not have a specific word to indicate "suffering". Thus it defined as "evil" everything that was suffering. Only the Greek language, and together with it the New Testament (and the Greek translation of the Old Testament), use the verb *pascho* ("I am affected by . . ., I experience a feeling, I suffer"); and thanks to this verb, suffering is no longer directly identifiable with (objective) evil, but expresses a situation in which the human being experiences evil and in doing so becomes the subject of suffering. Suffering has indeed both a subjective and a passive character (*patior*). Even when the human being 'brings suffering on himself, when he is its cause, this suffering remains something passive in its metaphysical essence'.[20]

Suffering, the Pope is arguing, can be a lived metaphysics, the natural response of our humanity to the impact on consciousness of the reality of evil, a response that both discloses to us something of what it is to be human and something of the nature of evil, and at the same time challenges us to self-transcendence. The disclosure is not necessarily at the level of intellectual apprehension. Emotions (*pathemata*) have, as Aristotle points out in the 'Rhetoric', a cognitive dimension. John Paul is quite clear that evil and suffering extend far beyond sickness and disease. As well as moral suffering and the torment of incomprehension one can experience faced with the apparent welfare of evildoers and the sufferings of the upright, he instances also natural disasters, 'social scourges',[21] and war. Alert suffering is a mode of awakening to the moral and spiritual order of the *kosmos* that is violated by the evil we experience, an order which a mind clouded by the disordered passions is unable to perceive.[22] Implicit in the Pope's argument is a distinction between suffering as simply the experience of evil, and a more fully human mode of suffering which responds with awakened moral and spiritual sensibility to the nature and significance of the evil suffered.

The Suffering God

For Christian theology the salvation of humanity, and in Eastern Christian theology the salvation of the entire *kosmos*, is accomplished by God's descent into humanity, into the depths of human suffering, uniting God with our humanity at the very moment of our encounter with evil. In that encounter traditional Christianity asserts that the incarnate God himself suffers. Despite some vigorous opposition, the Theopaschite formula 'one of the Trinity suffered' was finally declared orthodox by Pope John II[23] in the sixth century.[24]

The Theopaschite formula expresses a central aspect of the doctrine of the Incarnation; the Divine Word chooses to put on human nature, and assumes with that nature our human capacity for suffering. His suffering is voluntary and purposeful; he suffers with and for humanity.

Sharing in the Saviour's suffering

Pope John Paul II argues it is possible for other human beings to share in the salvific sufferings of Christ, 'because he himself in his redemptive suffering has become in a certain sense a sharer in all human sufferings'. The human being, 'discovering through faith the redemptive suffering of Christ, also discovers in it his own sufferings; he rediscovers them through faith, enriched with a new content and new meaning'.[25] 'He is called to share in that suffering through which all human suffering has also been redeemed. In bringing about the redemption through suffering, Christ has also raised human suffering to the level of redemption.'[26]

Christianity proclaims not only the suffering and crucified Messiah, it proclaims the risen Messiah, '. . . the paschal mystery of the cross and resurrection, in which Christ descends, in the first phase, to the ultimate limits of human weakness and impotence: Indeed, he dies nailed to the cross. But if at the same time in this weakness there is accomplished his lifting up, confirmed by the power of the resurrection, then this means that the weaknesses of all human sufferings are capable of being infused with the same power of God manifested in Christ's cross.'[27]

This theme of sharing in the sufferings of Christ is a common heritage of Orthodox and Catholic theology and spirituality. It became vividly alive to the Radical Reformers,[28] the Anabaptist, Hutterites, Menonites and similar communities, whose bitter experience of persecution sensitised them to the price that loyalty to their faith might easily demand of them. In such communities discipleship was readily identified with and lived out as following Christ on his journey to the Cross. Interestingly, Christians of the Radical Reform frequently saw the suffering of animals as an image of the suffering of the innocent Christ.

The salvation accomplished by the incarnate Word of God has not abolished evil and suffering from human life. Rather faith in the suffering saviour enables a transformation of the meaning of suffering for an individual believer. Suffering, then, can be seen as offering opportunities for spiritual and moral growth and development. It can be accepted as a form of sacrifice, as a form of ascesis, and ultimately as a means of sharing in the salvific work of Christ. If we consider the situation of someone who is incapacitated in an extreme degree, the option to find a positive significance in the suffering that person is undergoing offers at least a possibility of creating a sense of meaning and even special vocation in life at the point at which it might seem reduced to utter passivity.

The value of suffering versus the resistance to evil

This positive evaluation of the role of voluntarily accepted suffering in the individual's spiritual life does not, however, extend to the point of licensing an inference that there is a duty to accept all forms of suffering. As Pope John Paul II points out 'It can be said that' the human being 'suffers whenever he experiences any kind of evil.'[29] There can be no general duty to accept and endure evils, except, perhaps in a situation where the evil in question is the least of evils and choice is limited to a choice amongst evils. The general duty is rather to strive to combat, abolish or at least mitigate evils. Indeed, the suffering we experience in the face of the evil afflicting another can be a powerful motivation to take action to combat that evil.

The positive evaluation of voluntary suffering applies primarily to three kinds of case; first when suffering is inevitable or only avoidable by extraordinary measures, or, for example at great hazard or cost to others, and second the suffering at knowledge of the evil befalling others which can be avoided only by self-deception, culpable ignorance or continual self-distraction and third the suffering it is necessary to accept as a means of self-training, such as the severe restraint of food intake needed to curb habitual gluttony, and in general the suffering it is necessary to endure to free oneself from vicious habits.

A certain caution is also required in applying patristic advice on the endurance of suffering to the modern period. In the early Christian centuries medicine did not have the same ability to effect cures that it has had since the introduction of modern drugs. Surgery was far narrower in range, exquisitely painful and limited in success. The Hippocratic writings show how often the most scientifically minded doctors were sentenced to record the symptoms of ailments they could not diagnose, watch the inevitable and unrestrainable process of the disease and offer condolences to the bereaved. In many cases a person living in the age of Cyprian or of Maximos the Confessor had no alternative faced with disease or injury other than to suffer it. The issue of voluntary suffering rose not in the context of a choice between pain and sickness or relief, but between a willing and a reluctant endurance of the pain and sickness.

Nonetheless, the doctors of the early Christian centuries had significant medical resources at their disposal. In many cases they could offer relief and healing. The spiritual teachers of the patristic period sometimes found it necessary to remind people that a disciplined and well-ordered life does not necessarily involve the rejection of medicine. Diadochos, Bishop of Photike in the late fifth century, having just advised his readers to avoid the enervating and immodest luxury of the baths, says this: 'There is nothing to prevent us from calling a doctor when we are ill. Since Providence has implanted remedies in nature, it has been possible for human experimentation to develop the art of medicine. All the same, we should not place our hope of healing in doctors, but in our true Saviour and Doctor, Jesus Christ. . . . Furthermore, they should not succumb to the conceit and temptation of the devil, which have led some of them publicly to boast that they have had no need of doctors for many years.'[30]

This advice is offered, he says, to those pursuing self-control 'in monastic communities or towns.'[31] To solitaries dwelling in the desert he has rather different advice to offer. They should approach the Lord in faith, since he can heal everything. And in any case a hermit always 'has the desert itself to provide sufficient consolation in his illness.'[32]

The value of health

Diadochos sees the use of the skills and knowledge of doctors as justified since the medical profession makes use of remedies that divine providence has provided in the natural world. He points, that is, to the divine will underlying all creation as the source of the efficacy of all medical remedies. Our healing, then, is due to the God who furnishes the remedies the doctor uses rather than to the doctor who uses them.

Not only is recourse to medicine justified, physical health is a positive value to be promoted. Opposing the Gnostics' contempt for the body, Clement of Alexandria defends the importance of physical health, and a healthy lifestyle. He writes: 'let them learn that the harmonious mechanism of the body contributes to the understanding which leads to goodness of nature. Wherefore in the third book of the Republic, Plato . . . says, that "for the sake of harmony of soul, care must be taken of the body, by which, he who announces the proclamation of the truth, finds it possible to live, and to live well. For it is by the path of life and health that we learn gnosis."'

Basing himself on contemporary medical science, Clement advises moderation in diet and a wholesome measure of physical exercise, 'these most decorous and healthful practices'.[33] He warns that lack of exercise leads to a state where 'the faeces are in excess . . . and other superfluous matters abound . . . and also perspiration, as the food is not assimilated by the body, but is flowing out to waste'.[34] This excess production of bodily waste has a further undesirable consequence, in that 'thence also lusts are excited, the redundance flowing to the pudenda by commensurate motions'.[35] Clement's specific medical analysis may sound a little odd to modern ears, but the fundamental argument he is advancing has not lost its relevance. He sees a moderate, balanced diet, matched with a degree of exercise that keeps the digestive system working effectively, as promoting bodily health, alertness of mind, the capacity for self-control and moral sobriety, and at the same time producing a natural physical beauty.

Clement opposes the use of cosmetics by those who are 'made "in the image and likeness of God"',[36] as dishonouring the archetype by 'preferring the mischievous contrivance of man to the divine creation'. He advises women not to 'smear their faces with the ensnaring devices of wily cunning'. He advises them to prefer 'the decoration of sobriety. For, in the first place, the best beauty is that which is spiritual . . . For when the soul is adorned by the Holy Spirit, and inspired with the radiant charms which proceed from Him, – righteousness, wisdom, fortitude, temperance, love of the good, modesty, than which no more blooming colour was ever seen, – then let corporeal beauty be cultivated too, symmetry of limbs and members with fair complexion. The adornment of health is here in place, through which the transition of the artificial image to the truth, in accordance with the form which has been given by God, is effected.'[37]

Clement's contempt for cosmetics is rooted as much in Plato's contempt for the false *techne*[a] which produces a mere appearance of health, as in Christian values, as is his emphasis on the truth of the beauty which proceeds from physical and moral health. 'Beauty is the free flower of health',[38] he says. It requires 'temperance in drinks and moderation in articles of food'.

Clement's advice is intended for anyone seeking to lead a Christian life. Most Christian spiritual writing, however, has been produced from within the monastic tradition in its varied forms. Monastic writers, not surprisingly, generally show less interest in physical beauty and more in the moral and spiritual effects of dietary moderation. Gluttony in all its forms is looked on as a particularly dangerous vice as it leads not only to physical lassitude and slothfulness, but also to dulling of the mind. The health of body and soul alike is promoted by moderation in food and drink. Fasting is recommended as a remedy for excess, as well as a means of self.training in restraint and moderation. Frugality in eating is recommended as leading to simplification of life, clarity of thought and acuity of insight. The emphasis shifts in the monastic tradition from orderly restraint to promote health, to ascetic self-control to promote clarity of mind, spiritual insight, the awakening of the spiritual senses, and training in virtue. Gluttony is feared as leading ultimately to a self-centred and uncontrolled lifestyle, to deluded and confused states of consciousness.

Clearly in the case of gluttony and all forms of intemperance vicious conduct becomes itself the source of physical, mental and spiritual ill health and a significant cause of suffering. Such suffering is not to be endured patiently, but rather its causes vigorously uprooted by ascetic practice – which itself requires a degree of voluntary suffering, since learning self restraint requires uprooting established habits of immoderate conduct and a shift in mind-set. The spiritual father or mother plays a therapeutic role in helping in this reordering and reshaping of habits and patterns of thought.

The doctor as image of the Saviour

The ancient world was as familiar with the arrogant and extravagant claims of the less reputable members of the medical profession as is our own age. Indeed, the Jewish scholar who produced the Septuagint translation of the book of Psalms took a startling liberty with the text of Psalm 88 (LXX 87) to rebuke the arrogance of Alexandrian physicians. Instead of reading verse 10 as 'Do the shades rise up to praise you?' he deliberately misreads the 'rephaim' (shades) of the verse as 'rophim' (doctors), and produces a piquant translation: 'Will you work wonders for the dead, or shall doctors raise them up to praise you?'[39]

Nonetheless, Christianity acquired a profound respect for the medical profession, provided doctors exercised their role in a humble and unmercenary spirit. Indeed, the doctor's healing function provides a theologically illuminative image of the salvific role of Christ. Clement of Alexandria expresses it well: 'For while the physician's art according to Democritus, "heals the diseases of the body; wisdom frees the soul from passion." But the good Instructor, the Wisdom, the Word of the Father, who made man, cares for the whole nature of His creature; the all-sufficient Physician of humanity, the Saviour, heals both body and soul.'[40]

Throughout Christian history there have been men and women who individually or as members of a religious order or institution have taken up the care of the sick and the ministry of healing in imitation of Christ. The Knights Hospitaller (founded in the 11th century) serving 'our lords the sick', the Hospitaller Brothers of St John of God (d. 1550), the Camillians (founded by St Camillus of Lellis, d. 1614), the many orders of nursing sisters and many of the secular nurses who followed the path laid down by Florence Nightingale (1820 to 1910) all share in different ways in this tradition.

The cult of the Unmercenary Healers

Eastern Christians hold in special reverence the Anargyroi,[41] the Unmercenary Physicians who refused payment for the healing they accomplished by prayer and by conventional medicine. Some worked as doctors to the poor, a number were healers of animals. Some founded hospitals for the sick and hostels for travellers. Interestingly, some of the Anargyroi were actually hospital managers and administrators rather than doctors. The Anargyroi, of whom about seventy are venerated as saints, have considerable prominence in the Orthodox calendar. Their icons with their traditional insignia, the spatula, medicine chest and loose doctor's mantle are seen in churches and houses. They furnish an important model of Christian sanctity, and their role in society provided an inspiring model for the social service of both Church and Empire.

The Church's healing ministry

The Christian Church itself exercises a healing role in a variety of ways. All Christian traditions have recourse to personal and group prayer to seek healing, and the use of the laying on of hands is a common practice. Traditional Churches maintain a very wide repertoire of special services and observances. The intercession of particular saints is sought to seek defence against or healing from specific diseases. For example, the blessing of Saint Blaise is given in Roman Catholic tradition to defend against diseases of the throat. Special services are used. Orthodox Christians sing the Paraclisis, the Office of Intercession to the Blessed Virgin, to seek healing and consolation in all forms of sickness and misfortune. Both Catholic and Orthodox traditions have services for the dying. Many Churches have services for the anointing of the sick, and for the blessing of holy oil with which the sick can be anointed or anoint themselves. Blessed water, drunk or sprinkled, and the oil from icon lamps are also used for healing. In Orthodox tradition a sick person is often blessed with the lance and spoon used in the Eucharist. Blessings with sacred relics or icons are used, especially at the shrine of a saint. Pilgrimages, for example to Lourdes or Tinos are a well known means of seeking healing.

Exorcisms are used in several Christian traditions as a means of healing from conditions attributed to demonic agencies. Eastern Orthodox prayer books also contain similar prayers to drive away infestations of noxious insects and to purify polluted wells. The prayers of purification are accompanied by thoroughly sensible instructions to remove all water from the well, and clean it thoroughly with fresh water and wine before the prayer is used.

Eastern Orthodox prayer books also contain a prayer to remove the effects of the evil eye, *baskania*. In Ethiopian tradition the *dabtara*, the cantor, has an important role in providing sacred objects to defend against illness and misfortune and to heal, a role not infrequently extended to the production of amulets and formulae of a less official nature.

Side by side with the Church's official functionaries, throughout history there have existed in many places healers, seers, wise-women, specialists in many varieties of healing which have never had the church's formal approval[42] and often faced its stern disapproval, but which have nonetheless survived. Folk prayers and incantations are found in many sources. Midwives, herb-wives and executioners were all regular sources of folk medicine.

In Eastern Christian communities it is not unusual for a priest to be called to hold a Paraclisis or an Euchelaion service at the house of a sick person. Friends will gather and take part in the service, and in the latter case will also receive the anointing with the blessed oil. In both Eastern and Oriental Christian houses it is common for holy water and blessed oil to be kept for use when someone is sick.

The sick are prayed for in the public services of Christian communities, and a charismatic ministry of healing is exercised in many communities. Communion is brought to the sick, prayer services held at the bedside, and hands laid on the sick for healing. Churches generally look to their clergy or to lay societies to visit and help the sick. In mediaeval Byzantium brotherhoods existed to bathe the sick. Christian communities have founded hospitals and hospices many of which have passed into secular hands.

What is probably the most extreme and extraordinary case of organised ministry still survives: in Belgium the shrine of the martyr, Saint Dympna, a seventh-century Irish princess who is patron saint of the mentally afflicted, has been since at least the thirteenth century the centre of a remarkable ministry to the mentally handicapped and the mentally ill in which all the town of Gheel shares to some degree, many extending the hospitality of their houses and family life as a part of that ministry.

Medical missions which combine service to the sick with the preaching of the gospel, either by accounting the service itself as proclamation of the gospel or by using the one activity to give impact to the other, have been a notable element in Christian missionary work in developing countries and sometimes amongst impoverished communities in the developed world.

Conclusion: suffering in Christian life

Suffering, as Pope John Paul II points out[43] arises when one 'experiences evil'. Suffering as such cannot, then, be something intrinsically desirable. Sickness and injury are not things to be desired.

John Climacus sees sickness as something hazardous to the spiritual life. 'We have to be particularly vigilant whenever the body is sick, for at such times the demons, observing our weakness and our infirmity and our inability to fight against them as usual, rush in to attack us. . . . the demons of anger and even of blasphemy may be found around those who live in the world. Those leading a religious life but having all they need of a material kind may suffer the onslaught of the demon of gluttony and fornication . . .'[44] Illness can lead to excessive self-involvement, obsessive thinking, febrile imaginings.

Disease and injury are things to be avoided. When we suffer from them it is normally wise and generally a duty to seek remedy or cure. The medical profession and the Church both offer means of healing, which should be seen as complementary, not as alternatives.

The sufferings of others speak to us: we are moved to pity, as Aristotle argues in the 'Rhetoric' by something happening to another with whom in general we can identify,[45] when we should fear the same thing happening to ourselves. The presence of the suffering other with whom I can identify calls to me for help and relief.

In some cases, however, I cannot avoid suffering except by measures that it would be unreasonable to take. In such a case I am challenged to find meaning in my suffering. Christian theology offers several ways of understanding suffering that makes the voluntary acceptance of it a point of spiritual growth and transformation of consciousness. Climacus speaks pungently of the spiritual healing suffering can effect: '. . . I saw men freed from their souls' passion by grave sickness, as though it were some kind of penance, and I could only praise and thank God who cleans clay with clay.'[46]

The Christian spiritual tradition enables suffering to be accepted as a gift, a transforming gift that temporarily or permanently reshapes the sufferer's life project.

NOTES

1. Cyprian: *On the Mortality* 14. The Ante-Nicene Fathers. Vol. II. In Christian Classics Etherial Library, Wheaton College. http:\\ccel.wheaton.edu/fathers.
2. Op. cit., 8.
3. Op. cit., 14.
4. There exist forms of Christianity which take the opposite view and see illness and poverty as a direct result of lack of faith.
5. Op. cit., 9.
6. Those who see the *Genesis* story of Adam and Eve as symbolic, metaphorical or mythical would find a problem in attributing real-world causality to a symbolic contruct or to a mythical person; in this particular case resolving the Adam and Eve story into a story about humanity or about the choices made or changes taking place early in human existence cannot salvage the explanation of suffering in terms of their Fall since the time-shape of Creation given in *Genesis* is lost.
7. This text is quoted by Aquinas in the *Catena Aurea* on Mark, Tr. J. D. Dalgairns, Oxford, John Henry Parker, 1862.
8. Graphically described in *2 Maccabees* 9, 5 to 28.
9. John 9. 2.
10. My own free translation.
11. Maximus Confessor, 'The Four Hundred Chapters on Love,' third century, 82, in *Maximus Confessor*. Tr. G. C. Berthold. New Jersey, Paulist Press. 1985.
12. In *The Philokalia* Ed. G. E. H. Palmer &c. Vol. II, London, Faber and Faber, 1981. p. 178.
13. Cf. F. G. Downing *Cynics and Christian Origins*, Edinburgh, T&T Clark, 1992: C. Stead, *Philosophy in Christian Antiquity*, Cambridge University Press, 1994.
14. In the Second Epistle of Peter, 1. 4.
15. Op. Cit., (*Philokalia*) p. 173.
16. Apostolic Letter *Salvifici Doloris*. February 11th (World Day of the Sick.) 1994.
17. *Salvifici Doloris*, 2.
18. His text is somewhat ambiguous. Here and elsewhere the Pope seems to imply not only that human nature involves suffering, but that suffering is restricted to human beings. The capacity of animals to suffer is surely something that should not be denied a priori. Perhaps a distinction is required which would clarify the different modes or kinds of suffering that become possible at different levels of sensation, cognition and affectivity.
19. Ibid.
20. Op. cit., 7.

21. Op. cit., 8.
22. In the Greek language in which many of the Church Fathers thought their Christianity, the same word *pathe* designates sufferings, including the sufferings of Christ, and the passions.
23. In his letter *Olim Quidem* to the Constantinopolitan Senate, 533 CE.
24. The Theopaschite formula is accepted as orthodox, but there exists also a Theopaschite heresy that attributes suffering to God *as God*.
25. *Salvifici Doloris*. 20.
26. Op. cit., 19.
27. Op. cit., 23.
28. cf. *Christian Spirituality* Vol. II. Ed. Jill Raitt. London: SCM Press. 1989. Chapter 15.
29. *Salvifici Doloris*. 7.
30. Clement of Alexandria, *Stromatesis*. IV. 4. In 'The Ante-Nicene Fathers.' Vol. II. Electronic Edn. Christian Classics Etherial Library. Wheaton College. http:\\ccel.wheaton.edu/fathers.
31. Ibid.
32. Ibid.
33. Clement of Alexandria. *The Instructor*. (*Paidogogos*) III. xi. In 'The Ante-Nicene Fathers.' Vol. II.
34. Ibid.
35. Ibid.
36. Ibid.
37. Ibid.
38. Ibid.
39. I owe this information to Archimandrite Ephrem Lash. Schleusner's *Novus Thesaurus* records an identical translation in a very similar context in Isaiah 26. 14.
40. Clement of Alexandria, *The Instructor*. I. ii. ANF. v.s.
41. I draw much of my information about the Anargyroi from an unpublished paper kindly made available to me by Dimitri Brady, Chaplain to Overseas Students in Higher Education in Manchester.
42. An excellent study of the relation between the formal and informal structures of the sacred in a society is presented in *From Bishop to Witch*, by David Gentilcore. Manchester UP, 1992.
43. v.s.
44. John Climacus. *The Ladder of Divine Ascent*. tr. C. Lubhaid and N. Russell. London: SPCK. 1982. p. 232 f.
45. I do not pity Herod, however, when he is riddled with worms. Nor is pity the response the early Christian felt to the sufferings of the great martyrs.
46. Ibid.

CAN GOD INFLICT UNREQUITED PAIN ON HIS CREATURES? MUSLIM PERSPECTIVES ON HEALTH AND SUFFERING

Abdulaziz Sachedina

As we explore Muslim perspectives on health and suffering it is important to keep in mind that in the absence of an officially organized and recognized theological body, resembling, for instance, the Pope or Vatican Council in Catholicism, it is impossible to think of Islam in monolithic terms on any theological matter. In fact, plurality in belief and practice is inherent to Islam which, like Rabbinical Judaism, invests the power of interpretation and decision-making not in an institution like a church, but in the person of experts in religious matters, the 'ulamā'. Hence, in our search for Muslim views on health and suffering, there will be very little attempt made at identifying particular views as being strictly Sunni or Shi'i. As I shall demonstrate in this paper, it is not unusual to find contrary views about freedom of will and predetermination within a single school of thought that have ramifications for the way suffering is accounted for. Moreover, although it is not impossible to identify certain theological trends as being generally espoused by the Sunnis or Shi'is, it is rather misleading to insist on their dogmatic uniformity even within the same school.

In general, the Arabic term *muṣība,* which signifies suffering or affliction caused by events that lead to some form of harm or loss (*ḍarr* or *ḍurr*) is discussed in the light of Muslim belief about the omnipotent and omniscient God. Closely related to the issue of affliction and the ensuing harm is the everyday expression in Muslim culture which connects the occurrence of suffering to God's 'permission' (*idhn*) . It is very common to express one's sympathy for a loss or illness that you or someone you know suffers by saying: *bi idhni-llāh* or *bi mashiyyati-llāh,* that is, it happened with God's permission or God's will. However, such a statement creates a theological problem of imputing evil to God. It implicates moral

God in the dispute about the authorship of an action that is objectively described as evil.

There are contradictory responses in the foundational sources of Islamic thought to the question about the existence of evil in the world. Its positive or negative estimation among Muslims has depended upon the way pertinent texts are interpreted by various scholars representing different schools of thought. But it is also the cryptic nature of some of the scriptural language about God's role in creating or permitting evil in the world that lends itself to the problems of explication about the purpose of evil. Additionally, one can detect some kind of an unofficial state theology at work in furthering unquestioning submission to the all-powerful God, reaching almost psychological numbness in dealing with evil in the society in general. There is overwhelming historical evidence to show that under the Umayyad rulers (CE 660–748) the state policy was to perpetrate belief in the absolute will of God that predetermined all human action, including the evil conduct of those in power, to contain growing discontent and opposition to the dynasty. On the basis of selective verses of the Qur'an people were made to believe that human suffering as a form of God's punishment was caused by the divine will to which a good believer should submit without questioning.

In the Qur'an

To be sure, for Muslims the Qur'an is a foundational source for their belief system. Accordingly, what the Qur'an says about any religious or ethical issue is regarded as an authentic perspective on Muslim creed. A careful examination of the Qur'an in its natural context, on the one hand, reveals the vulnerability of human life in the threatening conditions of living near the desert; and, on the other, it shows the complex interaction between the divine and human wills to overcome the effects of the actual instances of suffering. In other words, the Qur'an juxtaposes a realistic treatment of suffering as part of what it means to be alive under severe life situations with suffering as a problem of theodicy in which it is ultimately faith in the transcendent God rather than the rational understanding of the philosophy of evil that can bring about confidence in the divine wisdom. Suffering in various forms through physical and mental tribulation is introduced in the Qur'an to demonstrate the all-encompassing power of God. It is the

Almighty Creator who causes it and it is 'He who answers the constrained, when he calls unto Him, and removes evil.' (27:61) The Qur'an is engaged in treating suffering as a divinely ordained temporary situation, rather than in estimating it as an ethical problem for the just and compassionate God that needs vindication and rationalization.

In some passages it clearly imputes the cause to humans who have been visited by 'an affliction for what their own hands have forwarded,' (4:63) requiring them to assess the positive role it plays in sharpening human awareness of God's continuous presence. In other passages it implicitly suggests that God has the foreknowledge of suffering because 'no affliction befalls in the earth or in yourselves, but it is in a Book, before We create it.' (57:22) Most of the commentators of this latter verse regard the affliction in general to be neutral in value, that is neither good nor evil. However, they differentiate natural catastrophe that befalls in the earth from the harm that reaches human beings through injury, illness, death and so on. The latter occur in order to call humans to heed to the call of faith, which requires them to spend in the path of God and to strive physically to make God's purposes on earth to succeed.

The theological problem arises about that affliction which is written in a Book before it is created. In both cases, their being written in a Book seems to suggest that the reference is to God's omniscience. Does this omniscience of God require Muslims to believe that God has knowledge concerning things before they existed, from eternity? God's omniscience certainly led to the creedal statement in majority of the Sunni works on theology that God has indeed decreed and ordained everything, including suffering as a form of evil, that nothing could happen either in this world or in the next except through His will, knowledge, decision, decree and writing on the preserved table (*al-lawḥ al-maḥfūẓ*).[1] However, this divine absoluteness was tampered with a declaration that God's writing is 'of a descriptive, not of a decisive nature.'[2]

In another verse the Qur'an admonishes human beings to endure patiently whatever visits them because 'no affliction befalls, except it be by the leave of God.' (64:11) 'By the leave of God' – *bi idhni-llāh* – seems to reinforce the Muslim cultural attitude of passiveness in the face of afflictions. But such an attitude also generates patience in the face of pain suffered by the occurrence of affliction because like all other things it comes from God and that also for a fixed period after which human beings must return to their Lord, the Creator of all Being. Muslim theologians have debated the adverse ramifications of the phrase 'by the leave of' if understood in terms of all suffering being written on the finite preserved table in eternity, whereas human conditions are supposed to be governed by the laws of causality. Does it imply that God's foreknowledge is the real cause of suffering? Or, does it mean that God controls the power of removing of the cause(s) that impede the realization of His salutary plan for humanity? Suffering, as the Qur'an asserts time and again, is in some sense purposeful.

Yet, God's foreknowledge about imminent affliction raises a serious ethical problem about God's willing an affliction to occur despite His omnipotence to prevent it. If He creates affliction before it is inflicted, then divine authorship of evil contradicts God's justice and boundless benevolence. Reasonable people, as these commentators argue, do not regard the Being who has the power to prevent the evil and still does not do so as just and good God. On the other hand, other scholars argue that there is some question as to whether evil exists in the world in the real sense of the word. In fact, they maintain that the evil of things is not a true attribute; it is a relative one. On many occasions when we encounter unpleasantness in our lives, we become unjustifiably upset and we term the causes of our discomfort as 'evil'. Good and evil do not represent mutually exclusive categories or series in the order of creation. Goodness is identical with being, and evil is identical with non-being; wherever being makes its appearance, non-existence is also implied. Thus when we speak of poverty, ignorance or disease we should not imagine that they have separate realities: poverty is simply not having wealth, ignorance is the absence of knowledge, and disease is the loss of health. Wealth and knowledge are realities, but poverty is nothing other than the emptiness of hand and the pocket, and ignorance, the absence of knowledge. Hence poverty and ignorance have no tangible reality; they are defined through the non-existence of other things.

The same is the case with afflictions and misfortunes that we regard as evil and the source of suffering. They, too, are a kind of loss or non-being, and are evil only in the sense that they result in the destruction and non-existence of something other than themselves. Apart from this, as these scholars hold, nothing, insofar as it exists, can in any way be called evil or ugly.

If afflictions did not entail sickness and death, the loss and destruction of certain creatures, thus preventing their capacities from unfolding, they would not be bad. It is the loss and ruin arising from misfortunes that is inherently bad. Whatever exists in the world is good; evil pertains to non-being, and since non-being does not form a category independent of being, it has not been created and does not exist. The Qur'an regards the world as being equivalent to good. Everything is inherently good; if it is evil, it is so only in a relative sense and in connection with things other than itself. The malarial mosquito is not evil in itself. If it is described as such, it is because it is harmful to human and causes disease. That which is created is the existence of a thing in and of itself, which is a true existence; conditional existence has no place in the order of being and is not real. That which is real must derive its being from the Creator. Only those things and attributes are real that exist outside the mind. Relative attributes are created by the mind and have no existence outside it so one cannot go looking for the creator. From the vantage point of God's wisdom, either the world must exist on the pattern that is particular to it, or it cannot exist at all. A world without order or lacking the principle of causality, a world where good and evil were not separate from each other, would be an impossibility and a fantasy. It is for this reason that relatively speaking there are few references in the Qur'an to suffering and they appear as inevitable concomitants of the real entities that give rise to them. Thus the Qur'an sums its treatment of suffering in the following verse:

> Surely We will try you with something of fear and hunger, and loss of wealth and possessions, death, and the loss of fruits of your toil. Yet, give glad tidings to those who are patient who, when they are visited by an affliction, say, 'Surely we belong to God, and to Him we return.' Upon those rest blessings and mercy from their Lord, and those are the truly guided. (2:155–57)

In the *ḥadīth*

When one considers Muslim traditions collected in the books on the Sunna, that is, the prophetic paradigm, the treatment of suffering in general, and illness or loss of good health, in particular, appears to be treated in the light of certain theological positions maintained about the divine will and human will. Hence, there are traditions that speak of illness as a form of divinely ordained suffering based on the belief that God is the author of all that befalls human beings. In fact, such traditions have been the major source of skeptical attitude towards seeking medical treatment in some quarters of Muslim society because God is regarded as the only Healer on whom a true believer should depend. Moreover, in these traditions illness is evaluated as a form of divine mercy to expiate a believer's sins. According to a well known tradition, the Prophet is reported to have said: 'No fatigue, nor disease, nor sorrow, nor sadness, nor hurt, nor distress befalls a Muslim, even if it were the prick he received from a thorn, but that God expiates some of his sins for that.'[3]

On the other hand, there are traditions that contradict the attitude of passivity in confronting suffering in any form. Since God is just He cannot cause unrequited pain to His creatures. In fact, there is a strong emphasis on God's goodness and purposiveness in all that He does. He intends only benefit. Reconciling this tenet with the suffering of the innocent has not been easy in Islam. Even when the general trend in Muslim piety is to hold human beings accountable for their own suffering and to recommend undertaking to do righteous acts to rid the world of suffering, it has been specifically onerous to explain the suffering of infants and animals. The idea that some imperfect beings serve merely to ransom other perfect beings was not compatible with God's infinite benevolence and justice. Some Muslims tried to explain such sufferings as admonitions for adults. Since all God's acts are purposeful, nothing could be in vain, including the suffering of the children. In that sense, sufferings of the children served as a divine sign and a warning for the discerning. They provided a convenient means for putting the parents to test. However, God then made up for the unmerited sufferings which children underwent in this world in the hereafter.

The problem of infant suffering was difficult to resolve from juridical point of view also. In Islamic juridical doctrine children as minors are not regarded legally competent to assume any religious or moral responsibility (*mukallaf*) for God to inflict suffering upon them if they failed to carry out their obligations. More difficult was to justify the suffering of the animals, lesser beings, as an admonition for humans, higher beings. And, although there were views among some Muslims that animals will be rewarded lavishly in paradise and even in this world in ways we humans cannot understand, the intricacies related to the workings of divine justice in the case of the sufferings of the innocent was regarded as being beyond human comprehension.[4]

The *ḥadīth* literature overwhelmingly regards illness as an affliction that needs to be cured by every possible legitimate means. In fact, in these traditions, the search for cure is founded upon unusual confidence generated by the divine promise reported in one of the early traditions that 'There is no disease that God has created, except that He has also created its treatment.'[5] Hence, the purpose of medicine is to search for cure and provide necessary care to those afflicted with diseases.

It is also this confidence in being cured by human efforts that a physician's role as a healer is regarded as spiritually and morally commendable and a collective duty among the religious obligations, in that medicine is a religious necessity for society. Muslim physician, male or female, must treat illness not merely as a physical reality, but also pay attention to psychological causes, because in Islam medicine, hygiene, and regulations for healthy living together form the guidelines for good living according to God's will. In practice, Muslims have taken this responsibility very seriously. They were among the first in the world to build hospitals for more effective cure of the sick. Like all human activity, medical practice can be both an act of worship and a source of divine testing, if God's mercy is misused to evil purposes. Medical doctors are exhorted to work sincerely under the guidelines of the religious law, to avoid all temptations of personal arrogance or richness, and to resist all kinds of social pressures, be they personal, political, or military. Medical caring and curing should therefore be practiced in a climate of piety and awareness of the presence of God.[6]

The latter requirement raises questions concerning doctor-patient relations whether a male physician can treat a female patient, or vice versa, and whether a female nurse can take care of a male patient, or vice versa. Since the assumption is that the physician or the nurse is bound by professional ethics, the general rule that applies to all such cases is that necessity renders forbidden act legal and men and women may be treated by physicians and nurses of the opposite sex.[7]

Although some of the traditions attributed to the Prophet primarily serve as further elaboration of the Qur'anic views about suffering, a vast number of them function as prophetic directives about the proper etiquette in dealing with illness and when visiting the sick and bereaved. The following tradition provides the paradigm for the community to emulate the Prophet in what to say when visiting a patient. According to this tradition, the Prophet entered the home of a desert Arab to visit him – and it was his custom when he visited the sick to say, 'Don't worry. It is a purification, if God will' – and he said to him, 'Don't worry. It is a purification, if God will.' The man replied, 'Never! rather it is a fever boiling on an old man, which will send him on a visit to the graves!' The Prophet replied, 'Very well, then be it so.'[8] In another tradition it is related that when a person fell ill the Prophet used to rub him with his right hand and then pray to God saying: 'O Lord of the people, grant him health, heal him, for Thou art a Great Healer.'[9]

Other traditions recognize a religious purpose of illness and underline the reason for it, as for other forms of suffering, being God's trial of the people and the cleansing effect of illness. Hence, in a tradition the Prophet says that the patient earns merits under these trials and can attain the rank of a true believer. 'When God intends to do good to somebody, He afflicts him with trials.'[10]

Aṣābahu bi maradin: He (i.e. God) afflicted him with disease; or rendered him diseased, like its converse, *aṣābahu bi ṣiḥatin*, He rendered him healthy, is a common expression of God's activity in everyday human situation in the Muslim culture. In a Muslim thanksgiving prayer besides praising and thanking God for all the blessings a believer affirms: 'To You [o God] belongs praise for all the good affliction (*balā'*^{in} *ḥasan*^{in}) with which You have inured me.'[11]

The characterization of affliction as 'good' in the above prayer indicates that suffering as such does not create a theoretical problem in Islam. Rather, it is treated in direct terms as part of the divine plan for humanity. When it occurs it is identified and its impact is reversed by the education and the discipline of a person in a true affirmation and submission to the will of God (*islām*). The Qur'an and the traditions provide an uncommon interpretation of suffering as a concrete human experience, as an unavoidable condition of human existence. They do not regard suffering as an evil and hence a problem that needs to be explained or vindicated since its author is the good God.

In the Theology

As we move into theological evaluation of suffering we are in face to face with the problem of theodicy in Islam.[12] In view of its preoccupation with the malicious polytheism of the Meccans of the seventh century Arabia, it is reasonable to maintain that the Qur'an was more concerned with the question of belief and disbelief than the question of suffering in human society. To be sure, for the Qur'an abandoning faith in God is both sinful and evil and as such evil is nothing but the withdrawal of good, just as darkness is the withdrawal of light. In this sense evil is treated like sin which in itself has no essence. It is a state of moral inadequacy in varying degrees which manifests itself in the lack of the good relevant for a creature's well estate. If this explanation is applied to specific evil like illness it cannot be regarded as truly evil. Rather, illness as a trial from God, although a form of tribulation and suffering, fulfills a positive role in the life of a faithful, revealing God's power to cure and to show His limitless compassion. The question whether God can inflict unrequited pain on His creatures is central to any theodicy even in this day and age when we, as modernly educated men and women, claim to have found efficient causes through scientific progress to explain the perplexing problems of existence in human life rationally. The disharmony between the concept of a just God and the reality of human suffering constitutes one of the most crucial and perplexing problems in human history.[13] It is not only Muslims who bitterly complain about the various forms of extant evil that prevail in their society. One just needs to listen to the mass media to get some sense of different forms of suffering that afflict humanity across national and cultural-religious boundaries.

The problem of rationalizing God's justice with the fate of humanity faced with adversities, illnesses and all kinds of natural and human-caused afflictions is a major concern among the sensitive followers of Islam. Can one explain the suffering of the righteous or the prosperity of the wicked without losing faith in God's omnipotence, as emphasized by Sunni Muslims? Can one harmonize the unmerited suffering of the innocent with the concept of divine justice, as maintained by the Shi'ite Muslims? These questions are not merely academic concerns of Muslim theologians trying to explain the inscrutable ways of God. They are real issues among the majority of the Muslim peoples around the world.

Muslims, like their other Abrahamic cousins, the Jews and Christians, affirm God's goodness and the Divine Omnipotence and Almightiness over the entire creation. At the same time in the face of human suffering they are required to defend God's justice and the Divine absolute power. Why does not God, who is all-compassionate (*al-raḥmān*) and all-merciful (*al-raḥīm*), who is omnipotent (*al-qādir*) and omniscient (*al-'alīm*), prevent suffering insofar as

He is able? How can one interpret the apparent incompatibility between God's absolute goodness and the fact of suffering of the innocent?

To be sure, Islamic theodicy is very much a feature of its ethical monotheism which affirms God's goodness and almightiness while at the same time accepts suffering as part of the divine plan for humanity's betterment. Moreover, the religiously inspired ideals about a good society in Islam logically create an existential need to explain suffering and evil despite God's promises to the contrary. A theodicy is necessary in any religion where any god is regarded as invariably benevolent and omnipotent.[14] However, in Islam it would seem that its insistence on 'submission' (one of the essential meanings of the term *islām*) to the divine will would remove untenable contradictions inherent in Muslim belief about the benevolent and omnipotent God and would reduce the centrality of theodicy similar to the Hebrew Bible and New Testament. In fact, Islam's emphasis on God's transcendence from human moral judgement led Kenneth Cragg to observe that Islam 'ignores or neglects or does not hear these questions [about the wrongs in life] . . . . It does not find a theodicy necessary either for its theology or its worship.'[15]

This is an oversight of a theological problem that existed in Islam because of its rational theology founded upon human free will.

In Muslim theology, as we shall see below, the free-will theodicy was constructed on the Qur'anic references about human free agency and all-powerful divine will. The notion of evil as a necessary concomitant of good was an important theme in the theological, mystical and philosophical literature in Islam. Muslims, like the followers of other traditions, endeavored to understand the sources of specific evils that manifested in the form of suffering. The underlying concern in all these endeavors was: How to reconcile specific evils with God's attributes like All-knowing, All-powerful, and All-merciful? In view of God's regenerative mercy (*raḥma*) on all His creatures, regardless of whether they believe in Him or not, can one explain illness as a specific evil simply by contending that it is nothing more than the lack of the good state of being that is health?

The problem of disharmony between the concept of a God of justice and the evils present in the world, is encapsulated in the tradition in which after doing away with all secondary causality

God is made the sole agent of infectious disease. The Prophet is reported to have said:

> 'There is neither contagion nor augury nor jaundice nor bird of evil omen.' A bedouin asked: 'O Prophet of God, how is it then that my camels were in the sand [as healthy as] gazelles, and then a mangy camel mingled with them and made them mangy?' The Prophet replied: 'Who infected the first (camel)?[16]

In other words, God has Himself implanted the disease which causes suffering. There are verses in the Qur'an that could be cited as supporting a predestinarian theology of the later period that literally imputed evil to God.[17] However, there are opposing verses also in which God plainly delegates responsibility for suffering to free creature's abuse of their freedom.[18] These latter verses speak about free-will theodicy in which suffering can be traced back to the human agency. The Qur'an reminds human beings that 'God will not wrong so much as the weight of an ant.' (4:40) Moreover, the Qur'an, as previously discussed, also views suffering as a test of righteousness. 'Do the people reckon that they will be left to say, "We believe," and will not be tried?' (29:1)[19]

In the first half of the eighth century, the debates about the existence of injustices in the community, and its appropriate response to redress the situation, formed the rudiments of the earliest systematic theology of the group called Mu'tazilites.[20] Before them, some Muslim thinkers had developed theological arguments, including a doctrine of God and human responsibility, in defense of the Islamic revelation and the prophethood of Muḥammad when these were challenged by other monotheists. The Mu'tazilites, however, undertook to show that there was nothing repugnant to reason in the Islamic revelation. In defining God's creation and governance of the world, they sought to demonstrate the primacy of revelation. At the same time, their recognition of a substantial role for human reason in explaining the ways of God reflected Hellenic influences. From the ninth century on, translations of the full Greek philosophic and scientific heritage became available in Arabic. The result was the development of a technical vocabulary and a pattern of syntax that reflected theological terminology substantially similar to some familiar positions in the Judeo-Christian theodicy.[21]

The Mu'tazilites were the champions of human free agency and hence was the school that formulated the free will theodicy, insisting upon an inseparable link between free will and divine justice. The principle of divine justice was central to their theology and ethics in which human intellect was capable of recognizing good and evil without any aid from revelation. In other words, human intuitive reasoning was capable of discovering the rational aspect behind every circumstance and event. God has the best interest of His creatures at heart when He does not prevent their suffering. Since all God's actions have their ultimate object the specific well-being of individual creatures, it was necessary for human beings to discover, and defend, God's purposeful actions in the most apparently unseemly events.[22]

A reaction against Mu'tazili emphasis on free-will theodicy was bound to appear with the realization that it is not in human power to explain God's wisdom in apparently unmerited suffering of the just and the prosperity of the wicked. Even a vivid Qur'anic eschatology with the concept of the life to come, the Hereafter, where all the inequities will be corrected, the wicked punished just as the righteous rewarded, could not explain the tribulations suffered by the innocent. 'Whatever God does He does for the best' was a believer's way of accepting the hardships caused in this world, and it was this maxim that formed the Ash'ari theodicy based on predestinarian position.

The Ash'arites, reacting to Mu'tazilite free-will theodicy, limited speculative theology to a defense of the doctrines given in the *ḥadīth* reports attributed to the Prophet. These were regarded as more reliable than abstract reason in understanding individual doctrines. The Ash'arites emphasized the absolute will and power of God, and denied nature and humankind any decisive role. What humans perceive as causation, they believed, is actually God's habitual behavior. In their response to the Mu'tazilite view about the objective nature of good and evil, they maintained that good and evil are what God decrees them to be. This was the way they intended to preserve the effectiveness of a God, at once omnipotent and omnibenevolent, who could and did intervene in human affairs. Accordingly, good and evil cannot be known from nature but must be discovered in the sources of revelation, like the Qur'an and the Prophet's paradigmatic conduct, the Sunna. There are no inherently unchanging essences and natural laws that self-subsistent reason can discern.[23] God transcends the order of nature.

Hence, the notion of free will is incompatible with the notion of divine transcendence, which determines all actions directly.

Ash'arite theological views remained dominant throughout Islamic history, well into modern times, and had profound effects upon scientific and particularly medical theory and practice among the Sunni Muslims. The attitude of resignation, a by-product of belief in predestination, is summed up in the Sunni creedal confession: 'What reaches you could not possibly have missed you; and what misses you could not possibly have reached you.'[24]

To elaborate on this creedal declaration, the Ash'arites maintained that God directly wills whatever occurs in this world. He knows and it is the direct expression of His will. It is He, and only He, who causes actions. Hence, good and evil are what God decrees them to be and it is presumptuous for human beings to judge God on the basis of categories God has laid down for human beings. In some actions, however, God superadds a special quality of voluntary acquisition which by God's will makes the individual a voluntary agent and responsible. But, this limited human autonomy still leaves all responsibility to the divine agency which extends to all facets of human existence, such as sustenance, span of life, pleasure and pain. It is God who allots to a human being all that he/she has.

In summary, Ash'ari theodicy of determinism does not deny the evil aspects of pain, incapacity, illness or poverty. Nor does it ignore the painful realities of existence. They are evils but they are not the result of social inequity or accident or human wickedness. God intends poverty or pain or disbelief for certain individuals, just as He intends wealth, well-being, and belief for others. In fact, based on the doctrine of trust in God's will, a form of optimism underlies the belief that disease, destitution, social inequity, and the like are right and just.[25]

This belief in the overpowering destiny was bound to have negative implications in encountering adversities caused by illness and other forms of suffering in some sectors of Muslim society. The Shi'ite theological and ethical doctrines were, on the other hand, based on Mu'tazilite thesis about the Justice of God, and the objective nature of moral values. Hence, the religious evaluation of illness and suffering were regarded as caused by human excesses in the exercise of freedom of will. However, as a minority within a Muslim community, whose leaders had suffered martyrdom in their cause, Shi'ites saw tribulations as steps towards an eternal and blissful end. Their pious literature celebrating the martyrdoms of the Shi'ite Imams, especially the grandson of the Prophet Muḥammad, al-Ḥusayn and his family, describes the suffering of the innocent women and children in a very positive way as a divine blessing meant to become a source of self purification and preparation for the arduous spiritual journey towards God. For the pious, as the Shi'ites maintain, this world is a world of suffering and sorrow. But these trials of affliction are the means of attaining God's mercy and conform to His will. They are more than a mere discipline; they are an active choice made independently of rewards and punishments.[26] Suffering has its own merit with God. It is the road to salvation for the people of faith and it is good in itself as a means of purification of the soul. Humility before God can be most deeply expressed through patient endurance of suffering. The Shi'ites share this positive outlook to human suffering in any form with Muslim mystics, the Sufis.[27]

Muslim mystics, who, in general, shared the Ash'ari optimism about the divine wisdom in their understandings of human suffering, regarded it as a necessary part of their ascetic lifestyle. The inward life of the soul depended upon affliction to detach itself from the world and love God only. The goal was to gain control over one's passions which caused pain and suffering at the loss of anything to which one was attached or one has most desired. Among the Sufis to reach a level of consciousness where one could let one's entire life be guided by the immediate will of God meant giving up anything that did not bear the marks of divine blessing, however dire the consequences might be. This was their idea of trust in God. Hence, trials, afflictions, and pains are part of the journey towards the everlasting happiness that culminates in being blessed with the love of God.[28]

Ibn al-'Arabī (CE 1165–1240), one of the great mystics of Islam, sees human affliction as an expression of divine mercy caused by fluctuation in that mercy as the heart of the mystic goes through the inner purification in the hands of God:

> But the heart is between two fingers of its Creator, who is the All-merciful . . . . Hence He does not cause the heart to fluctuate except from one mercy to another mercy, even though there is affliction (*balā'*) in the various kinds of fluctuation. But there lies in affliction's midst a mercy hidden from man and known to the Real, for the two fingers belong to the All-merciful.[29]

In another place he regards affliction as an instrument used by God to measure a person's ability to reflect on the divine purposes in creation:

> God afflicted man with an affliction with which no other of His creatures was afflicted. Through it He takes him to felicity or wretchedness, depending upon how He allows him to make use of it. This affliction with which God afflicted him is that He created within him a faculty named "reflection." He made this faculty the assistant of another faculty called "reason." Moreover, He compelled reason, in spite of its being reflection's chief, to take from reflection what it gives. God gave reflection no place to roam except the faculty of imagination. God made the faculty of imagination the locus which brings together everything given by the sensory faculties.[30]

Concluding Remarks

Two contradictory evaluations about the purpose of suffering emerge within the context of theological discussions in Islam:

First, suffering is part of God's plan for the betterment of humanity. All forms of suffering, including illness, serve two purposes:

(a) As a form of punishment to expiate for a sin;

(b) As a form of a test or trial to confirm a believer's spiritual station.

Second, suffering is caused by human free will in choosing to believe or disbelieve and face the consequences of this choice. Disbelief then is treated as the source of human misconduct which results in suffering. Suffering in this situation serves educational function. It is instrumental in revealing the consequences of absence of faith in human life and the accruing evil in the form of afflictions.

Should one take upon himself to alleviate suffering where possible and endure otherwise?

Two responses are offered in the light of two above-mentioned positions, which have negative and positive implications for medical treatment, respectively:

(a) A passive response based on the belief that since God is testing human belief, one must endure suffering. A corollary of this belief is that, as reported in the words of Abraham in the Qur'an,

God is the only Healer on whom a believer should depend:

> '. . . Lord of all Being who created me, and Himself gives me to eat and drink, and, whenever I am sick, heals me, who makes me die, then gives me life . . . .' (26:80)

The statement 'whenever I am sick, heals me,' becomes a source for a skeptical attitude towards medical treatment. This skeptical attitude is not limited to any particular school of thought in Islam. Rather, it is commonly held in the culture without sometimes any reference to the aforementioned belief in God's sole power of healing.

(b) An active response based on the belief that since a human being is the cause of his/her own suffering, he/she should undertake to do righteous acts to rid the world of suffering. Good works negate suffering. Obviously, the latter belief generates a positive attitude to medical treatment and it derives its strength from the oft-quoted Prophet Muhammad's advice to his followers:

> 'O servants of God, seek the cure, because God did not create a disease without creating its cure, except for one disease . . . . senility.'

Theological-ethical debates on these two responses are based on the two forms of Islamic theodicy: the determinist and free-will theodicies based on the concepts of the divine omnipotence and the divine justice.

Ethical Decisions in Applied Islamic Medical Jurisprudence

Medical Treatment = Active Response to human suffering based on traditions that relate:

(a) Health is preferable to sickness.

(b) 'A powerful believer is preferred and better liked by God than a weak believer.'

(c) Seeking cure does not contradict the trust in God and submission to God's decision about humanity.

The place of Life-sustaining Treatment in Islam:

Fundamental criteria:

(a) There is an absolute obligation to save human life. In the case of a patient in the vegetative state ethical deliberations in Islam are not only concerned with determining the value of the patients life. The principle of public good (*maṣlaḥah*) demands that an individual's life must be weighed in the scale of general well estate of those who are horizontally related to the patient. End of life decisions require to take into consideration an individual's interpersonal relationship with his own family and society in general. If active medical intervention in the case of a severely brain-damaged patient leads to further suffering of the patient and those related to him in society, then the ethical judgement cannot ignore the ensuing general harm, including the rising cost of prolonging such life for the entire society. There is no obligation to prolong a persistent vegetative state in a patient through intensive care technology, as required by the principle that rejection of harm is necessary. In this case, Islamic jurisprudence views aggressive medical treatment as a source of harm and obstruction of nature's course to terminate human suffering through death. Moreover, necessity renders the prohibited permissible, which in this case will make it permissible to discontinue the life-sustaining equipment.

(b) Availability of affordable resources, both human and technological, to sustain a terminally ill patient's life must be assessed in terms of collective social needs founded upon the principle of distributive justice.

(c) Benefits of active medical intervention must be open to all.

Principles of 'justice' and 'utility' as known in the secular bioethics would be hard to implement in the case of inclusiveness and community-oriented nature of the Islamic ethics of medical treatment. Moral problems connected with the allocation of scarce resources in majority of Muslim societies in the Third World remain unanswered because of the authoritarian and paternalistic nature of health care in these countries. However, the requirement to adhere to the principle of equal worth of human life by a mere fact of being human suggests that no human life can be treated lightly when it comes to the distribution of limited medical resources.

Physician-Assisted Suicide and Euthanasia in Islam

As stated above, illness as a form of divinely ordained suffering serves two purposes:

First, as a form of punishment to expiate for a sin;

Second, as a form of a test or trial to confirm a believer's spiritual station.

Suffering is, thus, instrumental in revealing God's purposes for humanity. Should one take upon oneself to alleviate suffering where possible and endure otherwise? Obviously, the Qur'anic directives make it clear that death cannot be negotiated because life is a divine trust and cannot be terminated by any form of human intervention. Hence, the rulings are:

(a) 'Mercy killing' or 'Physician-assisted Aid in Dying' (PAID) of terminally ill patients is prohibited.

(b) Withdrawing or withholding necessary-to-life interventions is construed as murder, because a physician is responsible to maintain the process of life, not of deciding death. However, there is no obligation to continue these interventions if these simply prolong the imminent death of a terminally ill patient.

(c) Patient's own determination of death being a better outcome and physician assisting him/her to terminate life, both are committing an offense against God.

(d) 'Killing' and 'Letting die' carry equal moral consequences even if the person to be killed is competent to determine that death is a better outcome.

(e) In final analysis, there are no grounds for justifiable killing whether through voluntary active-euthanasia (VAE) or Physician Assisted Suicide (PAS) in Islam.

NOTES

1. For a sample of Sunni creed on this subject and its theological discussion see: A. J. Wensinck, *The Muslim Creed* (London: Frank Cass & Co. Ltd., 1965), pp. 188ff.
2. Ibid., p. 190.
3. *Ṣaḥīh al-Bukhārī, Kitāb al-marḍā* (Chicago: Kazi Publications, 1979), Vol. 7, pp. 371–2, *ḥadīth* # 545.
4. Eric L. Ormsby, *Theodicy in Islamic Thought: The Dispute over Al-Ghazālī's 'Best of All Possible Worlds'* (Princeton: Princeton University Press, 1984), pp. 241–5 discusses various views held by Muslim theologians regarding the suffering of children and animals in the context of God's 'doing the best for His creatures.'
5. *Ṣaḥīh al-Bukhārī*, Vol. 7, *ḥadīth* # 582.
6. First International Conference on Islamic Medicine, *Islamic Code of Medical Ethics*, Kuwait Document, Kuwait Rabi 1, 1401 (January 1981), pp. 16–23.
7. Vardit Rispler-Chaim, *Islamic Medical Ethics in the Twentieth Century* (Leiden: E.J. Brill, 1993), p. 63.
8. Ibid., *ḥadīth* # 566.
9. *Ṣaḥīh Muslim* (New Delhi: Kitab Bhavan, 1986) *ḥadīth* # 5432–8 report the various forms of the prayer for the sick.

10. *Ṣaḥīh al-Bukhārī*, Vol. 7, p. 373, *ḥadīth* #548.
11. 'Abbās Qummī, *Mafātīḥ al-jinān* (Tehran: Kitābfurūshī-yi 'Ilmiyya-yi Islāmiyya, 1381), pp. 405.
12. Ormsby, *Theodicy*, Chapters 3–5, provides a detailed examination of theodicy and the problem of evil in Islamic theology in the context of the scholastic debates in the classical age.
13. Article "Theodicy" in the *Encyclopedia of Religion*, ed. Mircea Eliade (New York: Simon Schuster Macmillan, 1995), Vol. 14, pp. 430–41.
14. Wendy Doniger O'Flaherty, *The Origins of Evil in Hindu Mythology* (Berkeley: University of California Press, 1976), p. 2 cites Gananath Obeyesekere, "Theodicy, Sin, and Salvation in a Sociology of Buddhism," in *Dialectical in Practical Religion*, ed. by E.R. Leach (Cambridge: Cambridge University Press, 1968), p. 8. See also Clifford Geertz, *Interpretations of Cultures: Selected Essays* (New York: Basic Books, 1973), p. 103 writes: 'There are few if any religious traditions, great or little, in which the proposition that life hurts is not strenuously affirmed, and in some it is virtually glorified.'
15. Kenneth Cragg, *The House of Islam* (Encino: Dickenson Publishing Co., Inc., 1975), p. 16.
16. There are different versions of this tradition in Muslim sources. The shorter version in *Ṣaḥīḥ al-Bukhārī*, Vol. 7, p. 409, *ḥadīth* # 608 simply states first part of the tradition in the section on leprosy. On the other hand, *Ṣaḥīḥ al-Tirmidhī* (Beirut: Dār al-Fikr, 1983), Vol. 3, p. 306, *ḥadīth* # 2230 mentions the detailed version which ends with the declaration by the Prophet: 'There is neither contagion nor jaundice. God created every person and then decreed his term, his sustenance and his afflictions (*maṣā'ib*).'
17. See the Qur'an, Sūra 6:125, which reads:

    Whomsoever God desires to guide, He expands his breast to Islam; whomsoever he desires to lead astray, He makes his breast narrow, tight . . .

    Or, 61:5

    When they swerved, God caused their hearts to swerve; and God guides never the people of ungodly.
18. See the Qur'an,sūra 2:24:

    He leads none astray save the ungodly.

    Or, 4:80

    Whatever good visits thee, it is of God; whatever evil visits thee is of thyself.
19. Article 'Theodicy,' in the *Encyclopedia of Religion*.
20. Marshall G. S. Hodgson, *The Venture of Islam: Conscience and History in a World Civilization* (Chicago: University of Chicago, 1977), Vol. 1, pp. 384–6.
21. Ibid., pp. 412ff., George F. Hourani, *Reason and Tradition in Islamic Ethics* (Cambridge: Cambridge University Press, 1985), Introduction.
22. Hourani, *Islamic Rationalism: The Ethics of 'Abd al-Jabbār* (Oxford: Clarendon Press, 1971), pp. 100ff.
23. Hodgson, *Venture of Islam*, Vol. 1, pp. 440–1.

24. *Fiqh akbar,* Article 3, cited by Wensinck, *The Muslim Creed*, p. 103. See also the *ḥadīth* reported in *Ṣaḥīḥ al Tirmidhī*, Vol. 3, p. 306, *ḥadīth* # 2231, which actually specifies that which unavoidably reaches human beings through the divine decree, namely, 'affliction'.
25. Ormsby, *Theodicy*, pp. 253ff.
26. Whether in Shī'ism there is a concept of 'redemptive' suffering, comparable to Christianity, is taken up in Mahmoud Ayoub, *Redemptive Suffering in Islam: A Study of the Devotional Aspects of 'Ashura' in Twelver Shī'ism* (The Hague: Mouton Publishers, 1978). However, at no point has the author connected the mourning rituals for the martyrdom of al-Ḥusayn, including the so-called self-flagellation, as a process of 'redemption' or 'self-mortification' in Shi'ite Islam. In some works by Western Christian authors a connection has been drawn between this Shi'ite practice and Christian monastic tradition where self-flagellation was regarded as necessary process of self-mortification. See, for instance, Sir Lewis Pelly, *The Miracle Play of Hasan and Husayn*, 2 Vols. (London: W. H. Allen & Co., 1879). My own studies in Shī'ite literature on martyrology has not found any support for the latter interpretation.
27. Ayoub, *Redemptive Suffering*, Chapter I, pp. 25ff.
28. Annemarie Schimmel, *Mystical Dimensions of Islam* (Chapel Hill: University of North Carolina Press, 1975), pp.136ff.
29. As cited and trans. by William Chittick, *The Sufi Path of Knowledge* (Albany, SUNY, 1989) p. 107.
30. Ibid.

RELIGION, HEALTH AND SUFFERING AMONG CONTEMPORARY TIBETANS

Geoffrey Samuel

The intention of this chapter is to complement Tadeusz Skorupski's primarily textually-based account with a more ethnographic description of religion, health and suffering in one particular Buddhist society, Tibet. What happens in an actual contemporary Buddhist society is more complex than one finds in the texts, for several reasons. In particular, (1) the texts are old, and are often far distant from current practice, and (2) other things are happening which are not reflected in the texts.

However, Buddhist societies do not all deal with these issues in the same ways. I will talk a little about the situation in Theravādin Buddhist societies before turning to the Tibetans, the main subject of this paper.[1] I will then talk about some recent field research on health among Tibetan refugees in India which I carried out with two colleagues in July and August 1996, before moving to some more general conclusions.[2]

Buddhism and Everyday Life

Suffering, as we know from the Four Noble Truths, is at the centre of the Buddhist analysis of life. It was Gautama's initial encounters with illness, old age and death, in the famous narrative, that spurred him on to his renunciation of his father's kingdom and his subsequent attainment of Buddhahood. The suffering of all ignorant and deluded beings, human and otherwise, within the endless cycles of rebirth that constitute the world we know, and the need to end that suffering through replicating the Buddha's achievement of Enlightenment, were central themes of the Four Noble Truths and of many other teachings of the historical Buddha.

Suffering and the transitoriness of life remain central themes of Buddhism to this day, but within the Theravāda tradition now dominant in Southeast Asia and Sri Lanka the attainment of Enlightenment long ago came to be seen as beyond the abilities of the human beings in these degenerate times. The ideal of the full-time religious career remained, but was seen in practice as achievable by only a small minority of mostly male monastics (*bhikkhu*).

The best that most lay people could aspire to was to improve their situation somewhat in the next round of rebirth through the practice of virtuous action. In other words, through performing good actions which would have positive consequences in a future life, and avoiding bad actions which would have negative consequences, Theravāda Buddhists could hope to be reborn as a human being with better opportunities to practise the Buddhist teachings, or at least hope to avoid being reborn in one of the lower realms – as an animal, a *preta* (hungry ghost) or a being in hell – or being born as a human being to a life of extreme poverty and suffering. This became the basis of what has been described by anthropologists working in Theravāda societies as an 'ideology of merit' (Tambiah 1968). Meritorious actions, apart from becoming a monk or nun[3] oneself permanently or temporarily, included in particular sponsoring one's son to become a monk, and making donations to monasteries and other Buddhist institutions. In this way Buddhism, with its normative stress on the rejection of *saṃsāra* (worldly life), and lay life, which is by definition grounded in *saṃsāra*, reached a kind of ongoing compromise.

The corollary to this emphasis on future lives in Theravāda Buddhist teachings is that Buddhism in these societies became primarily concerned with *karma*, death and rebirth. This again has been spelled out in great detail for Buddhist practice in Thailand (e.g. Tambiah 1968, 1970), Burma (Spiro 1967, 1982) and Sri Lanka (Gombrich 1971). In practice, dealing with death is today probably the most important area of specifically Buddhist activity in these societies. Theravāda Buddhist monks deal with death; this-worldly concerns are largely handled by other classes of religious practitioner. Marriage, for example, has traditionally never been a Buddhist ritual in any Theravāda society, and for that matter it is not one in Tibet either. The evolution of a specifically Buddhist marriage ceremony, as Richard Gombrich and Gananath Obeyesekere have noted (Gombrich and Obeyesekere 1990) is a twentieth-century development under Western influence. Similarly the consecration of rulers in Southeast Asia, and the whole area of court ritual, was carried out by hereditary families of Brahmin priests retained for this purpose within otherwise Buddhist courts, and some Brahminical functions continue to be carried out at the village level by lay ritual officiants (Brohm 1963, Tambiah 1970). In other words, Theravāda Buddhism is not officially concerned with the management, let alone the sacralization, of everyday life as such.

I say officially because in practice Buddhist monks with supernatural yogic powers and the magical use of Buddhist amulets and relics are of considerable significance in the everyday life of Theravāda countries (Spiro 1982, Tambiah 1984, Mulder 1992). Generally speaking, though, everyday life in Theravāda Buddhist countries, including the question of health and of medical treatment, is essentially a matter which falls outside the scope of Buddhism, though it may certainly involve the cult of non-Buddhist gods and spirits.

The details of these spirit cults vary from one place to another, and one can refer to the ethnographic literature for detailed accounts. The spirits concerned are often local in nature, associated with places within the landscape such as hills or lakes, and while they may have been more or less reshaped in terms of Indic imagery and ritual procedures they are still not Buddhist in the sense of sharing Buddhism's world-renouncing concerns, and are not on the whole addressed or dealt with by Buddhist monks. Illness may be attributed to these spirits being offended in some way, or to the action of lesser malevolent spirits, or to the loss from the body of some kind of spiritual substance or wandering soul such as the Thai *khwan* (Tambiah 1970). Priests, exorcists, spirit-mediums and shamans of various kinds can divine the origins of the problem and take curative action (Spiro 1967). One can also appeal for help at major deity shrines, often of high-status gods such as Kataragama (Skanda) in Sri Lanka (Gombrich and Obeyesekere 1990: 163-99) or of Brahmā in Thailand, deities who derive directly from the Indic pantheon. Whether one chooses to regard these areas of religion in Theravādin countries as constituting a separate religion to Buddhism, as Melford Spiro does (1967, 1982), or as forming part of a total and relatively integrated field of religious action within which Buddhism is also situated, as Stanley Tambiah does (1970), is to some degree a matter of emphasis, although my own tendency would be to stress interconnections and relationships rather than boundaries.

I have placed some stress on the situation in Theravāda Buddhist countries because it contrasts markedly with that in Tibetan societies.[4] In Tibetan societies too we find the local gods and malevolent spirits, the regional and state deities, and the high-level Indic guardian deities (Mahākāla, Palden Lhamo[5]). Yet interactions with all these kinds of gods form an integral part of the everyday practice of Tibetan Buddhist lamas and monks, whereas this is much less true in Theravādin countries. In Tibetan societies too we find village shamans and spirit-mediums, but their practice tends to be conducted very much under the authority of the lamas, who can themselves undertake all the ritual functions of these lesser practitioners. I mentioned that most Theravāda Buddhists hold that Enlightenment is beyond the reach of anyone now alive (or anyone who has been alive for maybe two thousand years). In Tibetan Buddhism, in theory at least, it is thought to be still generally accessible, and the lamas (Buddhist practitioners and teachers, but not necessarily monks) are seen as ways in which the miraculous powers associated with Enlightenment can be channelled and accessed. The ideology of merit and the concern with future rebirth is still important, but Buddhist practice has a much wider scope than dealing with death and rebirth.

This wider scope of Buddhist practice in Tibetan societies is certainly associated with the Vajrayāna (Tantric) Buddhism practised by Tibetans, but, as I have argued elsewhere, this is only in part a question of a special development within Tibet. It is at least as much a matter of the historical suppression by the state of the pragmatic, this-worldly, magical-ritual side of Buddhism in what are now the Theravādin countries (Samuel 1993). It should be remembered that Mahayāna and Vajrayāna Buddhism developed in India and were for many centuries an established part of religious life in all the regions where Theravāda Buddhism now prevails. Their absence from the contemporary scene is the result of a long series of state-imposed 'purifications' of the Saṃgha. The magical rituals of the Vajrayāna, centred around charismatic figures such as the Tantric *siddha* or the Tibetan lama, who was not necessarily a monk and could be directly engaged in lay life and political activity, were particularly problematic and were progressively eliminated in favour of the well-disciplined *bhikkhu* or monk with his much more limited sphere of activity and his institutional separateness from lay life. At the same time the practice of medicine, which seems to have been closely associated with the ascetic traditions of ancient India (Zysk 1991), became a lay rather than a monastic profession.

All this is significant in our present context, because wherever we find it the magical-ritual side of Buddhism is heavily involved in the area of healing. Buddhist ritual healing was never eliminated from the Theravādin societies, but it is undoubtedly less prominent and less sanctioned by official Buddhist authorities than in Tibetan societies. This has become particularly true in recent years, with the gradual development of 'modernist' versions of Theravāda Buddhism, first in Sri Lanka and then in other Theravādin societies (cf. Bechert 1966-73, Gombrich and Obeyesekere 1990). In these modernist versions of Buddhism, the magical and ritual elements have been further marginalized in pursuit of a Buddhism that can be presented as fully rational and scientific, an appropriate religion for the modern world. The remaining health- and prosperity-oriented activities of the Buddhist monks, such as the recitation of *paritta* chants (Gombrich 1971: 201–6, Spiro 1982: 265–71) or the consecration of amulets (Tambiah 1984: 155–229, 243–65; Gombrich 1971: 200), are still important at a practical level – almost all Thais wear such amulets, for example – but are increasingly problematic in relation to what Buddhism is now supposed to be all about.

Thus if we look at the area of health and suffering: in Theravāda countries, Buddhism gives answers to why suffering occurs – the classical answers, framed in terms of *karma*, of the three roots of existence, desire, hatred and ignorance, and of the craving which keeps the whole process of saṃsāra in motion – and it gives ways of dealing with death – through counselling the dying and through funerary ritual – but it has only a limited involvement in the this-worldly questions of health and pain – though it does have some, minimally via the *paritta* chants, consecrated amulets and the like. The same is true in the Mahāyānist Far East, as far as I can tell, though for somewhat different historical reasons.

In Tibetan societies, by contrast, we find quite a different picture. While the lamas and monks are, as in the Theravādin societies, particularly responsible for the area of death and rebirth, they are also very much concerned with issues of welfare and health in this life. A variety of ritual and medical specialists, concepts and procedures cover the general area of health, illness and suffering, and all as I have said are in some general sense under Buddhist auspices. In addition, the traditional Tibetan medical system remains closely linked to Buddhism. It is common for monks or lamas to practise as traditional Tibetan doctors. In addition, medicine retains strong associations with Tantric practice through such matters as the empowerment of medicines through Tantric ritual. In this procedure, lamas and monks invoke Tantric deities in order to give magical potency to pills compounded from herbal and other substances (Dhonden 1986).

Nevertheless, the basic Tibetan ideas about health, illness and fate are not really Buddhist derived. They include a range of concepts such as *la, ts'e, yang, trashi, sog, wangt'ang, lungta,* all referring to various kinds of energy, vitality, life-force or good fortune, and another range of concepts, such as *drip, dön, nöpa, barch'é* referring to obstacles, spirit-affliction and the like (see Glossary, and also Tucci 1980: 163–212; Samuel 1993: 186ff, 260ff; Lichter and Epstein 1983; Schicklgruber 1992; Rozario, *forthcoming*). This material exists in theorized and sophisticated versions, for example in the astrological context, where the state of many of these quantities is calculated in detail and available in printed almanacs (cf. Cornu 1990), but most people's ideas are much less formal and precise than this might lead one to expect.

The Tibetan Refugees of Dalhousie

What I have said so far has been at a fairly high level of generality, if based on the fieldwork of various scholars in various Buddhist communities. It may be useful if we turn now to look at a specific Tibetan community, the refugee community of Dalhousie in Himachal Pradesh, 6,000 feet up in the Himalayas in Northern India, where I spent some time in July and August 1996 researching health, healing and medical pluralism with Linda Connor and Santi Rozario, two colleagues from the University of Newcastle, New South Wales.

Dalhousie is a small Indian town, basically a holiday resort, with a Tibetan population of about 500. About half of the Dalhousie Tibetans work in the Tibetan Handicrafts Centre, mostly at carpet weaving, and live close by in the Tibetan settlement around 20 minutes' walk uphill from the Post Office. The other half live scattered around the town. The main other source of employment for the refugees is constituted by two small bazaars, one near the Post Office and the other at the Bus Stand, and each containing around 20 Tibetan-run shops. There is also a Tibetan school adjoining the main settlement. This has about 600 students, most of them boarders from other Tibetan refugee settlements in India.

Dalhousie was one of the first Tibetan refugee settlements, and was important in the early years of the refugees, but is now somewhat of a backwater, though it is only about six hours by bus from Dharamsala, the Dalai Lama's residence, head of the refugee administration and the centre of most aspects of refugee life. Many of the Tibetan refugees in India have attained a reasonable degree of prosperity, but the Dalhousie population are probably towards the bottom end of the income distribution. By the standards of the local Indian villagers, they are not badly off, but few have much money to spare, and their health choices are dictated in many ways by their income limitations.

When I first visited Dalhousie in 1971 it still had several large monasteries, but these were all gradually transferred elsewhere, and there are now only around 20 monks left, most of them in a small community at the other end of the town to the refugee settlement. The monks belong to the Gelugpa order, which is by far the dominant religious tradition in Dalhousie. One elderly lama, also Gelugpa, and formerly the head of one of the large monasteries which moved elsewhere, decided to stay on in Dalhousie when his monastery moved to Assam. This lama, whom I will refer to as the Rinpoche, is a reincarnate lama, a distinguished scholar and former abbot of a tantric college, who now lives a fairly simple life, catering to the religious needs of the community.

Our research was centred at a small clinic with one doctor (Doctor S.), a Buddhist monk who had been trained at the Men-Tsee-Khang,[6] the traditional Tibetan Medical and Astrological Institute in Dharamsala, and one pharmacist. This clinic, which is part of a network of clinics run by the Tibetan government-in-exile, dispensed traditional Tibetan medicine (*pö men*). We also spent some time with the previous doctor from this clinic (Doctor N.), a layman who now runs a similar clinic in Delhi.

During our stay in Dalhousie, which lasted around seven weeks, we spent several hours most days in the clinic. During this period around 135 patients, mostly Tibetans but also some Indians, visited the clinic, many of them several times. As these figures suggest, it was a fairly quiet clinic, and we had plenty of time to discuss cases with the doctor. We also interviewed eighteen of the patients at some length away from the clinic to get a picture of the total range of the medical resources they used and the way in which they saw them, and interviewed other major providers of health care within the community.

In fact, other specifically Tibetan health resources in Dalhousie are limited. Larger refugee settlements often have a substantial Tibetan-run community health centre. At the settlement of Bir, for example, a few hours away, there is a large Tibetan-run biomedical clinic which serves as the primary resource for most medical problems.[7] Dalhousie, by contrast, has one Tibetan community health worker and two school nurses, all linked to Delek Hospital, the main Tibetan refugee biomedical facility at Dharamsala. For biomedical treatment (*gyagar men*, literally 'Indian medicine') Tibetans are mostly dependent on local Indian resources, including a charity-run clinic a few minutes' walk above the settlement and two doctors in private practice in the town. They also buy medicines over the counter from local pharmacies. Dalhousie has a small Civil Hospital with limited facilities; serious cases are usually referred to the District Hospital three hours away by bus at Chamba, or the Zonal Hospital at Dharamsala. Other resources include private clinics at Pathankot, the rail-head for Dalhousie, four hours away by bus, and Delek Hospital at Dharamsala, but the private clinics are expensive, and the journey to Pathankot or Dharamsala may also be expensive, especially if the patient is too sick to travel by public transport. Āyurveda, homeopathy and other alternative healing modalities have little presence in Dalhousie. Tibetans do not appear to go to the one Āyurvedic doctor in town, and when they speak of 'Indian medicine' the reference is unambiguously to the biomedical system.

Healing Modalities in Dalhousie: Empowered Substances, Tibetan Medicine and Biomedicine

As I mentioned above, the basic Tibetan ideas about health, illness and fate are not Buddhist derived, and we saw relatively little of the more sophisticated versions of these ideas. There is a general shared understanding, though, that certain types of illness result from low vitality and/or spirit affliction of some kind, often associated with the state known as *drip* (perhaps best translated as spiritual contamination; cf. Schicklgruber 1992; Rozario *forthcoming*). Such problems are appropriately dealt with through the use of various *jinden* or sacred substances empowered by lamas or Buddhist deities. People may take these substances prophylatically if they feel in a vulnerable situation, for example if selling sweaters on the street in a dirty and polluted Indian city (a frequent winter occupation for Dalhousie Tibetans), or if going into an Indian hospital for the delivery of a child (Rozario, *forthcoming*).

In cases where spirit causation is suspected for an illness, people may try to confirm the nature of the problem through divination. In Dalhousie this would usually be by the Rinpoche or one of the couple of local lay diviners, but people would also go further afield in serious cases to visit a spirit medium at Dharamsala or a high-status lama elsewhere in India, such as Minling Terch'en at Clementtown or Sakya Gongma at Dehra Dun. Special Tantric rituals, such as the well-known *ts'ewang* (life-empowerment) ceremony, in which the power of healing Tantric deities is channelled and transferred to the participants (Samuel 1993: 259–64), might also be commissioned. Thus the Rinpoche conducted a *ts'ewang* during our stay for a small boy who had been suffering from fainting fits, and he provided a variety of other ritual services, such as supplying empowered water for purificatory purposes.[8]

Other kinds of illness are dealt with through traditional Tibetan medical treatment or through biomedicine. Tibetan medicine[9] has been mostly presented in Western descriptions in terms of its supposedly holistic theory of humoral imbalance, based on a system of three *nyepa* or 'humours' (*lung, tr'ipa, péken*) corresponding closely to the three *doṣa* of Āyurveda (*vāta, pitta, kapha* respectively, usually translated as 'wind', 'bile' and 'phlegm'). In practice, Tibetan medicine functions as an allopathic system, in that particular diseases are countered for the most part by specific drugs, mostly made from herbal or mineral substances. Some, but by no means all, of these diseases are explicitly associated with specific *nyepa*, so that diagnoses of *tr'ipa* and *lung* problems, corresponding roughly to 'jaundice' (hepatitis etc.) and 'hypertension' (high blood pressure) were quite common in the Dalhousie practice.[10]

The principal differences from Western medicine in practice are probably the modes of diagnosis (an elaborate system of pulse diagnosis, supplemented with urine analysis) and the emphasis on diet. As in Āyurveda, the digestive process is seen as central to much disease causation, and so control of diet is seen as very important. Most patients get at least some dietary advice (for example, to avoid chillis and sour foods) though it rarely receives great emphasis. The dominant mode of treatment is through drugs in the form of pills (*rilbu*) made from herbal and mineral ingredients.[11] Usually two or three different pills are prescribed, to be taken at different times of the day. The clinic had around 130

Table 1 Types of practitioner used by Dalhousie Tibetans

Type of practitioner	*Tibetan name*	*Local personnel*	*Function*
Traditional Tibetan doctor	*amchi*	Doctor N (until 4/96), Doctor S	Diagnosis and treatment with ordinary pills and Precious Pills (also moxibustion, cupping etc.)
Biomedical doctors, clinics, pharmacies	*[amchi]*	Various	Diagnosis and biomedical treatment
Lama	*lama*	The Rinpoche	Diagnosis and advice; Tantric ritual (life-empowerment etc.)
Lay Diviner	*mopa*	Several	Diagnosis and advice
Spirit Medium	*lhapa*	None in Dalhousie; patients went elsewhere	Diagnosis and advice, especially in cases of spirit-attack such as *tsadrip*

different medicines, generally named for the principal ingredients and total number of ingredients (e.g. *kyuru 25* has a total of 25 ingredients, with *kyuru* or emblic myrobalan, *Phyllanthus emblica* L., as the principal one). The price is uniform and relatively low, though by no means negligible in terms of the average income; some patients receive medicine at a free or subsidized rate. Some doctors also employ other techniques, such as *metsa* (gold needle moxibustion),[12] cupping or bloodletting.

Table 1 lists the various kinds of Tibetan practitioners consulted by Dalhousie Tibetans.

Attitudes to traditional Tibetan medicine and to biomedicine varied among Dalhousie Tibetans. Some people claimed only to use Tibetan medicine, while others said that they found it difficult to take the often bitter herbal pills, which are chewed with hot water, but most people we spoke to appeared to use both Tibetan medicine and biomedicine. By and large people saw them as complementary and as each having their own sphere of usefulness. A frequent opinion was that biomedicine acted quickly but did not cure the underlying problem and often had side-effects, while Tibetan medicine took much longer, had no side-effects and eventually cured the problem.[13] In fact, patients often seemed oriented as much to maintenance as to eventual cure; another common comment was that at least with traditional Tibetan treatment the problem would not get worse. In practice, a number of specific problems, such as jaundice, high blood pressure and *tsadrip* (see below), were frequently treated by Tibetan medicine, while others (e.g. fevers, tuberculosis) were routinely treated by biomedicine.[14]

While biomedicine is clearly distinct from *jinden*, the ritually-empowered substances obtained from lamas and monasteries, this is not necessarily the case with the mainly herbal pills given by the traditional Tibetan doctor. These pills are, in theory at least, also ritually empowered, if not so elaborately as the *jinden*, so that their effect is due to the empowerment as well as to the substances contained (cf. Dhonden 1986). The picture is complicated by an intermediate category, the *rinch'en rilbu* or *rilbu tsach'enpo*, usually referred to in English as Precious Pills. These are also obtained from the Tibetan doctor, and are both more expensive and thought to be more powerful than the ordinary pills. Sometimes the doctor will prescribe them for a particular problem, but patients may also ask for them, and many people take them annually or more frequently as a kind of general tonic. The *rinch'en rilbu* are ritually empowered to a higher degree than ordinary *rilbu*, and they are supposed to be taken in a ritualized manner which involves taking the pill where possible on an auspicious day of the lunar calendar such as full moon, avoiding certain foods for some days before and after, staying up late at night to uncover the pill (which is enclosed in a cloth wrapping) in the dark and dissolve it in water, then getting up in the early morning, while it is still dark, to drink the water after reciting the mantras of the Buddha of Medicine (Bhaiṣajyaguru) and Avalokiteśvara.[15] Most Dalhousie Tibetans seem to use *rinch'en rilbu* at least occasionally, and in fact the demand for these pills is so high that they are rationed. Table 2 summarizes the three varieties.

We encountered a variety of opinions about this range of remedies (ordinary Tibetan medicine, *rinch'en rilbu* and *jinden*

Table 2 Types of traditional Tibetan remedies

Type	*Tibetan name*	*Description*
Ordinary Tibetan medicine	*rilbu (pö men)*	Pills supplied by traditional Tibetan doctor, mostly made from herbal and mineral substances
Precious Pills	*rinch'en rilbu, rilbu tsach'enpo*	Special, ritually empowered pills also supplied by traditional Tibetan doctor, mostly made from herbal and mineral substances, taken with special ritual
Empowered substances	*jinden*	Various substances (e.g. empowered grain, empowered pills) obtained from monasteries and lamas

supplied by lamas). One person told us that all three types were *jinden*, since all were empowered. Most people we spoke to treated the *rinch'en rilbu*, the Precious Pills, with considerable respect. They claimed to follow the directions closely, though nobody we asked knew or used the Bhaiṣajyaguru mantra, and several added prayers to the Dalai Lama or other deities. A couple of people, young and Indian-educated, treated the *rinch'en rilbu* as ordinary medicine, and took them without the food avoidances and night-time ritual. For most people, though, it seemed that both kinds of Tibetan medicine had at least some association with the powerful realm of Buddhist Tantric ritual.

It is important, too, that both these types of medicine are very clearly Tibetan. Tibetan identity is a complex and sensitive area among these long-term refugees. Tibetan thought very frequently categorizes into inside and outside; for example, Buddhism is inside (the usual Tibetan term for Buddhist is *nangpa*, literally 'insider'), other religions outside. In these terms, both Tibetan medicine and *jinden* are clearly inside, while biomedicine is outside.

Tsadrip Problems: Healing Modalities in Practice

To illustrate the actual employment of this range of resources, I shall focus on a particular set of problems, those described by the term *tsadrip*. *Tsadrip* problems, although quite common, are not necessarily typical of health problems in general among the refugees, since they, unlike many other categories of illness, explicitly involve spirit causation of some kind. However, precisely for this reason they are one of the categories in relation to which specifically Buddhist healing resources are most elaborately brought into play, so revealing some of the complexities and ambiguities of those resources.

The term *tsadrip* is actually a combination of two terms; *tsa(kar)* (literally 'white channels', usually equated with the nervous system by modern writers on Tibetan medicine) and *drip* (spiritual contamination). In fact it is a kind of euphemism. *Tsadrip* cases are generally held to be caused by the *sa* spirits (Skt. *graha*),[16] but people much prefer not to name these dangerous beings directly. *Tsadrip* cases are generally characterized by some degree of paralysis, temporary or long-lasting, partial or total, on one side of the body. They vary from near-total paralysis of one side of the body to facial tics on one side of the face or temporary feelings of numbness in one arm. Whatever the case, they are immediately recognizable by lay people without any medical diagnosis.

The Tibetan doctors we worked with seemed on the whole ready to support the patient's diagnosis of *tsadrip*, but in milder cases at least often described the illness in their records as *tsakar* rather than *tsadrip*. By doing this they avoided direct reference to spirit-causation, since it is the *drip* or contamination which lays the patient open to spirit attack, or actually causes the spirit attack.[17] This creates a certain ambiguity as to treatment, since in the Tibetan medical classic *tsakar* and *sa* are distinct diseases, although there is some overlap between their treatment regimens.[18] As we will see, these differences, which few patients are likely to be aware of, are evaded in practice, since Doctor S. treated all the cases in terms of *tsakar*, but used drugs that were said to be good for *sa* also. However, they perhaps help contribute to the general feeling of a complex disease which needs to be approached through a variety of diagnostic and healing techniques, without any assurance that any of them will be successful.

I will now look at five of the dozen or so *tsakar* cases we encountered in Dalhousie in a little detail. The accounts come primarily from interviews with the patients in their homes, augmented by some material from the doctor. The reader should note that these accounts are largely based on the speaker's recollections some months or years after the event, occasionally supported by a friend or spouse. They are thus not necessarily precise as to chronology or treatment, but they do serve to illustrate attitudes to various available healing modalities. It may be helpful to refer back to Table 1, which lists the various types of practitioners consulted by Dalhousie Tibetans.

* * *

Case One[19] is a 45-year-old woman, who runs a small restaurant with her husband. She has had neck pain since she was 25 years old. When it first came, it was associated with shivering and trembling, so that she knew that it was a case of *drip*. She went to a well-known female spirit medium (*lhapa*) in Dharamsala who confirmed this while not giving any particular explanation for how it had happened. The spirit medium said that she should arrange for some monks to recite prayers for her.

A few years ago she had gold needle moxibustion from Doctor N., the previous Tibetan doctor in Dalhousie. This had cured the shakes and shivers, but not the neck pain. While in Jaipur for sweater-selling, she went for biomedical treatment. The doctor sent her to a physiotherapist who told her to wear a neck collar and do exercises. However, she was unwilling to do the exercises, since she knew that it was a *tsa* problem and they wouldn't help, so she keeps going to Doctor S. She also takes *drangjor*, the most expensive and powerful of the Precious Pills, once a month. She is not sure if it is doing any good. (Her husband, present at the interview, commented that it must be helping.)

* * *

Case Two,[20] a 32-year-old woman who also works in a small restaurant with other members of her family started suffering from pain and loss of sensation in her left arm and leg last year. She went to the same spirit medium as Case One. The spirit medium said that she had *tsadrip*, from sitting on green grass,[21] and should be treated with Tibetan medicine. She also went to the Rinpoche, who again diagnosed *tsadrip* and told her to stay 'clean'. She went to Doctor N., who confirmed that the case was *tsadrip* and advised her to avoid 'dirty' foods (pork, garlic and eggs). She can't always avoid eggs because they are cooked into noodle dishes. On his recommendation, she also took *chumar 25*, another of the Precious Pills.

The problem reoccurred last March in her arm and upper back. She was visiting Dharamsala at the time so she went to a well-known privately-practising Tibetan doctor there. He suggested gold needle moxibustion but she came back to Dalhousie and didn't have it. The Dharamsala doctor also gave her the same medicines as the Dalhousie doctor.

Last month, her problem reoccurred, so she went to Doctor S., the new Tibetan doctor in Dalhousie. The problem got better, but occurred once more, and she went back for more treatment.

* * *

Case Three.[22] This is a 59-year-old woman whose husband sells second-hand clothes in the bazaar. She is fairly overweight, and was primarily identified by the Tibetan doctor as suffering from high blood pressure (i.e. *lung* disorder). She had undergone six months' biomedical treatment for high blood pressure from the local charitable clinic, but was currently employing a mixture of Tibetan medicine, Precious Pills and *jinden*. She was also trying to control the problem through diet, and was taking milk and fruit because people had told her that this helped to reduce blood pressure. However, she continued to drink large quantities of buttered, salted Tibetan tea, despite pressure from Doctor S. and his pharmacist to avoid it.

She had developed a facial tic in which her mouth sometimes became twisted on one side. This is a sure sign of *drip*. Recently, she had consulted the same spirit medium as Cases One and Two. The medium confirmed that this was a case of *drip*, and was due to her having come into contact with raw meat, but said she should take Tibetan medicine for *lung*. She had also consulted a lama at Dharamsala who had apparently confirmed the diagnosis of *drip*. She feels that the *jinden* she is taking helps with the *drip*.

* * *

Case Four.[23] This is a 76-year-old woman whose husband works as a *chowkidar* (janitor) for lodging but no pay, earning a little money by working as a coolie (porter) in the winter months. Sixteen years ago she collapsed while carrying water in a bucket downhill. She felt as if struck by lightning. Since then she has been paralysed all down the left side of her body. She tried biomedical treatment for one month with one of the local doctors, but it did not help. She took Tibetan medicine for 15 years, and got the medicine without payment because of their poverty, but her record book got lost when Doctor N. left, so she can no longer get free medicine and has stopped taking Tibetan medicine. She has taken numerous Precious Pills and they help a little. Sometimes she is unable to speak, but recovers after taking Precious Pills for one or two days.

They never had any kind of divination for the problem; her husband commented that it was obviously *drip* so they knew that she wouldn't get much better whatever they did.

* * *

Case Five.[24] This is a 67-year-old woman who used to work as a carpet weaver. Seven years ago, she was working in the carpet workshop when she had a sudden fall. She felt as if a stone had struck the upper right side of her head. When she regained consciousness some time later, she was paralysed. She learned later that a divination had been done by a local lay diviner, which said that she would suffer some illness but would not die.

Her daughter and son-in-law came the next day and took her to Dharamsala, to the *labrang* (religious establishment) of her grandson, who had been recognized as a reincarnate lama. There she was treated with Tibetan medicine only at the Men-Tsee-Khang clinic; the diagnosis was *tsadrip* combined with *lung*. She also had regular massage from a Western woman who was studying at the Men-Tsee-Khang, and took five Precious Pills which had been made by her grandson's previous incarnation. While she was at the *labrang*, they also performed rituals for her recovery.

After a couple of weeks she regained some movement, and she is now quite mobile, but her left arm is still not very strong and she has been unable to resume carpet-weaving. Since she came back from Dharamsala, she has continued taking Tibetan medicine, and also occasionally taken Precious Pills, sometimes *drangjor* but now usually *retna samp'el* since Doctor N., the previous doctor at Dalhousie, had told her that these were best for her condition. She takes them on auspicious days. She also takes *jinden*, particularly when there are a lot of colds around.

* * *

These cases illustrate the complex interplay between different kinds of diagnosis (self-identification, consultation of spirit-mediums, lamas and doctors) and therapy (ordinary pills, Precious Pills, *jinden*, diet, ritual, massage) on the one hand, and the various expectations, understandings and resources of the patients and their families on the other. Case Four, the poorest of the patients, would probably have continued with Tibetan medicine had she been able to afford it, and still uses Precious Pills. Case Five, because of her family connections to the *labrang* in Dharamsala, had access to kinds of ritual treatment not readily available to the others. Cases One to Three all consulted the spirit medium, and each was told to continue Tibetan medical treatment. All the patients and their families seem to share a common body of understanding of what *tsadrip* or *sa* is and what the expectations are for its treatment. Most of them tried biomedicine, but apparently without much expectation of its being helpful, and they gave up on it fairly quickly.[25]

Table 3 Medicines prescribed for five *tsadrip* cases

Patient	*Visit*	*Medicine 1*	*Purpose*	*Medicine 2*	*Purpose*	*Medicine 3*	*Purpose*
1	1	*dali 18*	*tsakar*	*sengdog 11*	headache	*agar 20*	*tsakar*
1	2	*dali 18*	*tsakar*	*sengdog 11*	headache	*agar 20*	*tsakar*
2	1	*dali 18*	*tsakar*	*agar 20*	*tsakar*	*chumar 25* on alternate days	*tsakar*
3	1	*kyuru 25*	*lung*	*gurky'ung*	deafness	*agar 20*	*lung*, also good for *tsakar, sa*
3	2	*kyuru 25*	*lung*	*gurky'ung*	deafness	*agar 20*	*lung*, also good for *tsakar, sa*
3	3	*kyuru 25*	*lung*	*gurky'ung*	deafness	*agar 35*	*lung* only
5	1	*kyuru 25*	*lung*	*ruta 6*	*p'owa* (stomach pains)	*dali 18*	*tsakar*
5	2	*kyuru 25*	*lung*	*samnor*	*tsakar*	*dali 18*	*tsakar*
5	3	*kyuru 25*	*lung*	*agar 20*	*lung, tsakar, sa*	*dali 18*	*tsakar*

Four of these cases consulted Doctor S. one or more times during our visit, and it is worth looking at what he prescribed for them. The medicines are listed in Table 3.

As can be seen, Doctor S. generally prescribed a mixture of drugs for *tsakar* and for any other problems the patient presented with, for example deafness or *lung*. At least one of the drugs he selected is also good for *sa (tsadrip)*. He often changes the prescription slightly at each consultation, depending on the patient's response to the previous prescription. Other doctors probably have different prescribing routines for *tsakar/tsadrip*, though we have no real comparative information here except for three days of notes on the Delhi clinic, which had a rather different clientele with different problems.

Conclusion

While our Dalhousie research was primarily concerned with healing and medicine, it may be useful in conclusion to put the various healing procedures we have seen here in the wider context of Tibetan Buddhism. Does it make sense to speak of a characteristically Buddhist perspective on health and suffering within which people approach the various Tibetan and biomedical healing resources?

This is a difficult question to answer. Most lay Tibetans in Dalhousie do not have a sophisticated understanding of Buddhist teachings, although the younger members of the community (those under 40 to 45 years in age), who have mostly been educated in the Tibetan refugee school system in India, are at least literate in Tibetan and will have learned standard Buddhist prayers and some elementary religious history. What these lay Tibetans are familiar with is what could be called practical or everyday Buddhism. All households have some kind of domestic shrine, at which daily offerings (water, incense, light) are made before a collection of photographs and images of lamas and Buddhist deities, which always includes at least one photograph of the Dalai Lama. Who precisely they are making offerings to is not necessarily sharply defined. For most people, the offerings are perhaps more to deity in a generic sense (*Chomdendé* = Skt. *Bhagavān*), the Buddha, Avalokiteśvara and Dalai Lama combined into a single protective figure, than to a highly differentiated pantheon. Prayers may be recited, as they are at the school, to specific guardian deities.[26] In the mostly Gelugpa settlement of Dalhousie these would most usually be to the Dalai Lama's two principal protectors, Palden Lhamo and Nech'ung.

Dalhousie Tibetans do occasionally hear Buddhist teachings, typically in the context of an empowerment, where they will generally be presented with the characteristic graded path approach deriving from the eleventh century Indian teacher Atiśa, emphasizing the need for refuge in the lama and Buddhist deities, for virtuous action and for the development of altruistic motivation (*bodhicitta*) as part of a gradual approach to Enlightenment.[27] Do they understand much of what they hear on such occasions? This is hard to say. The Buddhist scriptures are in Tibetan, and teachings are given in Tibetan, but my impression is that the language of the teachings, with their sophisticated technical vocabulary, is much too difficult for most lay Tibetans to follow in detail. Their recitation is at least as much a ritual act as a pedagogical one.

However one can perhaps speak of a characteristic lay Tibetan Buddhist perspective on healing and its limitations among the people we met in Dalhousie. For one thing, contact with the positive power of the Tantric Buddhist deities is clearly important. People use *jinden* regularly, they seek the lama's divinations when faced by difficult choices, they go to *ts'ewang* and other rituals when the opportunity arises.[28] But beyond this, people's expectations about the limited possibilities of healing perhaps reflect a wider and recognizably lay Tibetan Buddhist orientation towards the possibilities of success and happiness in this world.

Some years ago David Lichter and Lawrence Epstein argued that lay Tibetans sought happiness, health and success in this world, but with a Buddhist-derived awareness that their attainment was uncertain and impermanent. Lichter and Epstein speak of Tibetans characteristically keeping a kind of ironic distance from these worldly goals at the same time as they pursue them (Lichter and Epstein 1983; see also Samuel 1993: 213–22). This seems to me to be quite a good description of what we found in relation to healing in Dalhousie. The Tibetan population of Dalhousie used whatever kinds of healing were available to them to deal with the unavoidable contingencies of human suffering, but they were oriented towards living with a fair degree of ongoing pain and discomfort. This comes out both in their ambivalence towards biomedicine, with its often limited effectiveness in the local environment, and in their attitudes towards Tibetan medicine, Precious Pills and *jinden*, which emphasize lengthy treatment and avoidance of further deterioration rather than the rapid attainment of a complete cure. Whether Buddhist-derived or not, given the general situation of healing and medical care in Dalhousie, and the limited resources of most of the people we met, these expectations are probably all too realistic.

NOTES

1. I know much less about the other major region where Buddhism is practised in modern times, the East Asian societies of China, Korea, Japan and Vietnam, so I avoid discussing these societies here.
2. I would like to acknowledge the support of the Australian Research Council, who funded the project, and the assistance of my colleagues, Linda Connor and Santi Rozario, as also of Kylie Monro, who has been carrying out doctoral research in a nearby settlement (Bir, H.P.) as part of the same project.
3. Strictly speaking, one cannot become a fully-ordained nun in a Theravādin society today, since the ordination lineage no longer exists, but various roles are available as female religious practitioners.
4. I prefer to speak of Tibetan societies rather than Tibet both because of the variety of social and political forms within which Tibetans have lived and live today, and because of the ambiguity in current usage of the term Tibet (see Samuel 1993).

5. Tibetan names and terms are given in a simplified Romanization. For formal spellings in Wylie system, see Glossary at end.
6. This is now the official name of the Institute (see Glossary).
7. Kylie Monro, a Ph.D. student working on the same project, has carried out several months' fieldwork at Bir.
8. Field notes on *ts'ewang* and interview with Rinpoche, 24/7/96.
9. Most of the by now quite substantial Western literature on traditional Tibetan medicine (e.g. Clark 1995, Parfionovitch *et al.* 1992, Dhonden 1986, Clifford 1989, Meyer 1984; see Aschoff 1996 for a general bibliography) is based closely on the Gyü Shi or Four [Medical] Tantras. This is a body of texts probably dating from the eleventh century and themselves adapted in part from Āyurvedic texts translated into Tibetan though also including material from (probably) Chinese, Islamic and indigenous sources (Emmerick 1977, 1987, Karmay 1989, Meyer 1984). I found that this literature, and the general image of holistic medicine conveyed within it, did not prepare me very well for Tibetan medicine in practice, on which very little has been written (Janes 1995, on Tibetan medicine in Chinese-controlled Tibet, and Kuhn 1988, 1994 on Ladakh are the only substantial items known to me so far).
10. English equivalents of this kind for Tibetan disease categories are frequently offered by English-speaking Tibetans but need to be treated with considerable caution. *Tr'ipa* patients may or may not have had hepatitis. *Lung* patients regularly had their blood pressure taken and recorded by the doctor, but the figures often seemed quite moderate. Blood pressure (*tr'agshé*), though freely used by Tibetan doctors and patients alike, is of course a biomedical category, not a traditional Tibetan one.
11. The traditional recipes include animal ingredients as well, but the Men-Tsee-Khang at Dharamsala, where the medicines used in the Dalhousie clinic are made, claims to be eliminating these as far as possible in favour of herbal substitutes.
12. This procedure, as we saw it in Delhi, involved a heated gold-tipped rod being applied momentarily to one or another specific point on the body.
13. This verdict on biomedicine may not be so unrealistic given local conditions. As elsewhere in South Asia, poor patients are likely to take the shortest possible course of antibiotics in order to reduce expense, so increasing the likelihood of recurrence, while a combination of poor general health and use of inappropriate drugs probably leads to high levels of side-effects and iatrogenic illness.
14. In the specific case of tuberculosis, which is common among Tibetan refugees, public health announcements from the Dalai Lama and the Dharamsala refugee administration have emphasized that biomedical treatment is appropriate, and Delek Hospital has developed a special adaptation of the standard WHO protocol for local conditions. Tibetan medicine is however now seen as appropriate for dealing with residual problems after 'third line' biomedical treatment.

15. A leaflet distributed with these pills gives these directions in Tibetan and English. The clinic pharmacist explained the directions to patients unable to read, but in any case most people seemed to know the procedure.
16. *Sa* in the medical sense, which is the subject of Chapter 80 of the Men-ngag Gyü or Oral Commentary Tantra (the third and longest of the Gyü Shi or Four Medical Tantras), is often translated as 'epilepsy' in Western books on Tibetan medicine. This identification, which appears to stem from Jäschke's dictionary of 1881 (1968: 492) and Das's of 1902 (Das 1989:1102) is misleading; Emmerick (1987) is I think correct in regarding *jé* [brjed] = Skt. *apasmāra*, the subject of the previous chapter (79) as corresponding much more closely to epilepsy.
17. My impression is that people were not really clear which of these was the case. I hope to provide a more extended treatment of *tsadrip* in a future paper, where I will also consider the wider context of *drip* in Tibetan culture.
18. In the Men-ngag Gyü, *tsakar* is the subject of Chapter 60, *sa* of Chapter 80.
19. P91, interview 31/7/96; clinic visits 29/7/96 and 8/8/96.
20. P96, interview 3/8/96; clinic visit 31/7/96.
21. She had no idea why this should cause *tsadrip*, and neither have I, unless perhaps this was a place belonging to a spirit who was offended.
22. P55, interview 29/7/96; clinic visits 18/7/96, 29/7/96, 6/8/96.
23. Q1, interview 29/7/96.
24. P4b, interview 9/8/96; clinic visits 2/7/96, 18/7/96, 5/8/96.
25. Of course, patients who used biomedicine exclusively would not have come to the clinic, and so to our notice, in the first place. All but one of the cases presented above were clinic patients; the exception was a relative of a clinic patient we were interviewing. However, clinic patients with other kinds of problems (i.e. not involving spirit causation) seemed more willing to continue with biomedical treatment, irrespective of whether they were also using Tibetan medicine.
26. The guardian deities (*ch'ökyong*, Skt. *dharmapāla*) are either Buddha-forms or high-status Indic or Tibetan deities bound to the protection of particular Tibetan Buddhist traditions. They are invoked extensively in monastic ritual.
27. At the Rinpoche's *ts'ewang* there was also considerable emphasis on the Dalai Lama as earthly representative of Avalokiteśvara, perhaps reflecting recent controversy over the Dalai Lama's role among some conservative Gelugpa monastics.
28. Thus the *ts'ewang* mentioned above was attended by around thirty people, mostly relatives and friends of the child's family, all of whom received the empowered substances prepared for the *ts'ewang*, while a more public Tantric empowerment performed by Serkhong Rinpoche, one of the Dalai Lama's Assistant Tutors, during my stay in Dalhousie in 1971 was attended by virtually the entire lay Tibetan population of the town at that time.

References Cited

Aschoff, Jürgen C. (1996) *Annotated Bibliography of Tibetan Medicine* (1789–1995). Ulm: Fabri Verlag and Dietikon, Switzerland: Garuda.

Bechert, Heinz (1966-73) *Buddhismus, Staat und Gesellschaft in den Ländern des Theravāda Buddhismus*. Vol.1, 1966, Dietikon, Switzerland: Alfred Metzner; vols. 2 and 3, 1967 and 1973, Wiesbaden: Alfred Metzner.

Brohm, John (1963) 'Buddhism and animism in a Burmese village'. *Journal of Asian Studies* 22: 155–67.

Clark, Barry (1995) *The Quintessence Tantras of Tibetan Medicine*. Ithaca, NY: Snow Lion Publications.

Clifford, Terry (1989) *The Diamond Healing: Tibetan Buddhist Medicine and Psychiatry*. Wellingborough, Northants: Crucible.

Cornu, Philippe (1990) *L'astrologie tibétaine*. Collection Présences.

Das, Sarat Chandra ([1902] 1989) *A Tibetan-English Dictionary with Sanskrit Synonyms*. Reprinted. New Delhi and Madras: Asian Educational Services.

Dhonden, Yeshi (1986) *Health Through Balance: An Introduction to Tibetan Medicine*. Edited and Translated by Jeffrey Hopkins. Ithaca, NY: Snow Lion Publications.

Emmerick, Ronald E. (1977) 'Sources of the rGyud-bzhi'. (Supplement, Deutscher Orientalistentag vom 28. Sept. bis 4. Okt. 1975 in Freiburg i. Br.). *Zeitschrift der Deutschen Morgenländischen Gesellschaft* (Wiesbaden) III, 2 (1977), p. 1135–42.

Emmerick, Ronald E. (1987) 'Epilepsy according to the *Rgyud-bzi*'. In G. Jan Meulenbeld and Dominik Wujastyk (eds) *Studies on Indian Medical History: Papers Presented at the International Workshop on the Study of Indian Medicine held at the Wellcome Institute for the History of Medicine, 2–4 September 1985*. Groningen: Egbert Forsten.

Gombrich, Richard F. (1971) *Precept and Practice: Traditional Buddhism in the Rural Highlands of Ceylon*. Oxford: Clarendon Press,.

Gombrich, Richard and Gananath Obeyesekere (1990) *Buddhism Transformed: Religious Change in Sri Lanka*. Delhi: Motilal Banarsidass.

Janes, Craig R. (1995) 'The transformations of Tibetan medicine'. *Medical Anthropology Quarterly* (Arlington/VA) 9, 1 (1995), pp. 6–39.

Jäschke, H.A. ([1881] 1968) *A Tibetan-English Dictionary with Special Reference to the Prevailing Dialects*. London: Routledge and Kegan Paul.

Karmay, Samten G. (1989) 'Vairocana and the rGyud-bzhi'. *Tibetan Medicine* (Dharamsala) Series No. 12 (1989), pp. 19–31.

Kuhn, Alice S. (1988) *Heiler und ihre Patienten auf dem Dach der Welt. Ladakh aus ethnomedizinischer Sicht*. (Medizin in Entwicklungsländern. 25.) Frankfurt/M.: Peter Lang.

Kuhn, Alice S. (1994) 'Ladakh: A pluralistic medical system under acculturation and domination'. In Dorothea Sich and Waltraud Gottschalk (eds) *Acculturation and Domination in Traditional Asian Medical Systems*. pp. 61–74. Stuttgart: Franz Steiner.

Lichter, David and Lawrence Epstein (1983) 'Irony in Tibetan Notions of the Good Life'. In Charles F. Keyes and E. Valentine Daniel (eds) *Karma: An Anthropological Inquiry*, pp. 223–60, Berkeley: University of California Press.

Meyer, Fernand (1984) *Gso-ba rig-pa, le système médical tibétain*. Seconde édition revue et corrigée. Paris: Éditions du Centre National de la Recherche Scientifique.

Meyer, Fernand (1990) 'Théorie et pratique de l'examen des pouls dans un chapitre du rGyud-bzhi'. In Tadeusz Skorupski (ed.), *Papers in Honour and Appreciation of Professor David L. Snellgrove's Contribution to Indo-Tibetan Studies*, pp. 209–56. Tring/UK: The Institute of Buddhist Studies. [Buddhica Britannica, Series Continua II].

Mulder, Neils (1992) *Inside Thai Society: An Interpretation of Everyday Life*. (3rd rev. edn.) Bangkok: Duang Kamol.

Parfionovitch, Yuri, Fernand Meyer and Gyurme Dorje (1992) *Tibetan Medical Paintings: Illustrations to the Blue Beryl Treatise of Sangye Gyamtso (1653–1705)*. London: Serindia.

Rozario, Santi (*forthcoming*) Indian medicine, *drib*, and the politics of identity in a Tibetan refugee settlement in north India. In L. Connor and G. Samuel (eds) *Healing Powers and Modernity in Asian Societies*.

Samuel, Geoffrey (1993) *Civilized Shamans: Buddhism in Tibetan Societies*. Washington, DC: Smithsonian Institution Press.

Schicklgruber, Christian (1992) 'Grib: on the significance of the term in a socio-religious context'. In Shōren Ihara and Zuihō Yamaguchi (ed) *Tibetan Studies: Proceedings of the 5th Seminar of the International Association for Tibetan Studies, Narita 1989*, pp. 723–34, Narita: Naritasan Shinshōji.

Spiro, Melford (1967) *Burmese Supernaturalism: A Study in the Explanation and Reduction of Suffering*. Englewood Cliffs, NJ: Prentice-Hall.

Spiro, Melford E. (1982) *Buddhism and Society: A Great Tradition and its Burmese Vicissitudes*. 2nd, expanded edn. Berkeley, CA: University of California Press.

Tambiah, Stanley J. (1968) 'The ideology of merit and the social correlates of Buddhism in a Thai village'. In Edmund Leach (ed) *Dialectic in Practical Religion*, pp. 41–121. Cambridge: Cambridge University Press.

Tambiah, Stanley J. (1970) *Buddhism and the Spirit Cults in North-east Thailand*. Cambridge: Cambridge University Press.

Tambiah, Stanley J. (1984) *The Buddhist Saints of the Forest and the Cult of Amulets: A Study in Charisma, Hagiography, Sectarianism and Millennial Buddhism*. Cambridge: Cambridge University Press.

Tucci, Giuseppe (1980) *The Religions of Tibet*. London: Routledge and Kegan Paul; Berkeley and Los Angeles: University of California Press.

Zysk, Kenneth G. (1991) *Asceticism and Healing in Ancient India: Medicine in the Buddhist Monastery*. New York: Oxford University Press.

Glossary

Agar 20 [a gar nyi shu] a traditional Tibetan medicine for *lung* and *tsakar*, also a medicine for *sa* diseases.

Agar 35 [a gar so lnga], a *lung* medicine, with no action for *tsakar* or *sa*.

Barch'é [bar chad] 'obstacle', 'obstruction', as determined by divination and countered by ritual.

Ch'ökyong [chos skyong, Skt. *dharmapāla*] guardian deities.

Chomdendé [bcom ldan 'das = Skt. *Bhagavān*] supreme deity, in a generic sense.

Chumar 25 [rin chen byur dmar nyer lnga] Precious Coral-25, one of the *rinch'en rilbu*.

Dali 18 [dwa lis bco brgyad] a Tibetan medicine for *tsakar*.

Dön [gdon] harmful spirits, illness etc. caused by harmful spirits (generic term).

Drangjor [rin chen grang sbyor ril nag chen po] Great Precious Cold Compound Black Pill, the most expensive and powerful of the *rinch'en rilbu*.

Drip [grib], contamination, state of vulnerability to spirit attack.

Gelugpa [dGe lugs pa] the largest of the Tibetan monastic and religious orders; the Dalai Lama is its most senior reincarnate lama.

Gurky'ung [gur khyung] a traditional Tibetan medicine for deafness.

Gyagar men [rgya gar sman], biomedical treatment, literally 'Indian medicine'.

Gyü Shi [rgyud bzhi] the four 'Medical Tantras', classic text of traditional Tibetan medicine.

Jé [brjed] a disease category in the Gyü Shi, corresponding to Skt. *apasmāra* and (approximately) to the Western category of epilepsy.

Jinden [byin rten] sacred objects or substances empowered by lamas or Buddhist deities.

Kyuru 25 [skyu ru nyer lnga] a traditional Tibetan medicine for *lung* problems.

La [bla] soul or life-force; an attribute of the individual which can be lost from the body, thus causing illness or misfortune.

Lhapa [lha pa] spirit medium.

Lung [rlung] one of the *nyepa* (q.v.), corresponding to the Āyurvedic *doṣa* of *vāta*, usually translated as 'wind'.

Lungta [rlung rta] literally 'wind-horse'; good fortune, vitality; an attribute of the individual which can decrease, causing illness and risk of death.

Mangjor [rin chen mang sbyor che mo] Great Precious Accumulation Pill, a type of *rinch'en rilbu*.

Men-ngag Gyü [man ngag rgyud] the third and longest of the four 'Medical Tantras', consisting of detailed descriptions of diseases and their treatment.

Men-Tsee-Khang [sman rtsis khang] literally Medicine and Astrology House; the Tibetan Medical and Astrological Institute in Dharamsala, also its predecessor in Lhasa and its branch clinics around India and Nepal.

Metsa [gser khab me btsa'] gold needle moxibustion (see note 12).

Minling Terch'en [sMin-ling gTer-chen] lama at Clementtown, known for his magical and divinatory power.

Nech'ung [gnas chung] Tibetan protective deity.

Nöpa [gnod pa] injury, harm, especially caused supernaturally by envious people or spirits; 'evil eye'.

Nyepa [nyes pa] the three so-called humours (*lung, tr'ipa, péken*) corresponding closely to the three *doṣa* of Āyurveda (*vāta, pitta, kapha* respectively, usually translated as 'wind', 'bile' and 'phlegm').

Palden Lhamo [dPal-ldan lha-mo] Tibetan protective deity.

Péken [bad kan] one of the *nyepa* (q.v.), corresponding to the Āyurvedic *doṣa* of *kapha*, usually translated as 'phlegm'.

Pö men [bod sman] traditional Tibetan medicine.

P'owa [pho ba] stomach (more precisely the epigastric area); *p'owa* pains are a common complaint among Dalhousie Tibetans.

Retna Samp'el [rin chen ratna bsam 'phel] one of the *rinch'en rilbu*.

Rilbu [ril bu] pills; the form in which most traditional Tibetan medicine is administered.

Rilbu Tsach'enpo [ril bu rtsa chen po] alternative name for *rinch'en rilbu*.

Rinch'en Rilbu [rin chen ril bu] These pills, usually referred to in English as 'Precious Pills', are also obtained from the Tibetan doctor, and are both more expensive and thought to be more powerful than the ordinary pills.

Ruta 6 [ru rta drug pa] a traditional Tibetan medicine for *p'owa* complaints.

Sa [gza' = Skt. *grāha*] class of spirits causing paralysis; also the disease itself. See *tsadrip*.

Sakya Gongma [Sa-skya Gong-ma] lama at Dehra Dun, known for his magical and divinatory power.

Samnor [bsam nor] a traditional Tibetan medicine for *tsakar*.

Sengdog 11 [gser mdog bcu gcig] a traditional Tibetan medicine for headache.

Sog [srog] life (breath); an attribute of the individual which can decrease, causing illness and risk of death.

Tantra [Skt. = Tib. rgyud] generic term for ritual and meditational traditions in Tibetan Buddhism and other Asian religions. Tantric Buddhism (also known as Vajrayāna) involves invocation of and identification with deities who are aspects of Buddhahood in order to acquire their enlightened qualities and exercise their powers.

Tr'agshé [khrag shed] blood pressure.

Trashi [bkra shis] good fortune; an attribute of the individual, etc. which can be increased, recovered or guarded from loss by appropriate ritual.

Tr'ipa [mkhris pa] one of the *nyepa* (q.v.), corresponding to the Āyurvedic *doṣa* of *pitta*, usually translated as 'bile'.

Tsadrip [rtsa grib], a disease characterized by some degree of paralysis, temporary or long-lasting, partial or total, on one side of the body. Equivalent to *sa*.

Tsakar [rtsa dkar, literally 'white channels'] channels within the body, usually equated with the nervous system by modern writers on Tibetan medicine.

Ts'e [tshe] life (duration); an attribute of the individual which can decrease, causing illness and risk of death.

Ts'ewang [tshe dbang] life-empowerment; a ritual to purify and strengthen the life-force (*tse, la,* etc.) within an individual.

Wangt'ang [dbang thang] force, vitality; an attribute of the individual which can decrease, causing illness and risk of death.

Yang [g.yang] good fortune; an attribute of the individual, family etc. which can be increased, recovered or guarded from loss by appropriate ritual.

SIKH PERSPECTIVES ON HEALTH AND SUFFERING: A FOCUS ON SIKH THEODICY

Pashaura Singh

I.

The purpose of this paper is to examine the central teachings of the Sikh Gurus pertaining to the problem of pain and suffering. The basic source for understanding those teachings is the sacred scripture of the Sikhs, the Adi Granth, which contains the writings of the Sikh Gurus along with the writings of certain medieval poet-saints of Sant, Sufi and Bhakti origin. In Sikh usage, the Adi Granth is normally referred to as the 'Guru Granth Sahib', which implies a confession of faith in the scripture as Guru. According to well-established tradition, the tenth and the last human Guru, Gobind Singh, terminated the line of personal Gurus before he died in 1708, and installed the Adi Granth as 'Guru Eternal for the Sikhs.'[1] As such, the Adi Granth carries the same status and authority as did the ten personal Gurus from Guru Nanak (1469–1539) through Guru Gobind Singh (1666–1708), and, therefore, it must be viewed as providing the authoritative response to the problem of evil and suffering. It should, however, be emphasized that each generation will have its own view of that authoritative understanding based on its particular interpretation of the text.

Before proceeding to examine the Sikh perspectives on health and suffering, however, we need to make a few preliminary remarks with respect to the basic issues and key terms. The challenge of evil and suffering is normally posed in the form of a dilemma: if God is perfectly loving, God must wish to abolish all evil; if God is all-powerful, God must be able to abolish all evil. But evil exists; therefore God cannot be both omnipotent and perfectly loving.[2] Thus the basic question is: how do believers in a good and powerful God explain the reality of suffering, especially of the innocent? The principal response to this question comes from an enquiry into the meaning of 'theodicy' (a term which comes from Greek *theos* 'god', and *dike*, 'righteous') and produces a doctrine which attempts to solve the theological problem of evil. John Hick has defined theodicy as 'an attempt to reconcile the unlimited goodness of an all-powerful God with the reality of evil.'[3] From a purely theological perspective theodicy is an exclusively defensive strategy. It is thus the 'vindication of the beneficent care of God in the context of the existence of evil.'[4] From the Christian point of view theodicy is therefore the religious response to the problem of pain and suffering. In the same way traditional Sikh theodicy offers the solution to this problem from the Sikh point of view. However, the phrase 'theodical solution' will be used in this study to refer to the religious response to the problem of evil and suffering.

In the context of the present discussion, the key term used in the Adi Granth is *dukkh*, a term which refers to 'pain, grief, sorrow, suffering.'[5] Although there is no exact word or phrase in English to capture the full significance and meaning of the Punjabi term *dukkh*, it does convey a sense of spiritual, mental and physical suffering. In order to understand the exact shade and meaning of its particular usage, however, we need to examine the actual context in which the term *dukkh* appears in the works of the Gurus. Moreover, the term *dukkh* has a rich historical and cultural background in the Indian religious traditions. In particular, it occupies a central place in the Four Noble Truths of Buddhist teachings where it means anything 'unsatisfying or frustrating.' In the classical Indian philosophy, all suffering (*dukkh*) is related to *karam* and hence deserved, being 'conditioned by the maturation of *karmic* residues laid down by actions in previous lives or in earlier portions of this one.'[6] Thus the doctrines of *karam* and *sansar* (rebirth, transmigration) form the basis of theodicy in Indian religious traditions, a theodicy that stresses the retributive theme.

It is important to note that human relationship to pain and suffering is affected by one's beliefs as well as by the context of differing philosophical or religious backdrops.[7] Undoubtedly, we come across different responses to the problem of evil and suffering in different religious traditions, and even we encounter diversity of views within one single tradition. This is not only true of the Sikh tradition, but it is also true of any of the traditions one might name. In order to understand the various dimensions of suffering in the world from the Sikh perspective, we must address the following questions: Is suffering an inevitable part of life? What is the root cause of suffering? What is the Sikh religious response or 'theodical solution' to the problem of evil and suffering? What happens to evil and suffering in a mystical experience? Is there any pessimism in the Sikh approach towards life on the issue of suffering? Is there any therapeutic value of suffering in Sikh teachings? What is the relationship between Sikh spirituality and healing? In the light of these preliminary remarks, let us now try to find answers to these questions.

II.

The themes of 'health' and 'suffering' are given a rich treatment throughout the Adi Granth, and good physical and spiritual health is regarded paramount to a devout Sikh. In this context, it will be useful to consider the following celebrated hymn of Guru Nanak in the *Malar* mode:

> First, there is pang (*dukkh*) of separation [from the Beloved];
> then there is pain (*dukkh*) of hunger.
> Again, there is anguish (*dukkh*) of tyranny and death;
> then there is affliction (*dukkh*) of bodily ailments.
> Prescribe no medicine, O ignorant physician! (1)
> Prescribe no medicine, O ignorant physician!
> If there is pain (*dard*) in the heart,
> there will be continued suffering in the body.
> Such medicine [as you have], brother,
> cannot remove this pain. (1). Refrain.
> [When] one indulges in carnal pleasures by forgetting the Lord,
> then one's body contracts many ailments.
> The wicked *man* (heart-mind-soul) is then punished.
> Prescribe no medicine, O ignorant physician! (2)
> As sandal is useful when it spreads its perfume:
> So man is useful as long as he has breath in his body.
> When the breath departs, the body crumbles away
> and becomes useless. No one takes medicine after that. (3)
> One's body becomes like gold and one's soul is made pure,
> when one possesses the essence of the divine Name.
> Thus all pains and diseases shall be dispelled;
> and one will be saved, Nanak, by the True Name. (4)
>
> (M1, *Malar* 2, AG, p. 1256)

The context of this hymn, according to the *janam-sakhis*, was the occasion when Guru Nanak lapsed into silence and inactivity, and his parents felt that he might be suffering from some ailment[8]. Thus a physician was called to cure him of his ailment. When the physician grasped his wrist to feel his pulse, Guru Nanak withdrew his arm and recited this hymn. Whether or not this tradition is historically accurate is not relevant to our present purpose. Rather, the most significant point is that this hymn provides us with an understanding of the concept of suffering (*dukkh*) in the Sikh tradition.

Here, Guru Nanak diagnoses different types of suffering (*dukkh*) such as pang of separation from the Beloved, pain of starvation, anguish of tyranny and death, affliction of bodily ailments, and torment of mental and spiritual diseases. All these pains, in fact, make suffering universal. They highlight different aspects of spiritual, mental and physical suffering. Indeed, Guru Nanak acknowledges two levels of suffering, one which is innate to all human beings by virtue of their entanglement in the cycle of existence (*sansar*) and the other which is encountered in everyday life as a result of hunger, distress, tyranny, and so on.[9] Elsewhere, he proclaims that the 'whole world is groaning in suffering.'[10] In fact, suffering is an inevitable part of the human situation. To wish it were not there, is to be oblivious of the divine Order (*Hukam*): 'Nanak, idle it is for one to ask for pleasure when pain comes. Pleasure and pain are like robes which one must wear as they come.'[11] Thus suffering is not some kind of 'illusion', but a stark reality of life.

The second major theme in this hymn deals with the origin of human suffering. In Guru Nanak's view suffering begins with separation (*vicchora*) from the divine Beloved: 'What terrible separation it is to be separated from God and what blissful union to be united with Him!'[12] Guru Nanak maintains that it is *haumai* or the sense of self-centeredness which is the root cause of one's separation from Akal Purakh ('the Timeless Being', God). The term *haumai* has a special meaning in Sikh theology. It is a compound of two personal pronouns, *hau* and *mai*, each meaning 'I', and thus *haumai* means 'I, I.' As such it signifies the powerful impulse to succumb to personal gratification so that a person is separated from Akal Purakh, and thus continues to suffer within the cycle of rebirth (*sansar*).[13] Under the influence of *haumai* a person becomes *manmukh* ('self- willed')[14] who is so attached to his passions for worldly pleasures that he forgets the Divine and wastes his entire life in evil. This is quite evident from the following verse of Guru Nanak's hymn: '[When] one indulges in carnal pleasures by forgetting the Lord, then one's body contracts many ailments.'[15] It is no wonder that the 'wicked *man* (heart-mind-soul) is then punished.' Guru Nanak thus holds human agents responsible for their miserable condition. Elsewhere he is more explicit on this point: 'Do not blame others, for you receive the reward or retribution for what you yourself do.'[16] Guru Nanak further maintains that 'divine justice takes virtue and vice into account, and in accordance with people's actions, some are brought near to the divine presence, while others are banished afar.'[17] Here the law of *karam* is invoked to explain the free-will and the retributive aspects of Sikh theodicy.

The third important theme that emerges from the *Malar* hymn is the relationship between *man* (heart-mind-soul) and body (*sarir*): 'If there is anguish (*dard*) in the heart, there will be continued suffering in the body.' Here Guru Nanak is employing the Persian term *dard*, a term which must be distinguished from *dukkh*. It has a rich connotation in Sufi terminology where it stands for 'pang of separation' from the divine Beloved. Guru Nanak repeatedly asserts that the ignorant physician who is unaware of the pain in the heart cannot successfully cure the disease.[18] Although medicine for bodily ailments may or may not be prized, the *Vaid* ('one who is learned', physician) who heals the pangs of a divinely afflicted heart is worthy of veneration.[19] Sometimes, the type of suffering which afflicts us by tormenting our heart, mind or soul is much more distressful than any corporeal suffering. Thus an in-depth analysis of the relationship between mind and body is absolutely necessary to reach to the bottom of any disease. One's capacity for enduring pain and suffering is also affected by moral courage and the spirit's control over the body. In fact, will power and heroism play an important role in an individual's physiological capacity to resist.[20]

The final theme in Guru Nanak's hymn deals with the solution to the problem of suffering. It provides a spiritual prescription in the form of the meditation on the divine Name that makes one's 'body like gold' (*kanchan kaian*) and one's soul like *hansa*-bird ('swan'). In this context, gold symbolizes 'purity' while the *hansa*-birds symbolize the liberated souls. Thus, with the transforming power of the divine Name, the liberated souls are cured from all kinds of maladies and suffering. We will return to this theme in the fifth section

III.

It is important to note that the most effective theodicies tend to justify suffering in terms of the realization of a higher purpose that necessitates the existence of evil and suffering in the world. These are frequently referred to as teleological theodicies, themes that do not reconcile evil in the present context, but look to the future for such justification.[21] The notions of *karam* and *sansar*, however, seem to provide an effective theodical solution to the problem of evil and suffering even in the present context. *Karam* is popularly understood in Indian thought as the principle of cause and effect. This principle of *karam* is logical and inexorable, but *karam* is also understood as a predisposition which safeguards the notion of free choice.[22] In Sikh doctrine, however, the notion of *karam* undergoes a radical change. For the Sikh Gurus, the law of *karam* is not inexorable. When Guru Nanak asserts that 'one cannot achieve spiritual-realization without the True Guru in spite of one's actions', it becomes clear that the traditional notion of *karam* is set aside.[23] In the context of his own theology, *karam* is subject to the higher principle of the 'divine Order' (*Hukam*). The divine Order in Guru Nanak's thought may be defined as an 'all-embracing principle, the sum total of all divinely inspired laws; and it is a revelation of the nature of God.'[24]

Guru Nanak maintains that 'all pains and pleasures are in accordance with the divine Order',[25] and that Akal Purakh graciously looks upon the suffering of mankind. He further says: 'Many endure constant suffering or hunger, yet even these are your gifts, O Lord.'[26] It clearly implies that even the suffering comes from the divine source. To overcome suffering one must interpret everyday occurrences as the will of the divine, and bear such suffering in a spirit of cheerful resignation.[27] However, there is no fatalism nor any passive acceptance of a predestined future in Guru Nanak's view of life. He proclaims: 'With your own hands carve out your destiny.'[28] Indeed, personal effort in the form of good actions has its place in Guru Nanak's view of life. His idea of 'divine free choice' on the one hand, and his emphasis on the life of activism based on human freedom on the other, reflect his ability to hold in tension seemingly opposed elements. In Guru Nanak's view, however, all human actions presuppose the functioning of divine grace. Thus the primacy of divine grace over personal effort is always maintained, and divine grace even breaks the chain of adverse *karam*.

In order to respond to the issue of the suffering of the innocent, let us turn to Guru Nanak's four hymns, collectively known as *Babar-vani* ('Utterances concerning Babur').[29] These hymns provide an eye-witness account of Babur's invasion of India and throw considerable light on the devastation caused by his army. Guru Nanak was pained to see the suffering of the innocent who had little to do with politics and war:

> You spared Khurasan but
> yet spread fear in Hindustan.
> Creator, you did this, but to avoid the blame
> you sent the Mughal as the messenger of death.
> Receiving such chastisement, the people cry out in agony
> and yet no anguish touches you. (1)[30]
> Creator, you belong to all.
> If the mighty destroy only one another,
> one is not grieved. (1) Refrain.
> But if a mighty lion falls upon a herd of cattle,
> then the master is answerable.[31]
> The wretched dogs (Lodhis) have spoiled the priceless jewels;
> when they are dead no one will regard them.
> You alone unite and you alone divide;
> thus is your glory manifested. (2)
> If anyone assumes an exalted name
> and indulges always in whatever his mind desires;
> He becomes as a worm in the sight of the Master,
> regardless of how much corn he pecks up.
> Die (to self) and you shall truly live.
> Remember the Name, Nanak, and you shall receive a portion. (3)[32]
> (M1, *Asa* 39, AG, p. 360)

Evidently, the actual context of this hymn is the battlefield when Babur's army invaded India. Here, the principal theme is related to the question of why the weak and innocent should suffer unmerited torment at the hands of the strong and in this respect this hymn has obvious affinities with the Book of Job. God is called into account, just as Job summons him.[33] Guru Nanak makes it quite explicit that it was the Creator who sent Babur as the messenger of death to destroy the Lodhi Sultanate. With a firm belief in Akal Purakh's omnipotence, however, he offers the theodical solution to the problem of suffering as follows: 'You alone unite and you alone divide; thus is your glory manifested.' He thus stresses the absolute nature of divine *Hukam* ('Order') which is ultimately beyond human comprehension. A similar response appears in certain other *Babar-vani* verses: 'To whom can one complain when the Creator himself acts and causes others to act? To whom can one go and weep when You yourself dispense suffering and happiness through your will?'[34] Here,

Guru Nanak is looking at the historical events from a mystical dimension.

It should, however, be emphasized that Guru Nanak's response to war and suffering is not limited to his personal anguish. He is responding to an actual life situation with his profound inner experience. In tune with Akal Purakh, he reflects on the situation at hand from various perspectives. In this context, J.S. Grewal argues that there is a moral dimension which restrains Guru Nanak from an outright condemnation either of the conqueror or the conquered.[35] Nevertheless, Guru Nanak describes the Lodhis as 'wretched dogs' for their moral failure to protect their sovereignty and the innocent (*ratan*, 'jewels') people. They had acted in a manner contrary to the divine intention and were responsible for the ultimate overthrow of their dynasty. In the *Tilang* hymn, on the other hand, Guru Nanak refers to Babur's army as the 'marriage-party of evil'[36] (*pap ki janj*), and thus charges them for their moral failure to demand a 'dowry' (*dan*) forcibly from the suffering people.

Elsewhere, Guru Nanak holds the heedlessness of Akal Purakh on the part of the general public as responsible for bringing about this retribution. Indeed, the greater part of human suffering is caused by those people who freely choose to act against the divine will. In the case of the rape of women, for instance, Guru Nanak makes the following observation:

> The wealth and sensual beauty which intoxicated them
> became their enemies.
> The messengers (of Death), under orders to persecute,
> strip them of their honour and carry them off.
> Glory or punishment, either we gather,
> as God in his purpose declares.
> Had they paused to think in time,
> then would they have received the punishment?
> But the rulers paid no heed,
> passing their time instead in revelry;
> Now that Babur's authority has been established
> the princes starve.[37]
>
> (M1, *Asa Astapadian* 11, (4–5), AG, p. 417)

Clearly, all the suffering involved in war and rape was not wholly undeserved. It was caused by the senseless pursuit of worldly pleasures and heedlesness of Akal Purakh on the part of the rulers and the ruled alike. For all his sympathy with the suffering people, however, Guru Nanak is fully cognisant of the situation of the poor women. Their agony, in fact, reminds him of a religious truth that 'God's justice cannot be ignored, that the divine Order (*Hukam*) cannot be defied, that unrighteousness will be punished.'[38] Those who have committed the unpardonable crimes will certainly receive punishment in the future. Here, we have a theodical solution to the problem of evil and suffering, a solution that stresses both the free-will and the retributive themes. Nevertheless, these themes cohere into the higher purpose of divine Order.

In sum, it is absolutely necessary to look at Guru Nanak's various utterances in their proper perspectives. When he is offering a theodical solution to the issue of suffering from a mystical dimension, he sees the divine Order at work behind all happenings. This is the ultimate state of liberation when the spirit ascends to the 'realm of Truth' (*sach khand*), a state where there is perfect and absolute accord with the divine Order (*Hukam*): 'As the *Hukam*, so too the deed!'[39] In this state one transcends the duality of joy and suffering. In this context, Guru Tegh Bahadur (1621–75) proclaims: 'They who are free from joy and sorrow, from greed, passion and pride: Says Nanak, they indeed are, my mind, the image of the Supreme Being.'[40] The issue of suffering is then seen as part of the higher divine purpose. However, when Guru Nanak addresses this issue from a moral perspective, he then offers all the possible causes of suffering, laying the blame where it is due and holding human agents responsible for their suffering. People suffer because they freely choose to act against the divine Order. At that time his theodical solution reflects both the free-will and the retributive themes, although these themes call for teleological reference in order to cohere. In particular, the law of *karam* and the divine Order (*Hukam*) are invoked simultaneously to explain the mystery of the suffering of infants. That is, the innocent children suffer in the present life because of the actions of their past life, but their suffering is intended for a higher divine purpose which will be realized in the future life according to the divine Order.

IV.

In this section, we will address the issue of 'pessimism' from the perspective of Sikh theodicy. Here it will be instructive to examine the works of the medieval Sufi poet, Shaikh Farid, preserved in the Sikh scripture. These works are collectively referred to by their Sikh title of *Farid-bani* in the Adi Granth. A careful examination of *Farid-bani*, for instance, suggests that its dominant theme is linked with the 'gloomy view' of life in the world.[41] In fact, Guru Arjan took special pains to 'restore social sanity to the views of Shaikh Farid where they touch borders of nihilism and total denial of life here and now.'[42] Several shaloks of the Sufi poet have received direct comments from the Sikh Gurus. For instance, let us consider the following two shaloks of Shaikh Farid in which the pessimistic tone finds its highest expression:

> Farid, if my throat had been cut on the same day
> as my navel string,
> I should not have fallen into such trouble
> nor undergone such hardship. (76)
>
> Farid, I thought I alone was in pain,
> but actually the whole world is in pain.
> I went up on the roof and
> looked on every house in flames. (81)
>
> (Shaikh Farid, *Shaloks* 76 and 81, AG, pp. 1381–2)

Here Shaikh Farid seems to be cursing human life as worthless. His attitude towards it is comprehensively negative. For him the life in the world is devoid of joy, containing and terminating in suffering (*dukkh*). This is, indeed, contrary to the life-affirming principles of the Sikh Gurus.

In responding to the issues raised by Shaikh Farid, Guru Arjan offers his solutions from the Sikh perspective. His comments are interjected into his own *Var Ramakali* and then repeated in Shaikh Farid's shaloks in the epilogue of the Adi Granth to reiterate the Sikh viewpoint:

> Mahala 5 (Guru Arjan)
> This lovely world is like a garden, Farid,
> in which some poison-bearing plants also grow.
> But they for whom the Master cares
> do not suffer at all. (82)
>
> Mahala 5 (Guru Arjan)
> How sweet is life, Farid,
> with health the body blooms!
> Yet those who love their dear, sweet [Lord],
> are rarely ever found! (83)
>
> (M5, *Shaloks* 82 and 83, AG, p. 1382)

Here, Guru Arjan employs the 'signatures' of 'Farid' since he is directly addressing the issues raised by the Sufi poet. In fact, he is actually addressing those issues being debated between the Sikh community and the contemporary followers of Shaikh Farid.[43] In his first comment, Guru Arjan asserts that just as poison-bearing plants also grow in a beautiful garden, so suffering is an inevitable part of life. Joy and suffering are two aspects of worldly life which make life worth living. The Guru further provides the hope that one may find the way through the grace of the Master (*pir*) to accept pain and pleasure with equanimity. Whereas Shaikh Farid regards the world with indifference or as a place of suffering, Guru Arjan likens it to a 'beautiful garden' (*bhum rangavali*, 'colourful earth'), thus emphasizing for the Sikh community a positive attitude towards life in the world.

In his second comment, Guru Arjan maintains that human life is the most delightful (*suhavari*) experience that one can have with the gift of this beautiful body (*suvannari deh*). Elsewhere human being has been called the epitome of creation: 'All other creation is subject to man; man reigns supreme on this earth.'[44] Although the existence of physical deformity and ugliness in the world is sometimes explained as the result of previous *karam*, it is intended for a higher divine purpose which is beyond human comprehension. This situation can, however, change through the functioning of divine grace: 'The cripple can cross over a mountain and the blockhead can become an accomplished preacher. The blind can see the three worlds through the grace of the Guru.'[45] Guru Arjan further proclaims that human life provides an individual with the opportunity to remember the divine Name and ultimately to join with the Lord.[46] But rare (*virle*) are the ones who seek the divine Beloved while participating in worldly actions and delights. Thus in contrast with Shaikh Farid, Guru Arjan places a positive value on human life and seeks to ignite a spirit of optimism among his followers. Whereas Shaikh Farid focuses on the suffering of the world, Guru Arjan's accent falls on the beautiful side of creation.

The dominant spirit of the Guru Arjan's works is remarkably exuberant. He speaks time and again of keeping the spirit of optimism in the midst of the trials and tribulations of life. In *Var Basant* ('Song of Spring'), for instance, he sings of the joys of living: 'Ponder devoutely the Name of Akal Purakh and bloom like the flowers in spring.'[47] Although Guru Arjan frequently acknowledges the woes of life, he enkindles the spirit of optimism by stressing the divine Name as their infallible remedy. For instance, there are numerous references in his compositions to real-life incidents about the detractors' campaign against him. His immediate response is always one of hope and reassurance: 'Those who are protected by the hand of Akal Purakh cannot be killed by anyone. Akal Purakh helps his saints, he has done away with their illusion. There is none but the Creator who can be one's support.'[48]

The theme of optimism is indeed a constant refrain in the teachings of the Sikh Gurus, a theme which evolved into the Sikh ethical virtue of *charhdi kala* or 'high spirits.' Literally, the Punjabi word *charhdi* is a verbal adjective meaning 'rising,' 'ascending' or 'soaring,' while the Sanskrit word *kala* predominantly means 'energy.' Together, the phrase *charhdi kala* means 'an intensely energized, ever-ascending state of the spirit of an individual or a group.'[49] In Sikh usage, *charhdi kala* is characterized by 'unwavering confidence in divine justice, absolute certainty which overrides all doubts, [and] supreme bravery which rises above any thought of defeat.'[50] Also, persistent cheerfulness (*sada vigas*) is the hallmark of *charhdi kala*, a virtue which has always inspired the Sikhs to maintain a perpetual readiness to act in the face of the most trying situations. In this context, Guru Nanak has emphasized that spiritual suffering is much worse than any type of physical punishment that can be inflicted by an oppressor.[51] Thus the spirit of *charhdi kala* has inspired the tradition of martyrdom among the Sikhs. In fact, the memory of Sikh martyrs is invoked in the daily recitation of the Sikh prayer, Ardas ('petition'). Those who sacrificed their lives for the faith are remembered along with the Gurus. This acknowledgement of their sacrifice is indicative of the esteem that the Sikh Panth ('community') associates with the Sikh martyrs.

Here, it will be useful to take a note of Clifford Geertz' argument that 'as a religious problem, the problem of suffering is, paradoxically, not how to aviod suffering, but how to make of physical pain, personal loss, physical defeat, or the helpless contemplation of others' agony something bearable, supportable – something, as we say, sufferable.'[52] There is, however, certain glory in the spirit of *charhdi kala*, which is marked not only by the stoic acceptance of suffering, but also by the spirit of bravery which prepares one to face up to all hardships and handicaps with courage and determination. In fact, during the tumultuous period of eighteenth century the Sikhs forged a new set of vocabulary (*singh bole*), eulogizing their privations and ridiculing their misfortunes. One who had nothing better to eat than a mouthful of gram would say that he/she was eating almonds, while a person with an empty stomach would declare himself/herself to have gone mad with prosperity. Death in the battlefield would be regarded as an expedition to the next world.[53] Even in the writings of Guru Nanak physical pain has been likened to 'immortal nectar' (*amrit*) which the devotees of Akal Purakh drink to remain spiritually alive: 'When one possesses the essence of the divine Name, then one's body becomes pure (*nirmal kaian*) and one's soul bright (*ujjal hansa*). That person drinks all sufferings as though these were the immortal nectar (*amrit*). Suffering does not attach itself to this person.'[54]

V.

Historically, the Sikhs have been preoccupied with the understanding of the relationship between spirituality and healing since the beginning of their tradition. Early Sikh reflections on pain and suffering are traditionally Indian, and they can be understood within the context of the major system of indigenous Indian medicine, popularly known as Ayurveda, the 'knowledge of enhancing life.' The Ayurvedic teachings embodied an understanding of illness as a lack of balance among three elements: air, phlegm, and bile. For cures, Ayurveda used diet and certain prescriptions of an impressive repertory of medicinal plants and minerals.[55] In particular, there was an emphasis on preparations using mercury as the means toward enhancing life. In this context, it is important to note a significant entry in the blank folios of the original manuscript of the Adi Granth (written in 1604 CE), popularly known as the Kartarpur manuscript, where there is a reference to the indigenous process of preparing mercury oxide, a medicinal preparation from mercury (*para ras rakhasu*).[56] In other words, this is a recipe for converting mercury into 'medicinal ash' (*kushta or bhasam*) to make it serve as panacea for several diseases. This entry is not part of the Adi Granth text itself, but its presence in the extra folios of the manuscript clearly indicates the preoccupation of the early Sikh community with health issues.

Although the Adi Granth is certainly not a treatise on medicines, there are numerous references to alchemy (*rasayana*) and the metaphorical use of the method of preparing indigenous medicines (*aukhadh*). In this context, Guru Nanak employs the metaphor of alchemy to diagnose the problem of suffering how 'lust and wrath destroy the body as flux (*sohaga*, 'borax') melts the gold.'[57] In his *Malar* hymn, he prescribes how the daily practice of meditation on the divine Name removes all suffering:

> Pain is poison
> but the divine Name is the antidote.
> Let patient contentment be the stone on which you pound it
> and let your hand be that of charity.
> Take it daily and your body shall not waste away,
> and at the end Death itself will be struck down.
> Take this medicine,
> for the consuming of it will purge the evil in you.[58]
>
> (M1, *Malar* 8, AG, pp. 1256–7)

Here, Guru Nanak is employing the metaphor of 'poison' for suffering (*dukkh mahura*), a lethal substance which is converted into a useful Indian medicine through the process of transmutation. The divine Name acts as an antidote (*maran harinamu*) in that process, and it makes suffering a useful medicine for the cure of evil inclinations in life. In *Var Asa*, Guru Nanak explicitly describes suffering as medicine (*dukkh daru*) and pleasure as disease (*sukh rog*), since 'pleasure seduces one's mind from the Master.'[59]

Indeed, Guru Nanak is offering a 'meaningful and creative approach' to suffering by stressing its therapeutic value. His assertion of 'suffering as medicine' may be better appreciated in the light of the psycho-physiological theory of sensibility. According to this theory, the habit of pleasure not only lowers one's strength, but it also makes one incapable of supporting the abrupt changes which the hazards of life can bring. The feeling of pain or suffering, on the other hand, contributes at times in strengthening the whole body; it instills more stability, balance, and equilibrium to the nervous and muscular system.[60] Thus the theme of 'the usefulness of pain' as an effective means to be employed in the struggle for life – which led to the therapeutic techniques using shock and stimulation – was part of a judicious calculation concerning the benefits which the patient can hope to expect from such treatments.[61] In this context, Teja Singh remarks that '[i]t is suffering that has intensified the Sikh character; and it is in this sense that, in Sikh Scripture, pain has been called a medicine, and hunger and affliction a blessing.'[62]

The central focus in Guru Nanak's *Malar* hymn, however, is on the discipline of meditation on the divine Name, a process that involves the cultivation of virtues like patience, contentment, charity, and forgiveness. Indeed, the list of virtues can be extended to include love, humility, fear of Akal Purakh, purity and true living. According to W.H. McLeod, the discipline of *nam simaran* ('rememberance of the divine Name') involves three levels:

> At one level this involves the practice of Nam Japan, or 'repeating the Name', a long-established convention whereby merit is acquired by devoutly repeating a sacred word or mantra. This helps the devotee to internalise the meaning of whatever he may be uttering and in this sense the practice is explicitly enjoined by the Gurus. The Gurus also insist that the discipline must be practised in corporate sense, with devotees gathering as a congregation (*satsang*) to sing hymns of praise (*kirtan*). A third level which is also required of the loyal disciple is meditation. God as expressed in the name is to be 'remembered' not merely in the repeating of auspicious words or the singing of inspired hymns but also in deep contemplation of the divine mystery of the Name. All three practices constitute legitimate and necessary forms of Nam Simaran.[63]

Here, McLeod aptly provides the standard theoretical framework in which the discipline of *nam simaran* can be understood. It ranges from the simple repetition of an appropriate word – such as 'Guru! Guru!' (ancient practice as evidenced in the *janam-sakhis*) or 'Vahiguru! Vahiguru!' ('Praise to the Guru', modern practice) – through the devout singing of hymns (*kirtan*) to sophisticated meditation on the nature of Akal Purakh. The actual practice, which may have varied in different historical periods among different sections of the Sikh Panth, has always been regarded as the only means of liberation from all types of suffering in the world.

A careful analysis of Guru Arjan's compositions reveals his constant concern to alleviate the pain and suffering of his audience. In his theology, Akal Purakh is frequently referred to as *Achint* ('Without anxiety'), *Dukkh-bhanjan* ('Pain-killer') and *Satr-dahan* ('Destroyer of enemies').[64] In fact, the divine Name is frequently described as 'panacea for all diseases' (*sarab rog ka aukhadhu namu*),[65] a theme which has indeed become the fundamental aspect of Sikh theology. Accordingly, Akal Purakh himself is the physician who removes all pain through the transforming power of his Name.[66] In the *Sorathi* hymn, for instance, Guru Arjan expresses his profound gratitude for his child's deliverance from a serious illness:

The True Guru is my Helper, my certain Protector,
my refuge and trustworthy aid.
By his grace Hargobind is saved from this illness,
saved by his merciful hand. (1) Refrain.
His fever subsiding, its heat has abated,
cooled by the grace of the Lord.
My honour is saved by the prayers of the faithful;
humbly I bow before the True Guru. (1)
Here and hereafter the Lord is my Keeper,
heedless of virtues and sins.
Says Nanak: Firm is your promise my Guru and Master;
blest be your merciful hand. (2)[67]

(M5, *Sorathi* 49, AG, pp. 620–1)

Here, Guru Arjan clearly describes the healing power of the prayers of the faithful. Elsewhere, he explicitly mentions how the child Hargobind recovered from smallpox (*sitala*) through the transforming power of the divine Name.[68] It will, however, be naive to claim that all Sikhs relied solely on the discipline of *nam simaran* to get rid of their diseases during different historical periods. The nineteenth-century data supplied by Harjot Oberoi, for instance, indicate that the Sikhs living in the rural areas of central Punjab widely worshipped Sitala Devi ('Cool One'), the goddess of pustular diseases, to get rid of their suffering.[69] Therefore, one must acknowledge the diversity of practices within a living religious tradition at the popular and elite levels.

In order to understand the relationship between Sikh spirituality and healing, it will be instructive to examine the recent clinical research on 'The *Sukhmani* and High Blood Pressure.' The *Sukhmani* ('Pearl of Peace' or 'Peace of Mind') is Guru Arjan's celebrated composition which 'stands out for the beauty of its expression and for the profundity of its thought.'[70] Its main focus is on the crucial significance of the divine Name in a person's quest for liberation. In particular, it addresses the problem of suffering and offers its solution. It emphatically declares that the sure and certain panacea is the divine Name. For instance, the last stanza of the last octave of the *Sukhmani* states:

He who nurtures the Name within
will find the Lord ever present there.
Gone forever the pain of rebirth,
his precious soul in an instant freed.
Noble his actions, gracious his speech;
his spirit merged in the blessed Name.

All suffering ended, all doubts, all fears;
renowned for his faith and his virtuous deeds.
Raised to honour, wonderous his fame!
Priceless the pearl, God's glorious Name! (8.24)[71]
(M5, *Gauri Sukhmani*, 8 (24), AG, p. 296)

Clearly, the sustained and faithful practice of *nam simaran* transmutes all suffering into bliss and makes a person virtuous in thoughts, words and deeds. Such a person is indeed the *brahamgiani* of Guru Arjan's conception, the one who possesses an understanding of Akal Purakh's wisdom and who has found enlightenment in the company of the devout.[72] Our main concern here is to understand the healing power of the recitation of the *Sukhmani*. That is why it enjoys a notable popularity among the vast majority of Sikhs and many Punjabi Hindus.

In 1978, clinical research was undertaken into the beneficial effects of reading the *Sukhmani* daily to the patients suffering from high blood pressure at Guru Tegh Bahadur Hospital in Amritsar. The project was undertaken by Ajinder Singh of Guru Nanak Dev University under the supervision of Harcharan Singh, Professor and Head of the Department of Medicine, Guru Tegh Bahadur Hospital. This study was intended to 'find (a) the incidence of hypertension in the regular reciters of the *Sukhmani*, and (b) the effects of its recitals on known cases of hypertension who are believers.' It produced statistics that 'proved scientifically that as a rule the incidence of hypertension among reciters of *Sukhmani* is decidedly lower than in the case of non-reciters.' The research concluded that 'regular recitation of *Sukhmani* is very effective, simple, easy and economical non-pharmacologic adjunct to the antihypertensive therapy and in some cases an alternative to antihypertensive drugs.'[73]

In this context, it will be useful to take notice of parallel developments in the Western world with respect to the physiological effects of meditation. For more than twenty-five years laboratories at the Harvard Medical School have systematically been studying the benefits of mind/body interactions. The research established that when a person engages in a repetitive prayer, word, sound, or phrase and when intrusive thoughts are passively disregarded, a specific set of physiological changes ensue. Decreased metabolism, heart rate, and rate of breathing, along with distinctively slower brain waves are observed. These changes are in opposition to those induced by stress and are part of an effective therapy for a number of diseases, among which are hypertension, cardiac rhythm irregularities, many forms of chronic pain, insomnia, infertility, symptoms of cancer and AIDS, premenstrual syndrome, anxiety and mild and moderate forms of depression. In fact, the extent in which any disease is caused or made worse by stress is comparable to the extent in which this physiological state is an effective therapy.[74]

In Punjab, an institution by the name of Sarab Rog Ka Aukhadh Nam Mission Trust ('The Divine Name is the Cure of all Diseases' Mission Trust) was opened at Chandigarh and Ludhiana in August 1987. It has been organizing residential camps each of five days duration at different places, inviting patients from all walks of life and providing them with free accommodation, balanced diet, and 'Nam Therapy.' I myself attended one meeting on 24 May 1990 at Ludhiana when I was on my research tour in India. The press brief on that day stated: 'During Nam Therapy, the recitation of God's name is done in the form of group singing by the patients and the rest of the congregation. This method has been found very effective and quick. Reason alone cannot explain this phenomenon. It is an experience, which is highly rewarding and works in a unique, sure and subtle manner.'[75]

The brief report released by the Sarab Rog Ka Aukhadh Nam Mission Trust then provided four success stories of patients who were completely cured of chronic diseases. In the first case of a male Sikh patient suffering from Hypertension, 'non functioning shrunk kidney with stones was restored to normal function and even size became normal. This is a unique cure through Nam Therapy.' In the second case of a female Sikh patient suffering from Chronic Diarrhea and loss of weight, she started Nam Therapy in 1989 and 'she has been completely cured of the ailment and she has gained over 8–9 kgs of weight in a year's time.' In the third case of a male Hindu patient suffering from Hypertension, Ischaemic Heart Disease and Congestive failure, 'Nam Therapy has given him a new lease of life.' In the final case of a female Sikh patient suffering from Juvenile Rheumatoid Arthritis, the report says: 'With this [Nam] therapy, not only the further damage to the bones and joint stopped, but her existing deformities were substantially set right. She can walk now and her deformed fingers are getting better.'[76]

All these studies suggest that there is a world of faith beyond medicine. They offer new data for consideration in the area of medical research. It is, however, important to note that such studies have not convinced everyone. Many doctors who follow the physical laws of nature frequently warn that it can be dangerous, even life-threatening, to rely on prayer or meditation alone if one is sick. Those who debate the quality of research on prayer agree on one piece of advice: 'Even if you believe in divine intervention, call your doctor and follow professional medical recommendations.'[77] Nevertheless, allowances must be made for the enthusiasm of the Sarab Rog ka Aukhadh Nam Mission. The experience of Nam therapy seems to confirm that there is a strong relationship between spirituality and the healing process. Although the Sikh experience of *nam simaran* is practiced in diverse ways, there has always been repeated emphasis on the conviction that the divine Name alone is the source of true bliss and the essential means of deliverance. As a 'panacea for all diseases', it has the efficacy to transform suffering into a blissful experience.

VI.

From the Sikh perspective, it may be concluded that the reality of suffering is acknowledged at two levels. At one level, suffering is encountered in everyday life as a result of hunger, distress, disease, tyranny and so on. In this case, Sikh theodical solution requires that one must interpret all such happenings as the will of Akal Purakh, and bear such suffering with the spirit of resignation. By submitting to the divine Order (*Hukam*) cheerfully one can gain confidence in coping with any situation of anguish and despair. Indeed, the submission to the divine Order becomes a means of release from the chain of *karam*. The issue of suffering in this case is seen as part of the higher divine purpose. Further, Guru Nanak addresses the issue of suffering from a moral perspective, thereby offering all the possible causes of suffering, laying the blame where it is due, and holding human agents responsible for their suffering. In this case, his theodical solution reflects the free-will and the retributive themes.

At the second level, suffering is innate to all human beings by virtue of their present situation in the cycle of existence (*sansar*). This is the given condition for all, and one can transcend this condition only when one has achieved liberation from the cycle of birth, death and rebirth. To achieve this ultimate state, one must practice the interior discipline of *nam simaran* to eradicate *haumai*, the sense of self-centeredness, and bring oneself into harmony with the divine Order (*Hukam*), thus earning for one the kind of *karam* which provides release. According to Guru Nanak, the ultimate state of liberation is achieved when one's heart, mind and soul ascend to the realm of Truth (*sach khand*), a goal which may be achieved during one's lifetime. This is the mystical dimension of Sikh experience in which one transcends the duality of joys and sorrows, and transmutes all suffering into blissful *sahaj* ('spontaneity').

Indeed, the Sikh Gurus have offered a 'meaningful and creative' response to the issue of pain and suffering. Their writings ignite the spirit of optimism in the face of trials and tribulations of life. Further, physical suffering has a therapeutic value in Sikh life. The divine Name has always been regarded as the 'panacea for all diseases.' In fact, the 'Nam Therapy' is gaining popularity in the healing process in this modern age of scientific and medical advancement. It is no wonder that people are rediscovering 'religious faith' in spite of their rational outlook in this post-modern world.

VII.

Here, it will be quite useful to make some brief comments on the religious issues for Sikhs that health-care workers should bear in mind while dealing with Sikhs. First of all, they should be sensitive to the Sikh customs and cultural traditions. In particular, they should understand the significance of the symbols of Sikh identity. For instance, all Sikhs initiated into the order of the Khalsa ('pure') observe the Rahit (code of conduct) as enunciated by Guru Gobind Singh and subsequently elaborated. The most significant part of the Rahit is the enjoinder to wear five items of external identity known from their Punjabi names as the five Ks. These are unshorn hair (*kes*), a wooden comb (*kanga*), a miniature sword (*kirpan*, literally this word is the combination of *kirpa* and *an*, meaning 'grace' and 'self-respect'), a steel 'wrist-ring' (*kara*), and a pair of short breeches (*kachh*). In Sikh self-understanding the five Ks are understood as outer symbols of the divine word, implying a direct correlation between *bani* ('inspired utterance') and *bana* ('Khalsa dress'). Putting on the five Ks along with the turban (in the case of male Sikhs) while reciting prayers symbolizes that the Khalsa Sikhs are dressed in the word of God. Their minds are thus purified and inspired, and their bodies girded to do battle with the day's temptations. They are prohibited from four gross sins: cutting the hair, using tobacco, committing adultery, and eating meat that has not come from an animal killed with a single blow (*jhataka*).

It is important to note that the *kirpan* worn by the Khalsa Sikhs is a religious symbol, not a weapon. In fact, it is neither designed as a weapon, nor it is intended to be used as an offensive weapon or in an offensive manner. But sometimes it is perceived to be a weapon by the hospital security personnel due to their ignorance of the Sikh traditions. In such cases, the hospital administration frequently invokes its policy which prohibits 'possession of an offensive weapon on the property.' If the health- care workers are properly informed about the religious significance of the *kirpan*, they can avoid a potential conflict between the Sikhs and the hospital administration. They should even discuss the meaning of the alleged 'dagger' with patients who complain about the wearing of the *kirpan* by the Khalsa Sikhs. Moreover, the *kirpan* is a symbol internal to the wearer; it does not have to be worn in such a way that it is visible to the outside world.

The health-care workers also need to know that there are other categories of Sikhs who do not formally belong to the Khalsa tradition. For instance, there is a large majority of Sikhs who retain their hair (*Kes-dhari*) and maintain a visible identity. In particular, the male Sikhs are easily recognized by their beards and turbans. They follow most of the Khalsa Rahit ('code of conduct') without having gone through the initiation ceremony. However, one should not assume that they will be wearing the sword (*kirpan*) too. Further, there are others who have shorn their hair and are less conspicuous, although their number is quite large in North America and the United Kingdom. They are popularly known as 'clean-shaven' (*Mona*) Sikhs. They are frequently confused with the so-called Sahaj-dhari ('slow-adopter') Sikhs who have never accepted the Khalsa discipline. Although the Sahaj-dhari Sikhs practice *nam simaran* and follow the teachings of the Adi Granth, they do not observe the Rahit and, in particular, cut their hair. This background knowledge about the various Sikh identities can be crucial in addresssing the various concerns that the health-care workers might have about Sikhs.

Finally, the health-care workers frequently deal with the religious issues associated with death. No rituals (derived from other religious traditions or of any other origins) should be performed when a Sikh dies in the hospital. The *Sikh Rahit Maryada* ('Sikh Code of Conduct') explicitly states that 'a dying person should not be taken from his bed and placed on the ground.' It is common practice for family members to recite Guru Arjan's *Sukhmani* or other hymns from the Adi Granth in the presence of a dying person. These devotional hymns are accessible on compact disk and can be played in the absence of a family member. In the case of the death of a Khalsa Sikh, the five Ks should be left on the dead body. Even if any of these five items (such as *kirpan*) were removed at the time of surgery, they should be restored on the body of the deceased. The hair should be neatly tied in a knot over the head (in the case of male Sikhs) and covered with a small turban. The health-care workers will earn the gratitude of family members if they are sensitive to these traditions. Moreover, it is always helpful to talk to the patients beforehand about specific instructions that they would like carried out in the event of their death.

Acknowledgements

I am grateful to Professor W.H. McLeod and Dr Louis Fenech for their valuable feedback on the earlier drafts of this paper. I would also like to thank the editors of this volume for their useful comments and suggestions.

NOTES

1. Harbans Singh, *Sri Guru Granth Sahib: Guru Eternal for the Sikhs* (Patiala: Academy of Sikh Religion and Culture, 1988).
2. John Hick, *Philosophy of Religion* (Englewood, N.J.: Prentice-Hall, 3rd edn., 1983), pp. 40–1.
3. John Hick, 'Problem of Evil,' in Paul Edwards, ed., *The Encyclopaedia of Philosophy*, Vol. 3 (New York: Macmillan, 1967), p. 136.
4. Michael Stoeber, *Evil and the Mystics' God: Towards a Mystical Theodicy* (Toronto: University of Toronto Press, 1992), p. 14.
5. C. Shackle, *A Guru Nanak Glossary* (London: SOAS, University of London, 1981), p. 156.
6. Karl H. Potter, 'Suffering in the Orthodox Philosophical Systems: Is there Any?,' in Kapil N. Tiwari, ed., *Suffering: Indian Perspectives* (Delhi: Motilal Banarsidass, 1986), pp. 1–2.
7. Roselyne Rey, *The History of Pain*, trans. by Louise Elliot Wallace, J.A. Cadden, and S.W. Cadden (Cambridge, Massachusetts: Harvard University Press, 1995; originally published, Paris: Decouverte, 1993), p. 2.
8. W.H. McLeod, *The B40 Janam-Sakhi* (Amritsar: Guru Nanak Dev University, 1980), pp. 16–17.

9. For details, see Louis Fenech, 'Playing the Game of Love: The Sikh Tradition of Martyrdom' (unpublished Ph.D. thesis, University of Toronto, 1994), p. 49.
10. M1, *Var Ramkali*, 1 (14), AG, p. 954.
11. M1, *Var Majh*, 2 (24), AG, p. 149.
12. M1, *Maru* 1, AG, p. 989. Cited in W.H. McLeod, *Guru Nanak and the Sikh Religion* (Delhi: Oxford University Press, reprint, 1976; originally published by Clarendon Press, Oxford, 1968), p. 148.
13. For an insightful analysis of key theological terms, see W.H. McLeod, *The Sikhs: History, Religion, and Society* (New York: Columbia University, 1989), p. 50.
14. McLeod uses the expression 'unregenerate man' for *manmukh*: 'This is the condition of pride of self-centredness, of sin, and so of death and transmigration. This is the condition which must be transcended if man is to attain release from transmigration.' See *Guru Nanak and the Sikh Religion*, pp. 177–8.
15. Ml, *Malar* 2, AG, p. 1256.
16. Ml, *Asa Patti Likhi* 21, AG, p. 433.
17. Ml , *Japu*, AG, p.8.
18. Ml, *Var Malar*, 1 (3), AG, p. 1279.
19. Ml, *Var Malar*, 2 (3), AG, p. 1279. Cited in J.S. Grewal, *Guru Nanak in History* (Chandigarh: Panjab University, reprint, 1979; 1st edn., 1969), p. 180.
20. Rey, *The History of Pain*, p. 2.
21. Stoeber, *Evil and Mystics'* God, pp. 11–12.
22. See Harold Coward, *Jung and Eastern Thought* (Albany: SUNY, 1985), pp. 95–107.
23. M1, *Sri Ragu* 1, AG, p. 72. Cited in Grewal, *Guru Nanak in History*, p. 264.
24. McLeod, *Guru Nanak and the Sikh Religion*, p. 203.
25. M1, *Basant Astapadian* 2, AG, p. 1188.
26. M1, *Japu* 25, AG, p. 5. Translation by W.H. McLeod, *Textual Sources for the Study of Sikhism* (Manchester: Manchester University Press, 1984; reprint, Chicago, Illinois: University of Chicago Press, 1990), p. 90.
27. G.S. Talib, 'Hukam – The Divine Ordinance', in Taran Singh, ed., *Teachings of Guru Nanak Dev* (Patiala: Punjabi University, 1973), p. 73.
28. M1, *Var Asa*, (20), AG, p. 473.
29. M1, *Asa* 39, *Asa Astapadi* 11, *Asa Astapadi* 12, and *Tilang* 5, AG, pp. 360, 417–8, and 722–3.
30. Translation of this verse is taken from W.H. McLeod, 'The Life of Guru Nanak,' in Donald S. Lopez, Jr. ed., *Religions of India in Practice* (Princeton, New Jersey: Princeton University Press, 1995), p. 455.
31. Translation of this verse is adapted from Grewal, *Guru Nanak in History*, p. 161.
32. Translation of final verse is adapted from McLeod, *Guru Nanak and the Sikh Religion*, p. 136, n. 2.
33. Ibid.
34. M1, *Asa Astapadi* 12, AG, p. 418.
35. Grewal, *Guru Nanak in History*, p. 163.
36. M1, *Tilang* 5, AG, p. 722.

37. Translation adapted from McLeod, *Guru Nanak and the Sikh Religion*, pp. 135–6.
38. Ibid., p. 136.
39. M1, *Japu* 37, AG, p. 8. Cited in ibid., p. 223.
40. M9, *Shalok* 13, AG, p. 1426.
41. For details, see Christopher Shackle, 'Early Muslim vernacular poetry in the Indus Valley: Its contexts and character', in Anna Libera Dallapiccola and Stephanie Zingel-Ave Lallemant, eds, *Islam and Indian Regions*, Vol. 1 (Stuttgart: Franz Steiner Verlag, 1993), pp. 268–78.
42. Attar Singh, ed., *Socio-Cultural Impact of Islam* (Chandigarh: Panjab University, 1976), p. 10.
43. For more details on the technique of textual commentary, see my 'Scriptural Adaptation in the Adi Granth', *Journal of the American Academy of Religion*, LXIV/2 (Summer 1996): 337–57.
44. M5, *Asa* 12, AG, p. 374.
45. M5, *Bilavalu* 37, AG, pp. 809–10.
46. M5, *Asa* 4, AG, p. 15: 'Precious this life you receive as a human, with it the chance to find the Lord (*Gobind*).'
47. M5, *Var Basant*, 1, AG, p. 1193.
48. Cited in Surjit Hans, *A Reconstruction of Sikh History From Sikh Literature* (Jalandhar: ABS Publications, 1988), p. 141. (Translations are slightly adapted.)
49. Harbans Singh, ed., *The Encyclopaedia of Sikhism*, Vol. I (Patiala: Punjabi University, 1992), p. 444.
50. W.H. McLeod, *Historical Dictionary of Sikhism* (London: Scarecrow Press, 1995), p. 61.
51. M1, *Var Majjh*, 3 (9), AG, p. 142. Also see, Fenech, 'Playing the Game of Love', p. 50.
52. Clifford Geertz, 'Religion as a Cultural System', in *The Interpretation of Cultures* (New York: Basic Books, 1973), p. 104. Also see Veena Das, *Critical Events: An Anthropological Perspective on Contemporary India* (Delhi: Oxford University Press, 1995), chaps VI and VII.
53. For details, see *The Encyclopaedia of Sikhism*, Vol. I, pp. 444–5.
54. M1, *Maru Solahe* 14, (6), AG, p. 1034.
55. For details, see Vasudha Narayanan, 'The Hindu Tradition', in Willard Oxtoby, ed., *World Religions: Eastern Traditions* (Toronto: Oxford University Press, 1996), pp. 62–3.
56. Kartarpur MS (1604 CE), ff. 21/2–22/1.
57. M1, *Ramakali Dakhani Oankaru* 18, AG, p. 932.
58. This translation is slightly adapted from the one given in McLeod, *Guru Nanak and the Sikh Religion*, p. 218.
59. M1, *Var Asa*, 1 (12), AG, AG, p. 469.
60. Rey, *History of Pain*, p. 115.
61. Ibid.
62. Teja Singh, *The Growth of Responsibility in Sikhism* (Calcutta: revised edn, 1951; 1st edn, 1919), p.36.
63. McLeod, *Textual Sources*, p. 40.
64. See Surjit Hans, *A Reconstruction of Sikh History*, p. 144.
65. M5, *Sukhmani*, 5 (9), AG, p. 274. Also see M5, *Asa* 32, AG, p. 378.

66. For more details, see my 'Nam da Sankalap te Marag', (unpublished M.A. thesis, Punjabi University, Patiala, 1973), pp. 93–6. Also see, Gurbachan Singh Talib, *Dukkh da Sankalap ate Samadhan* (Patiala: Guru Nanak Institute, Gurmat College, 1972), pp. 1–34.
67. Translation slightly adapted from the one given in McLeod, *Textual Sources*, pp. 52–3.
68. M5, *Gauri* 172, AG, p. 200. Also see, Surjit Hans, *A Reconstruction of Sikh History*, p. 149.
69. Harjot Oberoi, *The Construction of Religious Boundaries: Culture, Identity and Diversity in the Sikh Tradition* (Delhi: Oxford University Press, 1994), pp. 162–5.
70. W.H. McLeod, 'Sikh Hymns to the Divine Name', in Lopez, ed., *Religions of India*, p. 126.
71. Ibid., p. 131.
72. Ibid., p. 127.
73. Ajinder Singh and Harcharan Singh, 'The *Sukhmani* and High Blood Pressure: The Findings of a Clinical Enquiry', *Journal of Sikh Studies*, Vol. VI, No. 1 (February 1979), pp. 62–78.
74. See the course description of 'Spirituality and Healing in Medicine' offered by Harvard Medical School and The Mind/Body Medical Institute, Deaconess Hospital, under the direction of Herbert Benson, MD, Chief, Division of Behavioral Medicine. The course was offered on December 3–5, 1995 at Boston Marriot Hotel Copley Place, Boston, Massachusetts. For recent publications of this research, see Herbert Benson, with Marg Stark, *Timeless Healing: The Power and Biology of Belief* (New York: Simon and Schuster, 1997; originally published, Scribner, 1996) and Larry Dossey, *Healing Words: The Power of Prayer and the Practice of Medicine* (San Francisco: Harper, 1993).
75. Balwant Singh (Dr), *Press Brief* (Ludhiana: Sarab Rog Ka Aukhad Nam Mission Trust, Regd., 110 Model House, May 24, 1990), p. 1.
76. Ibid., pp. 1–4.
77. Gurney Williams III, 'The *healing* power of *prayer*', *McCall's* (April 1966), p. 89.

GLOSSARY

Adi Granth	(or *the Guru Granth Sahib*), the sacred scripture of the Sikhs compiled by Guru Arjan in 1603–4, consisting of the Sikh Gurus' compositions and selected hymns of *bhagats* or 'saints' of Sant, Sufi and Bhakti origin.
Akal Purakh	'The Timeless Being', Sikh concept of the divine Being; analogous to 'God.'
amrit	'nectar of immortality', the sanctified water used in the initiation ceremony of the Khalsa (q.v.).

Amrit-dhari — a Sikh who has 'taken *amrit*', viz. an initiated member of the Khalsa (q.v.).

Ardas — 'petition', the daily Sikh congregational prayer.

aukhad — 'medicine', an Ayurvedic medicine.

Ayurveda — 'knowledge of enhancing life', an indigenous system of Indian medicine.

Babar-vani — 'Utterances concerning Babur', four hymns of Guru Nanak in the Adi Granth (M1, *Asa* 39, *Asa Astapadi* 11, *Asa Astapadi* 12, and *Tilang* 5, AG, pp. 360, 417–8, and 722–3).

bana — uniform of the Khalsa: tight-fitting trousers, long outer shirt, sash, *kirpan* with belt diagonally over the right shoulder.

bani — the inspired 'utterances' of the Gurus or Bhagats recorded in the Adi Granth.

bhagat — (or *bhakta*), 'devotee', one who practices bhakti (q.v.).

bhakti — belief in, adoration of a personal God.

braham-giani — 'enlightened one', one who possesses an understanding of Akal Purakh's wisdom.

charhdi kala — 'the spirit of optimism.'

dard — 'anguish in the heart', a Sufi term which stands for 'pang of separation.'

daru — 'medicine.'

dukkh — 'pain, grief, sorrow, suffering.'

Farid-bani — 'utterances of [Shaikh] Farid' in the Adi Granth.

five Ks — five items (each beginning with the Punjabi letter 'k') which a Sikh of the Khalsa must wear. These are: *kes* ('unshorn hair'), *kangha* ('wooden comb'), *kirpan* ('a miniature sword'), *kara* ('a steel wrist-ring'), and *kachh* ('a pair of short breeches').

guru — a spiritual 'preceptor', either a person or the divine inner voice. The divine Guru became manifest in the form of ten human Gurus (from Guru Nanak to Guru Gobind Singh) and now persists in the form of the twin doctrine of Guru-Granth (scriptural Guru) and Guru-Panth (Sikh Community as Guru).

haumai — 'I-ness, my-ness', self-centered pride.

hukam — divine order.

janam-sakhi	'birth-testimony', traditional narrative of the life of Guru Nanak.
kanchan kaian	'body like gold', healthy body.
karam	(or *karma*), the destiny or fate of an individual, generated in accordance with deeds performed in one's present and past existences.
Kes-dhari	a Sikh who retains *kes* ('hair').
Khalsa	the religious order established by Guru Gobind Singh in 1699.
kirtan	devotional singing of hymns.
kushta	(or *bhasam*, 'ash'), a recipe for converting mercury into ash to make it serve as panacea for several diseases.
mahura	'poison.'
man	heart/mind/soul.
man-mukh	an unregenerate person, one who faces towards the uncleaned *man* (q.v.).
maran	'antidote.'
Mona	a Sikh who cuts his/her hair.
nam	the divine Name, a summary term expressing the total being of Akal Purakh.
nam-simaran	the devotional practice of meditating on the divine Name or *nam* (q.v.).
panth	'path' or 'way', system of religious belief or practice.
Panth	the key word refers to the Sikh community.
para	'mercury.'
pir	the head of a Sufi (q.v.) order; a Sufi saint.
Rahit	the code of conduct of the Khalsa (q.v.).
rasayan	'alchemy.'
rog	'disease.'
sach khand	the 'realm of truth', a goal which may be reached before death.
sahaj	the condition of ultimate bliss resulting from the practice of *nam-simaran* q.v.).
Sahaj-dhari	a non-Khalsa Sikh.
sangat	congregation, group of devotees.
sansar	(or *samsara*), transmigration.
sant	one who knows the truth; a pious person; an adherent of the Sant (q.v.) tradition.

Sant	one renowned as a teacher of a devotional school of North India.
sarir	human body.
Sikh	'learner', a follower of the Sikh faith.
Sikh Rahit Maryada	'Sikh Code of Conduct', the standard manual of Sikh doctrine and behaviour published in 1950 under the auspices of the Shiromani Gurdwara Prabandhak Committee (SGPC), Amritsar.
singh bole	'high-spirited words of the Khalsa Sikhs' of eighteenth-century.
Sitala	'Cool One', the goddess of pustular diseases.
Sufi	a follower of mystical Islam.
sukh	'pleasure.'
Sukhmani	'Pearl of Peace', a celebrated composition of Guru Arjan in the Adi Granth.
ujjal hansa	'bright soul', one having a clean *man* (q.v.).
Vahiguru	'Praise to the Guru', the modern name for God.
Vaid	'one who is learned', an Ayurvedic doctor.

HEALTH AND SUFFERING IN BUDDHISM: DOCTRINAL AND EXISTENTIAL CONSIDERATIONS

Tadeusz Skorupski

Overview

The nature, origin, and liberation from suffering stand at the very centre of the Buddha's teachings. Soon after his enlightenment at the age of thirty five, he set in motion the Wheel of Dharma and spent the rest of his life, some forty-five years, teaching his followers about suffering and the way of becoming free from it. After his demise, the Buddha's disciples continued to uphold his message in India, and eventually carried the torch of Dharma to other countries of Asia, and in the modern times to the West. During the course of some two and a half millennia, the teachings of the Buddha received a number of discordant doctrinal interpretations. The Abhidharma doctrines and practices of the early Buddhist schools, and the doctrines and practices introduced by the Mahāyāna and Vajrayāna adepts disagree between themselves, and often contradict the Buddha's primitive teaching as recorded in the Pāli Canon. However, despite all such disagreements and contradictions, the ultimate goal of all schools of Buddhism remains the same: liberation from suffering.

Taking into consideration the various categories of suffering, the primary preoccupation of Buddhism is with moral and spiritual suffering of living beings. Buddhism teaches that the entire spectrum of existence in its physical and sentient forms is impermanent (*anitya*), painful (*duḥkha*), and insubstantial (*anātma*). The primary source of such existence and the force that maintains and controls it are perceived in motivated actions (*karman*). It is a combination of positive and negative actions that brings about a variety of happy and unhappy lives all of which ultimately end in death. Intentional actions always lead to retribution, and consequently perpetuate existence but never bring complete freedom from suffering. The Dharma discovered by the Buddha at the time of his enlightenment constitutes the remedy or antidote to cure and liberate living beings from the woeful states of existence. The central theme of the Dharma set in motion by the Buddha in the Deer Park is the middle path[1] that leads to the appeasement and suppression (*nirodha*) of all actions motivated by desire, hatred, and delusion. The middle path starts amidst an 'ocean of suffering' and concludes in calm and tranquillity when its stormy waves become completely still. This state of calm and tranquillity which denotes freedom from suffering is expressed by the term *nirvāṇa*.

I. Doctrinal Considerations

Early Buddhism

The technical Sanskrit term for suffering is *duḥkha*. In its most general sense *duḥkha* denotes all kinds of mental and physical pain and misery in contrast to happiness termed in Sanskrit as *sukha*. Śākyamuni Buddha recognised that in the conventional sense the lives of living beings include various degrees of both happiness and suffering. He admitted that there is happiness experienced by people involved in worldly affairs and happiness of mendicants engaged in ascetic practices. There is happiness derived from attachment to the sense pleasures, and happiness arising from renunciation of all worldly pleasures. However, in the Buddha's perception both happiness and suffering experienced in this world fall under the heading of *duḥkha*. It is so because the whole of existence is pervaded by inherent imperfection and impermanence. The fragile and painful state of life was expressed by the Buddha in such words as: 'birth is suffering, old age is suffering, death is suffering; sorrow, lamentation, misery, grief and despair are suffering; association with those one does not cherish is suffering; separation from the loved objects is suffering.'[2] This encapsulates the Buddhist perception of suffering as suffering (*duḥkha-duḥkha*) which constitutes an existential reality consisting of all forms of physical and mental sensations.

A deeper notion of suffering is perceived in the constant change of things (*vipariṇāma-duḥkha*). The life of every being never remains constant but changes and rolls on in cycles of birth and death. All living beings remain in the clutches of Māra, the lord of death.

The third and most important notion of suffering is expressed by the Sanskrit term *saṃskāra* which is rendered as volitions, mental formations, or conditioned states.[3] In order to gain an insightful perception of what is meant by conditioned states, it is necessary to grasp the Buddhist interpretation of such terms as 'being' or 'individual'. Buddhism emphatically and relentlessly rejects the existence of a permanent entity defined by such terms as 'self' or 'soul' (*ātman*), or as 'person' (*pudgala*). Although Buddhism has encountered difficulties to explain the flow of existence without any permanent element, the doctrine of the non-existence of *ātman* does constitute the hallmark of Buddhist doctrines. It is a misconception,[4] according to Buddhism, to assume personality as a real entity. Buddhism admits that in terms of conventional truth (*saṃvṛti-satya*) there is personality but it rejects its existence in terms of ultimate truth (*paramārtha-satya*). All that exists represents a mere combination of ever-changing and mutually conditioned assemblage of material and mental conglomerates called the five aggregates or *skandhas*: matter (*rūpa*), sensation (*vedanā*), perception (*saṃjñā*), mental formations (*saṃskāra*), and consciousness (*vijñāna*).[5] The five *skandhas* represent a variety of configurations of physical and mental energies that are mutually conditioned and evolve in a stream of conscious life (*saṃtāna*). When pervaded by ignorance (*avidyā*) and defilements (*kleśa*), this stream of conscious life perceives itself as a living entity, and when it is purged from misconceptions it dissolves and ceases to function.

From the perspective of the various ways of rebirth, the entire spectrum of phenomenal existence is known as *saṃsāra* or the ever-revolving cycles of rebirths. The whole of *saṃsāra* contains infinite possibilities of being reborn but on the whole Buddhism recognises five or six pathways or destinies (*gati*) in which living beings endure the consequences of their actions.[6] Buddhism does not attribute the origin of *saṃsāra* to any agent or creator, but postulates that it evolves in cosmic cycles without a starting point in time (*anādikāla*). However, Buddhism does assert the arising of suffering. The primary source of suffering is perceived in craving (*tṛṣṇā*). It is the threefold craving for sense satisfaction (*kāma*), existence (*bhava*), and non-existence (*vibhava*), that constitutes the dominant condition for the arising and perpetuating of suffering. Craving as such is not the initial cause but constitutes the most powerful and all-pervasive factor, which in turn derives its driving force from sensations and defilements. There are no external causes of suffering but all causes and conditions of suffering are present within suffering itself. Suffering is existence which has no creator or any other externally controlling power.

Buddhism shares the basic doctrine of *karma* with Hinduism and Jainism but provides its own and quite different interpretation of *karma's* nature, function, and retribution. The nature of *karma* is explained within the context of mental formations (*saṃskāra*) which constitute the fourth *skandha*. The Buddha defined *karma* as volition (*cetanā*). 'Monks – he states in one of his discourses – *karma* is volition. Having willed, one commits an act with the body, speech, and mind.'[7] Volition constitutes a mental activity or tendency which influences the mind in the sphere of morally qualifiable actions. All intentional actions are good (*kuśala*) or bad (*akuśala*) and inevitably lead to their retribution or maturation (*karma-phala* or *karma-vipāka*). Thus the most important dimension of *karma* as volition lies in the mind pervaded by craving stimulated by desire, hatred, and delusion. The actual process in which craving is linked with *karma* and *karma* with rebirth is explained by the law of dependent origination.[8] It is the law that controls how all transient, painful, and impersonal phenomena understood as the five *skandhas* or *dharmas* arise and disappear in a constant series of events; the important stages in their flow being marked by death and birth.

The retribution of *karma* consists in the force that constantly regenerates phenomenal existence in the form of different categories of living beings experiencing specific pleasant and painful sensations. The living beings reborn in happy or unhappy destinies, their bodies and mental faculties, good and bad propensities, represent the actual retribution. Good actions alone never lead to deliverance but only to better or happy rebirths of limited duration. It is for this and other reasons given above that the whole of *saṃsāra* is described as an ocean of suffering.

Although the Buddha said that actions do not perish, and despite the fact that the force of *karma* runs its consistent and efficacious course, the process of *karmic* formations can be definitely eliminated and brought to a halt. The efficacy of *karma* is rendered ineffective by the suppression of all craving and motivated actions, and the emancipation from the cycles of rebirth. The detachment from all things, the suppression and appeasement of all *karmic* formations achieved through the practice of Dharma represent the state of *nirvāṇa*, which is the ultimate goal of all Buddhists. The state of freedom from all factors that lead to rebirth in this world and indeed freedom from phenomenal existence are expressed in such terms as *nirvāṇa*, arhatship, and Buddhahood. *Nirvāṇa* as arhatship fundamentally constitutes a complete purification from desire, hatred, and delusion, and an elimination of all future rebirths.

In contrast to phenomenal existence or *saṃsāra* which is conditioned (*saṃskṛta*), *nirvāṇa* represents an unconditioned state (*asaṃskṛta*) which is not subject to the laws governing phenomenal existence. *Nirvāṇa* has been described both in negative and positive ways. In negative terms it is, as stated above, the suppression of all desire and eradication of future rebirths. In positive terms it is described as tranquillity, peace and deathlessness. Since *nirvāṇa* is not subject to the law of causes and effects, it does not represent an effect of any effort or practice. It can be realised but not acquired. The final death or passing into *nirvāṇa* by the Buddha or arhats has been compared to an extinguished flame. The Buddha was questioned on several occasions about the state after his own death. He declined to give an answer on the grounds that it was one of the indeterminate or metaphysical questions (*avyākṛta*) that should not be posed or answered, mainly because it is not conducive to one's deliverance to know the answer.[9]

The practice that leads to the suppression of suffering has been set forth by the Buddha as the middle path which is described as the noble eightfold path. This path avoids the extremes of seeking happiness through indulgence in sense pleasures or through excessive self-mortification. The eightfold path includes three essential factors that constitute a trilogy of the Buddhist practice: ethical conduct (*śīla*), meditation (*samādhi*), and wisdom (*prajñā*). Morality purifies the body and leads to rebirths conducive to religious practices. Meditation purifies the mind and perfects inner dispositions, and wisdom that gradually unfolds induces the state of liberated awareness that penetrates the true nature of things. All three are considered as integral and essential to the Buddhist praxis, but it is wisdom that constitutes the dominant factor in the process of reaching the apex of the path. Although wisdom is expressed in terms of understanding and knowledge, its essential element constitutes a true perception of things combined with a kind of soteriological force that liberates from the bondage of existence permeated by ignorance.[10]

The Buddha's personal experience led him to teach that the best and most effective way to pursue the path to deliverance is to abandon the world and family life, and to become a recluse or mendicant. Soon after his enlightenment he established a monastic community known as Saṅgha and taught his monks (*bhikṣu*) how to practise the path in solitude and away from the worries and turmoils of worldly affairs. Everyone who entered monastic life was to pursue the path to deliverance. With regard to his lay followers (*upāsaka*) the Buddha taught that since it was very difficult to achieve *nirvāṇa* while living in the world, the lay followers should practise morality and accumulate merit (*puṇya*) with a view of gaining good rebirths in the immediate future, and eventually a rebirth enabling them to go forth from home to homeless life and pursue the practices leading to *nirvāṇa*.

The early Buddhist teachings, briefly summarised here, have been followed for centuries and still survive as the essential assumptions of Theravāda Buddhism practised in Sri Lanka, Burma, Thailand and other countries of Southeast Asia. Finally, before proceeding to the next section let us recapture the spirit of the early Buddhist teachings encapsulated in one stanza in Buddhaghosa's *Visuddhimagga*:

> There is suffering but no-one to feel it.
> There is action but no doer.
> There is *nirvāṇa* but no-one to experience it.
> There is a path but no-one to tread on it.[11]

Mahāyāna and Vajrayāna Buddhism

The Mahāyāna, which emerged some five hundred years after the Buddha's demise, accepted the Buddha's fundamental teaching on suffering, but it criticised as inferior the path leading to arhatship, and treated the doctrinal systematisations of the early schools, in particular those of the Sarvāstivāda, as largely misinterpretations of the Buddha's teachings. The Mahāyāna *sūtras* and the two major schools, Mādhyamika and Yogācāra, set forth new teachings in three major areas: Buddhology, doctrine, and religious ideal.

With regard to the Buddha, the Mahāyāna asserts that there are countless Buddhas who teach in equally countless worlds. While Gautama (or Śākyamuni) is the Buddha of this world system called Sāha Lokadhātu, there are other Buddhas who preside over and teach in other universes. All the Buddhas are considered as transcendent (*lokottara*) entities who become manifested in order to teach the Dharma for the benefit and happiness of living beings. Within the Mahāyāna context the Buddhas are supplicated not to pass into *nirvāṇa* but to remain in the world and teach.

Within the scope of their doctrines the Mahāyāna depts accepted the early teaching on the non-existence of a person (*nairātmya*) but they went further and drew logical conclusions that stem from it. Although the schools of early Buddhism rejected the existence of a permanent self (*ātman*), they did affirm the existence of the components of existence, which they systematised in their Abhidharma works into various categories of basic groupings such as *skandhas* and *dharmas*. The Mahāyāna undermined the Abhidharma structure by postulating that if there is no *ātma*, the elements (*dharmas*) of existence cannot be real and consequently do not exist either. The basic doctrines of Mahāyāna Buddhism became formulated mainly around a complex theory of universal emptiness (*śūnyatā*). All things were seen as illusory and devoid of self-existence and characteristics. In order to safeguard the value of religious life, the Mahāyāna adepts accepted that in terms of conventional truth there was suffering and that the law of dependent origination did function. However, viewed from the perspective of ultimate truth the things (*dharmas*) were unoriginated (*anutpāda*) and devoid (*śūnya*) of self-existence (*niḥsvabhāva*).

The religious goal of early Buddhism as portrayed by an *arhat* became replaced in the Mahāyāna by that of a Bodhisattva. The path to arhatship was degraded as limited in scope and understanding, and as focused on personal rather than universal deliverance. The attainment of *nirvāṇa* was retained as the ultimate but not immediate goal. The attainment of enlightenment (*bodhi*) and helping living beings became the immediate and central concern of Mahāyāna doctrine and practice. The Bodhisattva career became open to everyone and could be taken up by people of all walks of life. The Bodhisattva is characterised as the one who takes the vow to gain the supreme enlightenment and to work for the benefit and liberation of all living beings. He generates the thought of enlightenment (*bodhicitta*) and embraces compassion (*karuṇā*) as his motivation to help all living beings on the path to Buddhahood. The career of the Bodhisattva is outlined as the practice of the six or ten perfections (*pāramitā*) and the ten Bodhisattva stages (*bhūmi*). It is an arduous path which is said to last for some three incalculable aeons (*asaṃkhyeya*). On reaching the advanced stages of his career, the Bodhisattva becomes free from rebirth and the laws that control *saṃsāra*. He acquires wonder-making powers (*ṛddhi*) and the attributes similar to those of a Buddha. Abiding in wisdom and compassion, the two principal factors of his praxis, the Bodhisattva does not abandon *saṃsāra* and does not enter *nirvāṇa*. He abides in both but in two different ways. Having accomplished the perfections, in particular the perfection of wisdom, he partakes in the qualities of *nirvāṇa* but without actually passing into *nirvāṇa*. On the other hand he does not leave *saṃsāra* because of his compassion which commits him to pursue the benefit of living beings. Such a Bodhisattva being free from the law of *karma* is able to assume various manifested forms and employed appropriate skilful means and devices (*upāyakauśalya*) to aid and guide living beings.

The Mahāyāna texts abound in beautiful and moving descriptions of the salvific activities pursued by Bodhisattvas. As the activities of Bodhisattvas who have just begun their career are rather limited in scope and still subject to the law of *karma*, the texts predominantly depict highly advanced and idealised Bodhisattvas. A great number of such perfected Bodhisattvas is mentioned in Mahāyāna texts, and some of them such as Avalokiteśvara, Mañjuśrī or Kṣitigarbha, became objects of devotion and supplications for help.[12] The Bodhisattva ideal as portrayed in Mahāyāna texts is one of the most inspiring and perfected images of religious aspirations.

The two principal schools of Indian Mahāyāna Buddhism, the Mādhyamika and the Yogācāra (also called Vijñānavāda) explain the Bodhisattva career within the contexts of their respective doctrinal systems. While in the Mādhyamika school, headed by Nāgārjuna, the Bodhisattva practices centre on the realisation of the various categories of emptiness (*śūnyatā*), the Yogacāra doctrine and practice focus on the purification of the defiled mind (*citta*).

Although the Bodhisattva ideal stands at the centre of the Mahāyāna as a whole, certain Mahāyāna texts and schools also offer alternative and rather easier ways to deliverance. A number of Mahāyāna *sūtras* teach that the Buddha-nature (*tathāgatagarbha*) is inherently present in all sentient beings. Just as the honey in the comb or gold in ore, the transcendent and perfect Buddha embryo abides in all living beings who experience suffering only because they do not understand the true nature of things. The positive and appealing dimensions of this doctrine are apparent. Various degrees of this doctrine are found in all schools of Mahāyāna Buddhism, but they enjoy greater popularity in East Asia, in particular in China where they constitute the doctrinal focus of the Hua-yen, T'ien-t'ai, and Ch'an schools. The inherent and ever-present enlightenment within humanity as the Buddha-nature appealed to the Chinese mind which assumed the basic goodness and harmony of human nature, and which reacted rather negatively to the

Buddhist teachings on *karma*, the non-existence of the self, and the abandonment of one's family.

Some other Mahāyāna *sūtra* inspired devotional practices as the primary and almost exclusive means to attain deliverance. The *Sukhāvatī-vyūha* and related *sūtras* constitute the scriptural foundation for the Pure Land schools in China and Japan. The doctrine and practice of those schools centre on the Buddha Amitābha who in some remote past as the Bodhisattva Dharmākara took a series of forty-eight vows (*praṇidhāna*) and declared that he would not become a Buddha unless all his vows were fulfilled. He basically vowed to create a Buddha universe (*lokadhātu*) of unparalleled beauty and free from suffering. This universe (*lokadhātu*) called Sukhāvatī is described as a perfect realm free from the three evil destinies and any kind of suffering known in this world. He made it available practically to all beings on the condition that they profess faith in his salvific power, mainly by invoking his name. Except for people who committed the five heinous sins,[13] all beings who meditate on and invoke the name of Amitābha are assured of happiness awaiting them in the Sukhāvatī. There are other *sūtras* that offer similar ways of deliverance but the practices focused on the *Sukhāvatī-vyūha* are the most popular.

The Buddhist *tantras*, which emerged about a thousand years after the Buddha's death, represent the third and latest phase of Indian Buddhism. In addition to the Mahāyāna doctrines and practices which were accepted as the foundation, the *tantras* developed a large repository of meditational and *yogic* exercises, and made extensive use of ritual, devotion, magic, and other devices. The tantric path presented itself as the quickest and most efficient approach to gain Buddhahood. The *tantras* assert that the long and arduous path as portrayed by the Bodhisattva career lasting for three aeons can be shortened, and in some cases achieved within one single life. Tantric practices and rituals are incorporated into all schools of Tibetan Buddhism, and in Japan they are followed by the Shingon school.

Viewed as a whole, Buddhism offers a variety of doctrines and practices which can comfortably accommodate all kinds of religious needs and aspirations. This wide range of options has been often attributed to the Buddha's ability as the supreme teacher to device practices attuned to the intellectual and physical capabilities of all living beings. Having sketched the various methods of eliminating suffering as propounded in different schools, we shall now turn to specific questions pertinent to further understanding of suffering.

II. Existential considerations

Karma and retribution

The apparently inevitable and fatalistic implications inherent in the operation of *karma* do evoke questions about personal freedom and the validity to counteract the course of *karmic* force. There were in fact religious sects at the time of the Buddha which maintained fatalistic doctrines, and one finds a limited amount of deterministic tendencies in Buddhist texts, but in principle Buddhism firmly opposes fatalism.

As part of general Buddhist teachings, in particular those intended for the laity, the workings of *karma* have been extensively covered in many texts. In all periods of Buddhism, and in particular in early Buddhism, there are many texts which describe sufferings endured on earth or in various hells due to evil actions committed in previous lives. Even in the case of the Buddha and his disciples we find descriptions of various actions and their inevitable and painful consequences. One finds passages which speak of foolish beings reborn in evil destinies as having very small or no chances of doing good and consequently doomed for 'damnation'. Some texts depict evil actions and indicate specific types of suffering that are sustained for committing them. The five heinous sins, for instance, are said to require an immediate rebirth in the Avīci hell, which is the most painful of all Buddhist hells. There are also accounts which contain vivid and somewhat gruesome depictions of never-ending torments in various hells. The overall impression that one gains from such texts does insinuate a feeling of inevitability and helplessness. However, the primary purpose of such texts is to deter and discourage people from doing evil.

On the theoretical level the teachings relating to *karma* are an essential part of Buddhist doctrines. It is the doctrine of *karma* that provides the ultimate explanation of existence and the entire world, and it is in relation to *karma* that the Buddhist doctrinal edifice is constructed. The interpretation of *karma* has preoccupied Buddhist thinkers in all periods of Buddhist history. Viewed as a whole Buddhism does not have one coherent and universally accepted exposition of *karma*. There are serious disagreements between Buddhist schools in their interpretations. In fact all Indian religions accepting the doctrine of *karma* have problems in explaining it, and in Buddhism the non-existence of the agent of *karma*, which itself is problematic, adds further difficulties. However, our major concern here is to show that while affirming the doctrine of *karma*, Buddhism tries to guard itself against the fatalistic implications that can be imputed to *karma*. From the Buddhist position the force of *karma* does have an overwhelming control over the events in this world, but it is not admitted that this force functions in a merely mechanical manner and cannot be overcome.[14] Buddhism places an emphasis on ethical effort (*kriyāvāda*), and diligence (*vīryavāda*) as important factors to improve one's conditions in this world, and as part of practising the Dharma that definitely leads to freedom from *saṃsāra*. The texts consistently affirm that one is responsible for one's actions and must strive with diligence for deliverance.[15] It is affirmed that one has no control over the effects of the already committed actions, but also stressed that one does have control over the choice of actions in this life. There are certainly serious limitations and disadvantages in the case of mentally deranged people to accomplish good actions. Buddhism recognises this and other similar types of suffering as tremendous obstacles to spiritual progress, but it alleviates such hopeless situations by asserting that whenever such people have in store some good actions, they have the chance of gaining better rebirths.

In Buddhism *karma* and its own effect are not the same. While deliberate actions as causes have moral implications, the resulting effects or retribution are morally indifferent (*avyākṛta*) and do not lead to further retribution. Thus the bodily and mental conditions acquired at birth are without any moral stigma or imprint attached to them, and consequently there should be no discrimination against people who are born with bodily or mental defects. In addition to distinguishing between causes and effects, past and new deeds (*karma*), Buddhism also holds that the maturation and retribution of actions are not always achieved immediately: some actions are retributed in this life, some after death in the next life, and some in future rebirths. The actions committed during the present life and those that have not been retributed will eventually generate new existences. While recognising that one's actions are conditioned by the inborn mental and emotional dispositions, Buddhism at the same time affirms that one does have a choice to decide upon the course of one's actions.

As already stated above the workings of *karma* are perceived as the most prevailing cause of suffering. However, canonical and medical texts also recognise other causes of suffering. Counting *karma* as one, there are eight such causes which include pains that arise from the three bodily humours, changes of the seasons, adverse circumstances, and external intervention.[16] Buddhism also admits timely and untimely death. Just as the raw and the ripe fruits fall from trees, so do people die timely and untimely death. The *Milindapañha*, for instance, describes eight kinds of untimely death accidentally caused by such factors as famine, poison, fire, or inflicted wounds.[17] Similarly within the medical sphere, the various diseases are not attributed exclusively to *karma* but also to other causes. Viewed as a whole, the Buddhist teachings on *karma* do attempt to give a balanced and sustainable interpretation. It must be stressed that Buddhism reduces the operation of *karma* to this world alone and curtails its power by teaching that it can be completely eradicated by following the Buddhist path.

Although on the doctrinal level the position on *karma* is sustained with tenacity, in real life there exist certain practices in Buddhism which do not readily conform to the Buddhist teachings on *karma*. There are passages in the Pāli canon which say that one's *karma* is one's own, that one should strive for one's own deliverance,[18] and that one's meritorious actions are a treasure that is not shared with other people. We also find statements that prayers cannot advance or alter the *karmic* course of the departed people,[19] and a number of passages that firmly reject rituals. It is well established, however, that already in early Buddhism, and later in all forms of Buddhism there developed a practice of transferring merit and a great variety of rituals. In both Theravāda and Mahāyāna Buddhism monks perform funeral rituals and transfer merit to the dead, canonical texts are chanted, and various rituals performed for protection, blessing, and many other mundane and religious purposes. One also finds exorcism, fierce rites, and amulets. In the early layers of the Pāli Canon the Buddha rejected rituals as ineffective and illicit ways of earning livelihood. However, one also finds justifications for such activities in later Pāli texts in which the Buddha allows such practices, and in Mahāyāna and Vajrayāna traditions such practices are widely accepted as valid. Throughout the entire history of Buddhism one finds contrasting tendencies either to reject or to justify the use of prayers, rituals, magic, and exorcism.

The Buddha's personal afflictions

It is well attested in the canonical and later texts that the Buddha suffered from disturbances of the humours,[20] headaches, back pains, and dysentery.[21] He was also slandered by his adversaries and wounded by his cousin Devadatta. Since he was enlightened and liberated, the Buddha's pains evoked discussions in the canonical and later texts, and the explanations that are given in different texts disagree. Some passages in the Pāli canon conform to the Buddhist doctrine on *karma* and say that the Buddha indeed suffered in his last life due to certain adverse actions committed in his previous lives. Some texts suggest that he was only subject to pain resulting from the physical conditions,[22] and again other texts state that whatever happened to the Buddha he experienced only pleasant sensations.[23] The Abhidharma works do not offer one agreed interpretation. The Sarvāstivāda Abhidharma postulates that the Buddha's body born (*janmakāya*) from his mother was a retributed body (*vipāka-kāya*) and subject to impurities, passions, and pain. It also speaks of two other bodies: one which the Buddha could assume at will to visit different places (*nirmāṇa-kāya*), and one called *dharma-kāya* which consisted of pure *dharmas*. The Mahāsāṇghikas assumed that the Buddha was born in the world but remained completely unstained and unaffected by the world and worldly affairs, including suffering.[24] The Mahāyāna texts make a distinction between the absolute or truth body (*dharma-kāya*) and the fictitious or manifested body (*nirmāṇa-kāya*) which the Buddhas assume during their manifestations in different worlds.[25] There are many Mahāyāna texts which say that the Tathāgata's body is indestructible, infinite, pure, formless, and free of sensations. Putting aside the various disagreements and doctrinal disputes about the Buddha's body and suffering, all schools of Buddhism hold that the Buddha's body was endowed with the thirty-two bodily marks of a great man (*mahāpuruṣa*) and eighty minor bodily marks.[26] It is appropriate to mention that the Buddha's cremated remains are venerated as sacred in all Buddhist countries of Asia. The opinions put forward about the nature of the Buddha's body and whether it suffered or not clearly indicate that Buddhism does not have an agreed position on these issues.

Medicine and healing

In medical terminology happiness and suffering stand for health and disease. In one of his discourses the Buddha said that 'health (*ārogya*) is the highest gain (*lābha*), *nirvāṇa* the highest bliss; and of (different) ways (*mārga*), the eightfold (path) leads to peace (*kṣema*) and deathlessness (*amṛta*).'[27] While teaching the Dharma to heal the chronically ill living beings, the Buddha often gave examples from everyday experience. He demonstrated the efficacy of the Dharma by comparing it to medical treatment. A purge administered by a physician to check sickness is merely a purge but not a lasting cure. The Dharma is the true purge that releases beings from decay, old age and other sufferings.[28] When asked certain metaphysical questions, he indicated their utter irrelevance and danger by giving an example of a man struck by a poisonous arrow. One should not waste time on investigating who shot the arrow but offer an immediate help.[29] The Buddha himself has been referred to as a king among physicians (*vaityarāja*), and a supreme physician of sick living beings. Worldly physicians who do not know the supreme medicine are limited to curing ordinary diseases.[30] In Buddhaghosa's *Visuddhimagga*[31] the Buddha is referred to as the supreme physician, the Dharma as the medicine, and living beings as the patients. In Mahāyāna texts in addition to portraying the Buddha as a physician, we also have Bhaiṣajyaguru, the Buddha of Healing, and Amitāyus, the Buddha of Boundless Life.

Let us now consider some practical applications that Buddhism offers to remove suffering in addition to the practice of Dharma. There is evidence in Buddhist texts that the Buddha attached importance to maintain a healthy and well-functioning body. When the body is affected by diseases or temporary disorders, one has difficulties to meditate. There are sections in the Vinaya which deal specifically with medicine. The monks were to rely on the four resources: begging for food, robes of rags, lodging at the foot of trees, and medicine. Initially the Buddha permitted five kinds of medicine which included butter, oil, and honey. The monks were allowed to take them at any time in spite of the rule that solid food could be taken only between sunrise and midday. However, as various types of illness affected monks, further rules and regulations were laid down allowing herbal and other types of medicine. The Buddha instructed his monks that since they had no parents they should take care of one another at times of illnesses. In addition to the practice of medicine within the monastic compounds, we also learn of lay physicians who were skilled in medical knowledge, including the famous Jīvaka[32], who acted as physician to the king Bimbisāra, and the Saṅgha with the Buddha as its head. Ever since the Buddha's time the study and practice of medicine continued in Buddhist monasteries in India and later spread with Buddhism to other countries of Asia. In India itself Buddhism influenced and contributed to the Āyurvedic medicine.[33]

The causes of diseases discussed in Buddhist texts can be divided into two major categories: 1. diseases caused by previous *karma*, and 2. diseases arising from the factors in this life. The diseases caused or induced in the present existence are attributed mainly to demons, environment, intake of poisonous substances, and inappropriate habits and behaviour. The texts also speak of four hundred and four kinds of diseases which become manifested through the disorders of the primary elements and the three humours.[34] There is no assured way to establish with certainty which diseases are due to *karma* and which result from the factors in the present existence. The untimely kinds of death and seemingly accidentally acquired diseases and bodily harm can be also the fruit of *karma*. It is, however, maintained that no medicine of any kind can extend the lifespan or cure diseases acquired as part of *karma's* retribution. The diseases due to other causes can be checked and efforts should be made to cure them. The proper medical examination of the various bodily symptoms is frequently accompanied by the use of astrology and divination in order to determine the sources of diseases. The use of astrology and divination is attested in Buddhism from the very early period, and it still persists in all Buddhist countries of Asia. In addition to a wide range of proper medical remedies, Buddhism also offers a great variety of religious devices to prevent and heal diseases. Within this category we find meditation, moral conduct, recitations of Buddhist texts, rituals, exorcism, and amulets. It is well attested that for centuries all forms of Buddhism have offered such devices. In Theravāda countries monks perform a limited range of rituals which mainly consists of chanting a particular type of Buddhist texts known as *parittas*. Such texts are chanted to benefit the dead, to bring various blessings, for protection and healing. The various kinds of exorcism employed for healing are normally performed by lay specialists who are not monks.[35] In Mahāyāna and Vajrāyana countries where the use of rituals is doctrinally accepted, one finds an exceptionally wide range of rituals. Their use is not limited to healing and averting dangers, but also to gain mundane and transcendent benefits.

The human body and its value

From the doctrinal position the human body is rejected but at the same time it is highly appreciated as the best vehicle for attaining Buddhahood. It is maintained in all forms of Buddhism that in order to gain enlightenment and become a Buddha, one must posses a perfect body. In order to help one to develop aversion for sensual desires and detachment for the body, the texts suggest meditational sessions focusing on the impurities of the body[36] and decomposing corpses.[37] The body has been often described as full of suffering and diseases, as a ball of foam, a bubble of water, as arisen from defilements like a mirage, a magical illusion sprung from misconceptions, and a replica of previous actions. However, viewing it in a positive way, the majority of relevant texts explain in detail the functions of the body and mind, and provide guidance how one can counteract all bodily, emotional, and mental impediments which prevent one from gaining the final goal. In early Buddhism the human body was appreciated mainly as a vehicle of deliverance although the Buddha's body was considered as perfect in all respects. In Mahāyāna and Vajrayāna Buddhism, where aims were higher than just becoming an arhat, the state of spiritual perfection and enlightenment has been coupled with the acquisition of a perfect Buddha body. The Bodhisattva invests much of his effort to acquire such a body, and it is only in the final stages of the path that the Bodhisattva acquires such a perfect body. In the Vajrayāna where the long period of gaining Buddhahood and acquiring a Buddha body have been decreased, some new methods have been introduced to develop a Buddha body. The *tantric* yogins, although their minds and bodies are healthy, do not normally posses perfected Buddha bodies. In order to acquire such bodies, the *tantras* invented meditational exercises during which one gradually activates a subtle body which enables one to transcend the ordinary body and acquire a perfect Buddha body. The *tantras* also speak of the five *skandhas* as the five cosmic Buddhas. In addition to appreciation of the human body as a vehicle of deliverance, we find that in all Buddhist countries the remains of holy persons are venerated and considered as sources of spiritual powers. In Mahāyāna and Vajrayāna traditions, the remains of spiritual masters are often enshrined in temples or *stūpas*. An appreciation of the perfect body is also apparent in Buddhist iconography, where one finds idealised and beautifully proportioned images of Buddhas,

Bodhisattvas, female and male deities, and many lineages of spiritual masters.

Saṅgha and Society

The relationship between the early Saṅgha and the society was based on several principles which regulated their respective positions. The Buddha drew a firmly dividing line between mendicant and secular lives. He asserted that celibate and mendicant life was the most appropriate and effective course of action to execute the practice of the Dharma, and that the family and social life had serious obstacles and disadvantages to achieve *nirvāṇa*. He had no interest in worldly affairs, and like all mendicants of that time, the Buddha and his monks lived outside the mainstream of the Indian society. Initially all Buddhist monks lived homeless life and secured their food by begging, and their personal conduct and the internal life of the Saṅgha were regulated by the Vinaya or the code of monastic discipline. The Buddha and the Saṅgha have always considered themselves as being exempt from social obligations, and as not being subject to the control of secular rulers. With the rapid growth of the Saṅgha and the large numbers of people becoming lay followers, the Saṅgha and the laity were inevitably brought into closer contacts. The generosity on the part of the laity and several other pragmatic factors affected the mendicant life of the Saṅgha to the extent that already during the Buddha's life the Saṅgha became settled in permanently built monasteries. The spirit of mendicancy was retained but further rules had to be introduced to regulate the internal life of monasteries and their relationship with the lay communities. The basic division between monastic and secular lives remained unaffected but the interaction between the Saṅgha and the laity increased.

The Buddha made no class distinctions in admitting people to monastic life. However, not all people who joined the Saṅgha entered it with noble intentions. Branded criminals, absconded soldiers, non-believers, and slaves who entered monastic life caused the Saṅgha to take appropriate steps in order to safeguard its reputation and to prevent internal problems. Eventually some thirty-two sanctions were introduced to exclude unsuitable people from joining the Saṅgha. People who killed one of their parents, people with certain diseases[38] and mutilated bodies, eunuch, hermaphrodites, thieves and serious debtors were excluded from entering monastic life. It was of great importance for the Saṅgha to maintain a good reputation, and to assure that monks properly observed the Vinaya rules. The individual monks were forbidden by the Vinaya rules to accept gold and silver, and prohibited to earn their livelihood by means of any secular profession, including the practice of medicine. However, the Saṅgha as a whole could receive donations of any kind, including money and land. It needs no explanation that all material support could only generously flow into monasteries when monks behaved properly and complied with the spirit of their vocation, and expectations of their lay patrons. Although the material support came from the laity, the monks had no imposed obligations to reciprocate but as part of the Buddha's concern for the welfare of humanity, the monks were instructed to teach the Dharma and assist people's spiritual needs. Whenever asked they were to visit the sick and perform appropriate ceremonies. The lay followers were taught to practise morality and generosity, and to accumulate merit. The material support given to monks and monasteries was automatically rewarded in the form of spiritual merit. Thus the immediate spiritual concerns of the laity focused on living moral life and on gaining better rebirths through their merits. The Buddha never discouraged his lay followers to give alms to non-Buddhist mendicants but he did grade the meritorious value of donations on the grounds of the recipient's state of sanctity.[39]

Within the Mahāyāna context the Bodhisattva ideal which could be practised by monks and lay people provided a powerful impetus for an even closer interaction between the monastic and lay communities. The Vinaya followed by Mahāyāna monks is the same as the one for the monks in Theravāda Buddhism. However, the Mahāyāna altruistic doctrines enable the Mahāyāna monks to forge even closer links with the lay communities. The historical records available to us show that Buddhist monks acted as spiritual advisers to kings and emperors, and provided inspiration for many activities benefiting people in need of spiritual and mundane help. There is evidence that already during Aśoka's reign in India in the third century BC, and thereafter in all Buddhist countries appropriate actions were taken to help suffering people in various ways, including administering medicine and building hospitals. However, on the whole the Dharma dispensation always remained the main preoccupation of Buddhist monks. This was done by teaching the Buddhist principles and performing rituals to protect the state and people, to enhance spiritual dispositions, and to heal and alleviate all kinds of spiritual and worldly anxieties. In modern times both the Saṅgha and the laity try to keep up with the practice, but they face the same problems as other religions of the present age.

Conclusions

The Buddha told his disciples that what he taught them was like a handful of leaves picked up in the autumn but it was adequate to guide people to gain deliverance. He also compared the Dharma to a raft that carries one across to deliverance, but once the ocean of *saṃsāra* has been traversed, the Dharma serves no purpose. He further said that certain things including *karma*'s retribution were inconceivable.[40] The purpose of these and other similar statements was to indicate that the ultimate truth remains beyond ordinary human understanding. The true reality of things is accessible to mystic experience but it is difficult to express it in conventional language. The Buddha and his enlightened followers strove tirelessly to explain the Buddhist truths in words but at the same time maintaining that it is religious experience that brings the true wisdom and freedom from suffering, but never mere philosophical speculations or material wealth.

Finally, I shall quote some verses from a Mahāyāna text called *Vinayaviniścaya-Upālipariprṛcchā* to illustrate the basic spirit of Buddhism in terms of its complete detachment from the world, and also to indicate how much can be done to improve the world's suffering.

> Forever happy in this world are the men
> Who know the *dharmas* as inconceivable.
> There is no distinction into *dharmas* and *adharmas*.
> They all are invented through the mind's differentiation.[41]
>
> Since everything is inconceivable and unarisen,
> Invented is the knowledge of existence and non-existence.
> The simpletons subject to the power of the mind
> Endure suffering for many millions of lives.
>
> Though I have praised before the world the value of generosity,
> Yet the *dharma* 'avarice' cannot be conceived of.
> Likewise the *dharmas* of the Victorious remain inconceivable.
> They too cannot be apprehended or observed.

Though I've explained the practice of morality as pure,
Yet immorality is like a hand in (empty) space.
All wrong morality is like (empty) space.
That which is good morality, that too is the same.

I have taught and encouraged a holy alertness
In order to practise vigilance day and night.
And yet should one generate energy for hundreds of aeons,
It will remain neither augmented nor diminished.

Meditation, deliverance and concentration were taught
To the world as the appropriate portals of excellence.
Though here there are no *dharmas* whatever to suppress
One still teaches to analyse them into categories.

I have taught wisdom as the kernel of mystic insight,
Saying: 'Do learn the *dharmas* of wisdom.'
But again since existence is without self-nature,
Surely one must also teach that it cannot be known.

Though I have taught ascetic life to the wicked world,
Saying: 'Find contentment in solitude, delight in ascetic practices',
Yet the *dharmas* which do not bring contentment
Are mere suppositions in this world.

Though I have taught the terrors of hells
Which have terrified countless thousands of beings,
Yet the beings who die and fall into dreadful destinies
Do not exist in this world whatsoever.

The world invents through the power of imagination.
The simpleton differentiates through his adherence to perception.
Yet both the one who grasps and the one who does not, do not exist.
Indeed mental constructions are like illusions and mirages.

Though I have taught the most excellent and noble career,
Saying: 'Raise the thought of enlightenment for the good of beings',
Yet enlightenment does not exist as the object of thought.
The one who strives for it, he too does not exist.

The mind is radiant and stainless by its very nature.
It is spotless, without blemish, immaculate – This I have said.
Yet the simpleton who imagines the non-existing existent,
Becomes imbued with passion, hatred and delusion.

The one who applies his thought to the empty *dharmas*
Is indeed a simpleton following the wrong path.
The empty *dharmas* are proclaimed through verbal sounds,
And again they are explained through words as wordless.

NOTES

1. The Buddha's first sermon (called in Sanskrit *Dharmacakrapravartana*) encapsulates the basic Buddhist principles of the middle path (*madhyamapratipad*) under four headings known as the Four Noble Truths (*āryasatya*): the truth of suffering (*duḥkha-satya*), the arising of suffering (*duḥkhasamudaya*), the destruction of suffering (*duḥkha-nirodha*), and the path that leads to the suppression of suffering (*duḥkha-nirodha-gaminī-pratipad*).
2. Saṃyutta-nikāya, V, 420. An excellent exposition of suffering in early Buddhism is given in Buddhaghosa's *Visuddhimagga*, 591ff.
3. The difficult term *saṃskāra* basically denotes the activity of evolving mental formations or the state of their being already evolved and formed. In its active sense, it is identical with *karma* formations as a collection of good and bad volitional activities (*cetanā*) committed with the body, speech, and mind. In its accomplished state, it stands for all formed phenomena of existence. It is, however, more restrictive in scope than the term *dharma* which includes both formed or conditioned (*saṃskṛta*) and unconditioned (*asaṃskṛta*) phenomena. Within the classification into *dharmas*, the Theravāda school lists fifty-two mental activities, and the Sarvāstivāda school fifty-eight.
4. There are four such misconceptions (*viparyāsa*). 1. taking for eternal what is transient, 2. for pleasant what is painful, 3. for pure what is impure, 4. for *ātman* what is not *ātman* (namely the five *skandhas*). Aṅguttara-nikāya, II, 62.
5. In addition to the five *skandhas*, the phenomena of existence have been also classified into twelve bases (*āyatana*: the sense faculties and their objects), the eighteen elements (*dhātu*: the previous category is expanded by adding further six kinds of sense consciousness), and seventy-two (Sarvāstivāda school) or eighty-one (Theravāda school) *dharmas*.
6. Rebirths among human beings or among the various classes of gods are classed as happy destinies (*sugati*), and rebirths among animals, tormented spirits (*preta*) or in one of the hells are considered as evil destinies (*durgati*).The *asuras, niraya* and *pretas* are considered unhappy realms in the Theravāda but in the Sanskrit texts the *asuras* are treated as the lowest of the *sugati*.
7. Aṅguttara-nikāya, III, 415. For expositions and academic discussions of the Buddhist doctrine of *karma* see the bibliography under the following names: E. Lamotte, J.P. McDermott, B. Matthews, K. Fujita.
8. The law of dependent origination (*pratītyasamutpāda*) consists of twelve interactive links (*nidāna*): 1 . ignorance (*avidyā*), 2. karmic formations (*saṃskāra*), 3. consciousness (*vijñāna*), 4. name and form (*nāmarūpa*), 5. six bases (*ṣaḍāyatana*), 6. contact (*sparśa*), 7. feeling (*vedanā*), 8. craving (*tṛṣṇā*), 9. grasping (*upādāna*), 10. becoming (*bhava*), 11. birth (*jāti*), 12. old age and death (*jāramaraṇa*).
9. The questions which the Buddha refused to answer are: 1. Whether the world is eternal, or not, or both, or neither; 2. whether the world is

finite (in space), or infinite, or both, or neither; 3. whether the Tathāgata exists after death, or does not, or both, or neither; 4. whether the soul is identical with the body or different from it. Majjhima-nikāya, I, 426–32.

10. The practice and acquisition of wisdom is usually sketched in three progressive stages: wisdom acquired through hearing the Dharma (*śrutamayī-prajñā*), wisdom developed through reflection (*cintamayī-prajñā*), and wisdom matured through meditation (*bhavanāmayī-prajñā*). See T. Skorupski, 1987.
11. *Visuddhimagga*, 609.
12. The Bodhisattva Avalokiteśvara, who epitomises the Mahāyāna notion of compassion, is particularly popular in Māhayāna countries. Kṣitigarbha is seen in China as the one who helps the departed through the stages of the after-life judgement presided over by Yama, and in Japan as protector of aborted children.
13. Killing father, mother, or arhat, causing schism in the Sàngha, and acting with malice towards the bodies of the Victorious Ones (Buddhas).
14. According to *Milindapañha*, 268–9, two things in this world are not born from *karma* or any other cause, namely space (*ākāsa*), and *nirvāna*.
15. Saṃyutta-nikāya, III, 42.
16. Saṃyutta-nikāya, IV, 230; Aṅguttara-nikāya, II, 87; *Milindapañha*, 135–36: 1. bile (*pitta*), 2. phlegm (*śleṣman*), 3. wind (*vāyu*), 4. the union of the humours (*sannipāta*), 5. changes of the seasons (*ṛtu*), 6. stress from adverse circumstances (*viṣamaparihāra*), 7. external intervention (*upakrama*), 8. *karma* maturation (*karma-vipāka*).
17. *Milindapañha*, 302, first speaks of eight kinds of timely death (*kālakiriyā*). 1. (bodily) wind, 2. bile, 3. phlegm, 4. union of the humours, 5. change of seasons, 6. stress of circumstances, 7. accidents, 8. *karma*. Then having explained each item, the text repeats (page 304) the same list as causes of untimely death but with the following modifications and additions: 1. adventitious diseases, 2. (bodily) wind, 3. bile, 4. phlegm, 5. the union of the humours, 6. change of seasons, 7. stress of circumstances, 8. suddenly, 9. hunger, 10. thirst, 11. snake-bites, 12. poison, 13. fire, 14. water, 15. wounds. Just prior to these two lists the same text gives the following list of seven kinds of people who die untimely death although a portion of their life span remains to run. They are people who die from: 1. famine, 2. thirst, 3. snake-bites, 4. poison, 5. fire, 6. drowning, 7. injury. P. Demiéville, 1930, 256, gives a list of nine causes of premature death: 1. untimely food (eating when satiated); 2. immoderation in food; 3. unaccustomed food; 4. indigestion; 5. stoppage of inner heat (malfunction in passing urine and excrement); 6. violation of precepts (murder can lead to one's execution); 7. evil frequentations; 8. going to places at wrong times; 9. not avoiding what can be avoided.
18. Saṃyutta-nikāya, III, 42.
19. Saṃyutta-nikāya, IV, 311ff.
20. Vinaya, I, 278–80; Saṃyutta-nikāya, I, 174.
21. Digha-nikāya, II, 127.
22. Saṃyutta-nikāya, IV, 230–31; *Milindapañha*, 137–8.

23. Majjhima-nikāya, II, 227.
24. Meaning the so-called eight worldly *dharmas*: 1. gain (*lābha*), 2. loss (*alābha*), 3. glory (*yaśas*), 4. ignominy (*ayaśas*), 5. blame (*nindā*), 6. praise (*praśaṃsā*), 7. happiness (*sukha*), 8. suffering (*duḥkha*).
25. The Mahāyāna adepts, and in particular the Yagācāca school distinguish three Buddha Bodies (*trikāya*): absolute body (*dharmakāya*), rapture or celestial body (*sambhogakāya*), and manifested body (*nirmāṇakāya*).
26. The lists of the thirty-two bodily marks of a *mahāpuruṣa* given in various sources do not follow the same order and have significant variants. The list given here follows the order, but not always the exact wording, of the *Mahāvyutpatti* (236–67): 1. protuberance on the top of the head; 2. the hair on the head curled towards the right; 3. a prominent forehead; 4. a hairy mole between the eye-brows; 5. deep blue eyes and eyelashes like a cow's; 6. forty teeth; 7. even teeth; 8. well-spaced teeth; 9. bright white teeth; 10. a perfect sense of taste; 11. jaws like a lion's; 12. a long and slender tongue; 13. a voice like Brahmā's; 14. an evenly rounded bust; 15. seven prominences [hands, feet, shoulders, back of the neck]; 16. no indentation between the shoulders; 17. delicate and gold-like complexion; 18. hands reaching the knees while standing and without bending; 19. the front part of the body is like a lion's; 20. (bodily) symmetry of the *nyagrodha* tree; 21. one clockwise curling hair to each pore; 22. body-hairs growing upwards; 23. male organs concealed in a sheath; 24. well-rounded thighs; 25. concealed ankles; 26. soft and tender palms and soles; 27. webbed hands and feet; 28. long fingers and toes; 29. palms and soles marked with wheels; 30. well-positioned feet; 31. projecting heels; 32. legs like an antelope's. The list of the eighty minor marks is also given in the *Mahāvyutpatti*, 269–348.
27. Majjhima-nikāya, I, 508.
28. Aṅguttara-nikāya, 219.
29. Majjhima-nikāya, I, 430.
30. P. Demiéville, 1930, 225.
31. *Visuddhimagga*, 721.
32. For an account of his life see the Pali Vinaya, I, 268ff. See also E. Chavannes and K.G. Zysk in the bibliography.
33. In India there eventually emerged three major systems of medicine: Āyurveda followed by the Hindus, Yunānī among Muslims, and Siddha among Tamils. The Āyurvedic medicine is based on Sanskrit texts written during the past two millennia. It should be distinguished from medical practices pursued by exorcists, astrologers and types of healers related to magico-religious treatments of diseases. The Āyurveda basically understands the origin of diseases (*vyādhi*) as the imbalance of the three physiological principles or humours (*tridoṣa*). The Āyurveda is associated with the Atharva Veda. In the four Vedas medical matters are dealt with peripherally as part of their world view. They offer charms, prayers and various propitiatory rites to cure diseases which are often attributed to demons. The origin of the medical teachings is attributed to certain

deities (Indra) and sages (Ātreya). On the whole there are three great masters of the classical Āyurveda: Suśruta, Caraka and Vāghbaṭa. The texts attributed to Suśruta and Caraka are assumed to have been written during the first three centuries AD. Vāghbaṭa who lived in the 7th century AD is believed by some scholars to have been a Buddhist. There may be some truth in it as Vāghbaṭa's *Aṣṭāṅgahṛdayasaṃhīta* is the only representative work of Indian medicine included in the Tibetan Tanjur. On the involvement of Buddhism in the Āyurveda see A.L. Basham, 'The Practice of Medicine in Ancient and Medieval India', in C. Leslie, ed., *Asian Medical Systems*, Berkeley, 1976, 24.

34. According to certain sources there are four basic categories of diseases: 1. *karmic* diseases: one hundred and one disorders caused by *karma*. The diseases belonging to this category cannot be cured by ordinary medicine because the causes are spiritual and consequently their elimination must be achieved through spiritual divices. 2. one hundred and one diseases caused by evil spirits. They are treated with religious medicine and ritual; exorcism in combination with herbal medicines and other treatments such as oils. 3. current or immediate diseases or superficial disorders: self-terminating ailments. As they occur and subside by themselves they do not require medical treatment. They can be eliminated by proper diet and behaviour. 4. one hundred and one life diseases or disorders induced in this life. The causes of such diseases arise in the early stages of life and become manifested later in the same lifetime. They are treated by standard somatic medicine but when left untreated the patient may die. T. Clifford, 1984, 97. P. Démieville, 1930, 255.
35. For an informative study of various types of exorcism used for healing in Sri Lanka see P. Wirz, 1954.
36. The Buddhist texts list thirty-two parts of the body. One such list is given in the Dīgha-nikāya, II, 14, 293–4, where the parts of the body are said to be permeated by impurities and enclosed by the skin. The specific parts are: 1. head-hairs, 2. body-hairs, 3. nails, 4. teeth, 5. skin, 6. flesh, 7. sinews, 8. bones, 9. bone-marrow, 10. kidneys, 11. heart, 12. liver, 13. pleura, 14, spleen, 15. lungs, 16, mesentery, 17. bowls, 18. stomach, 19. excrement, 20. bile, 21. phlegm, 22. pus, 23. blood, 24. sweat, 25. fat, 26. tears, 27. tallow, 28. saliva, 29. snot, 30. synovic fluid, 31. urine, 32. brain.
37. This is presented in texts as the ten kinds of foulness: 1. the bloated, 2. livid, 3. festering, 4. cut-up, 5. gnawed, 6. scattered, 7. hacked and scattered, 8. bleeding, 9. worm-infested, 10. skeleton.
38. According to the Pāli Vinaya the person afflicted with one of the following five diseases must not be allowed to become a monk: leprosy, boils, eczema, consumption or epilepsy. The Mūlasarvāstivāda ordination manual called *Ekottara-karmaśataka* and composed in India in the seventh century by Guṇaprabha gives a much longer list of diseases. In addition to the five diseases given in the Pāli Vinaya, it includes such diseases as goitre, small pox, scabies, foot ulcers, excessive bodily leanness or dryness, excessive appetite,

jaundice, elephantiasis, fistulas on the private parts, different types of fever, indigestion problems, cough, asthma, abscesses filled with blood, rheumatism, chronic enlargement of the spleen, haemorrhoids, vomiting, weariness.

39. One such gradation of merit is given in the Majjhima-nikāya, III, 255. When a gift is given to an animal, it yields a hundredfold advantage; when to an ordinary person of poor moral habit, the yield is thousandfold; when to a person detached from sense pleasures, the yield is a hundred thousandfold of crores; when to a Buddhist recluse progressing towards the first level of sanctity (stream-winner), the yield is incalculable and immeasurable. So what can be said, the text asks rhetorically, about the advantages of giving to arhats and Buddhas?
40. It is said in the Aṅguttara-nikāya, II, 80, that there are four unthinkables (*acinteyya*), namely the range of Buddhas, the range of meditation, the fruit of *karma*, and speculations about the world (*lokacintā*).
41. Sanskrit *prapañca*.

SELECTED BIBLIOGRAPHY

Note: Unless specifically indicated all references to the Pāli sources such as Dīgha-nikāya or Aṅguttara-nikāya are given to the texts published by the Pali Text Society.

Basham, A.L., 'The Practice of Medicine in Ancient and Medieval India', in C. Leslie, ed., *Asian Medical Systems*, Berkeley, California Press, 1976.

Bowker, J., *Problems of Suffering in Religions of the World*, Cambridge, Cambridge University Press, 1970.

Burang, T., translated by S. Macintosh, *The Tibetan Art of Healing*, London, Robinson and Watkins Books Ltd., 1974.

Chandra, Lokesh, (ed.), *An Illustrated Tibeto-Mongolian Materia Medica of Ayurveda of 'Jam dpal rdo rje of Mongolia*, New Delhi, International Academy of Indian Culture, 1971.

Chavannes, E., 'Sutra prononcé par le Buddha au sujet de l'Avadāna concernant Fille-de-Manguier (Āmrāpali) et K'i-yu (Jīvaka)', number 499 in *Cinq cents contes et apoloques du Tripitaka chinois*, vol. 3, Paris, Ernest Leroux, 1911.

Clifford, T., *Tibetan Buddhist Medicine and Psychiatry*, Wellingborough, The Aquarian Press, 1984.

Dash, Bhagawan, *Tibetan Medicine with Special Reference to Yoga Śataka*, Dharamsala, Library of Tibetan Works and Archives, 1976.

Demiéville, P., 'Byō', in *Hōbōgirin*, Tokyo, Maison Franco-Japonaise, 1930, 224–5; translated by M. Tatz, *Buddhism and Healing*, Boston, University Press of America, 1985.

Filliozat, J., *La Doctrine classique de la médicine indienne: Se origines et ses parallèles grecs*, Paris, Imprimerie Nationale, 1949; translated by D.R. Chanana, *The Classical Doctrine of Indian Medicine*, New Delhi, Munshiram Manoharlal, 1964.

Filliozat, J., trans., *Yogaśataka: Texte Medical Attribué à Nāgārjuna*, Paris, 1979.

Fujita, K., 'The Doctrinal characteristics of karman in Early Buddhism', in L.A. Hercus, *et al.*, *Indological and Buddhist Studies, Volume in*

Honour of Prof. J.W. de Jong on his Sixtieth Birthday, Camberra, 1982, 149–59.

Gomez, L.O., 'Some Aspects of the Free-will Question in the Nikāyas', *Philosophy East and West*, 25, 1975, 81–90.

Gunawardana, R.A.L.H., 'Immersion as Therapy: Archaeological and Literary Evidence on an Aspect of Medical Practice in Precolonial Sri Lanka', in *Sri Lanka Journal of the Humanities*, 4, 1978, 35–59.

Huard, P. and Ming Wong, *Chinese Medicine*, New York, McGraw-Hill Book Co., 1968.

Jaworski, J., 'La section de la nourriture dans le Vinaya des Mahīśāsaka', *Rocznik Orientalistyczny*, 7, 1929, 53–124.

Jaworski, J., 'La section des remèdes dans le Vinaya des Mahīśāsaka et le Vinaya pāli', *Rocznik Orientalistyczny*, 5, 1927, 92–101.

Jayatilleke, K.N., 'The Buddhist Doctrine of Karma', *Mahabodhi*, 76, 1968, 314–20.

Lamotte, E., 'Le traité de l'Acte de Vasubandhu Karmasiddhiprakaraṇa', in *Mélanges Chinois et Bouddhiques*, 4, 1935–1936, 151–288.

Matthews, B., 'Karma and Rebirth in Theravāda Buddhism', in R.W. Neufeldt, (ed.), *Karma and Rebirth, Post Classical Developments*, Albany, State University of New York Press, 1986, 123–43.

Matthews, B., 'Post-Classical Developments in the Concept of Karma and Rebirth in Theravāda Buddhism', in R.W. Neufeldt, (ed.), *Karma and Rebirth, Post Classical Developments*, Albany, 1986, 123–43.

McDermott, J.P., 'Karma and Rebirth in Early Buddhism', in W.D. O'Flaherty, (ed.), *Karma and Rebirth in Classical Indian Traditions*, Berkeley/London, 1980, 165–92.

Milindapañha, translated by T.W. Rhys Davids, *The Questions of King Milinda*, Delhi, 1993.

Mitra, J., 'Lord Buddha: A Great Physician', in K.N. Udupa, (ed.), *Religion and Medicine*, Varanasi, Institute of Medical Sciences, 1974.

Nimalasuria, A., (ed.), *Buddha the Healer: The Mind and its Place in Buddhism*, Kandy, Buddhist Publication Society, 1960.

Nyanatiloka, Thera, *Karma and Rebirth*, Kandy, Buddhist Publication Society, 1959.

Obeyesekere, G., 'Theodicy, Sin and Salvation in a Sociology of Buddhism', in E.R. Leach, (ed.), *Practical Religion*, Cambridge, Cambridge University Press, 1968.

Rechung Rinpoche, J.K., *Tibetan Medicine*, Berkeley, University of California Press, 1973.

Skorupski, T., 'Prajñā', in *The Encyclopedia of Religion*, New York, 1987, vol. 11, 477–81.

Stablein, W., 'Tibetan Medical-Cultural System', in Dawa Norbu, (ed.), *An Introduction to Tibetan Medicine*, Delhi, Tibet Review Publications, 1976.

Visuddhimagga, translated by Pe Maung Tin, *The Path of Purity*, London, PTS, 1975.

Vogel, C., *Vāgbhaṭa's Aṣṭāṅgahṛdayasaṃhitā, The First Five Chapters of Its Tibetan Version*, Wiesbaden, Kommissionsverlag Franz Steiner GMBH, 1965.

Wayman, A., 'Buddhist Tantric Medicine Theory', in Dawa Norbu, (ed.), *An Introduction to Tibetan Medicine*, Delhi, Tibet Review Publications, 1976.

Wezler, A., 'On the Quadruple Division of the Yogaśāstra, the Caturvyūhatva of the Cikitsāśāstra and the "Four Noble Truths" of the Buddha', in *Indologica Taurinensia*, 12, 1984, 290–337.

Wirz, P., *Exorcism and the Art of Healing in Ceylon*, Leiden, E.J. Brill, 1954.

Zysk, K.G., 'Studies in Traditional Indian Medicine in the Pāli Canon: Jīvaka and Āyurveda', *Journal of the International Association of Buddhist Studies*, 5, 1982, 70–86.

Zysk, K.G., *Asceticism and Healing in Ancient India, Medicine in the Buddhist Monastery*, Delhi, Oxford University Press, 1991.

FROM FOLK MEDICINE TO BIOETHICS IN JUDAISM

Norman Solomon

This paper falls into two parts. In the first I shall indicate something of the range of approaches to medicine and healing to be found in traditional Jewish sources; in the second I shall illustrate how an issue in medical ethics might be decided, and why opinions might differ; and there will be a concluding reflection.

My title 'From Folk Medicine to Bioethics' suggests a progression, a diachronic survey of Jewish attitudes to healing from a primitive, 'folk' stage at some undetermined time in the distant past, to a sophisticated ethical system geared to advanced medical science and technology in the present.

But this is not at all what I have in mind. I wish to emphasise a synchronic rather than a diachronic perspective. There is continuity and also complexity within the Jewish tradition. Popular attitudes to health and sickness have existed and continue to exist side by side with strictly scientific approaches, and the two are bridged by theology. Three major trends – the popular, the scientific, and the religious – have persisted to the present.

Three Attitudes to Healing

Popular Medicine

The first trend is represented by the strong Jewish tradition of popular, folkloristic medicine, too easily dismissed as 'superstition'. The Babylonian Talmud, which is the main repository of ancient Jewish wisdom after the Bible, contains several collections of remedies introduced by the third-century teacher Abbaye with the words 'my mother told me' – an attribution to be taken not at its face value but as editorial semantics for 'popular tradition'. Some of the remedies are common sense, as for instance to turn the seam of a baby's swaddling cloth outwards so as not to injure him (*Shabbat* 134a[1]); others concern the formulae and repetition of spells (*Shabbat* 66b); many are to do with diet (*Ketubot* 10b) or the correct use of plants and herbs. In recent years numerous Hebrew amulets and incantation bowls from the first to fifth centuries have been recovered and studied by archaeologists; many of them were written by non-Jews evidently hoping to capture the efficacy of the 'Jewish magic' which was held in such high repute in late antiquity.

Allied with this are the widespread belief in alleged phenomena such as demons, possession, and the evil eye. Many readers will know the play *The Dybbuk* by the Yiddish writer S. Ansky (1863–1920), on the theme of possession, or will have read the novels of Isaac Bashevis Singer which conjure up the atmosphere of the Jewish *stetl* (village) of pre-World War Two Eastern Europe and convey something of the vividness with which people imagined themselves surrounded by invisible beings and forces which controlled or at least influenced our destinies.

In the middle of the twelfth century Moses Maimonides (1135/8–1204), one of the profoundest of mediaeval Jewish thinkers, wrote:

> And all these matters [*sc.* astrology, necromancy etc.] are falsehood and deceit, by means of which idolatrous priests in ancient times misled the people of the nations to follow them. It is not fitting that (the people of) Israel, who are wise and learned, should be attracted by such nonsense or entertain the possibility that there is any benefit in it; as it is said, 'Surely there is no divination in Jacob, and no augury in Israel' (Numbers 23:23), and 'Those nations whose place you are taking listen to soothsayers and augurs, but the Lord your God does not permit you to do this' (Deuteronomy 18:14). Whoever believes in such things, or anything like them, and thinks that they are true, though the Torah forbade them, is a fool, an ignoramus, and in the category of women and children whose comprehension is imperfect. But wise people, of perfect understanding, know through convincing proofs that all these things which the Torah forbade are not wisdom, but empty nonsense which attracts the ignorant and on account of which they abandon all the paths of truth; that is why the Torah states, in prohibiting this nonsense, 'You shall be perfect with the Lord your God' (Deuteronomy 18:13).[2]

Maimonides' enlightened view convinced few scholars in his time and had virtually no impact on popular belief. As late as the eighteenth century Elijah the Gaon of Vilna, a man of immense piety and vast erudition, sharply criticised the him for denying the existence of demons;[3] still today, many of the more reactionary orthodox leaders endorse such beliefs, as well as astrology, on the grounds that they were held by the rabbis of the Talmud.

Scientific Medicine

On the other hand, a more scientific attitude to medicine and healing has always prevailed in some circles. Even with regard to amulets, the Talmud in its legal sections distinguishes between those regarded as tested and reliable and those not so regarded, a distinction which could only have been established by experiment and observation.[4]

Several scholars in modern times, following the pioneering work of Julius Preuss (1861–1913),[5] have discussed Talmudic anatomy and physiology. This is not an easy exercise, for there is no Talmudic treatise on either of these subjects. To assess Talmudic anatomy, for instance, one has to work with literary material such as a list of body parts compiled in connection with laws of ritual purity,[6] or lists of defects which would render priests[7] or sacrificial animals[8] unacceptable for Temple service, or render an animal or bird impermissible for consumption;[9] such knowledge of physiology as is preserved in the Talmud has to do with matters such as childbirth and sexual relations which are regulated by the law, or is implied in random comments on nature, divine providence and the like. We know very little about the actual practice of medicine by Jews in the Talmudic era; the Talmud is concerned not with the art of medicine *per se*, but with the *halakha*, or law, and has preserved only those elements of medical science as are needed for correct interpretation and application of the law. Just as, today, one might learn quite a lot about issues in medical ethics from studying the law reports, but little of the relevant basic science, we are able to derive fundamental ethical principles from the Talmud though we are often in the dark as to the rabbis' finer understanding of anatomy and physiology.

A systematic scientific approach to medicine appears in Jewish sources only in the Middle Ages, when the influence of the Hippocratic School and of Galen is prominent; the earliest known medical works written by a Jew are the Arabic treatises of Isaac Israeli (*c.* 855–955). The *Book of Asaph or Book of Healing*, of which several versions exist, is the oldest Hebrew medical treatise, cited in some form perhaps as early as the tenth century.[10] Asaph ha-Rofé (Asaph the physician), the supposed author, to whom a version of the Hippocratic oath[11] subsequently in use by Jewish physicians is attributed, cannot be identified. The book – at least in one manuscript – contains 'treatises on the Persian months, physiology, embryology, the four periods of man's life, the four winds,[12] diseases of various organs, hygiene, medicinal plants, medical calendar, the practise of medicine, as well as an antidotarium, urinology, aphorisms, and the Hippocratic oath'.[13] It is interesting that it draws not on the ample medical material in the Talmud but on 'the books of the wise men of India' and a 'book of the ancients'; it ascribes the origin of medicine to Shem, son of Noah, who received it from angels. The contents clearly show dependence on Galen, Hippocrates and Dioscorides, indicating that the practice of Jewish physicians was modelled not on rabbinic sources but on 'scientific' medicine.

Many Greek medical works were translated into Hebrew, generally from Arabic rather than the original language, and often with the commentaries of leading mediaeval Muslim scholars. Opinions vary as to the originality of Jewish contributions to medicine, but there is no doubt that during the Renaissance Jews played a significant role in the transfer of ancient Greek medical knowledge, together with later Islamic insights, to the West. Sadly, the great European Universities which were formed at that time excluded Jews, so that although many individual Jews acquired medical knowledge and gained high reputations for their skills it was only converted Jews such as Amatus Lusitanus[14] who were able to play a full part in the development of the science before modern times.

But the systematic scientific approach created problems for traditionalists, since it implied the rejection of those folk elements and superstitions which had been included in the Talmud. Maimonides, in the short regimen of health he includes as a single chapter in his *Mishneh Torah*,[15] casts aside tradition in favour of Galen and his own contemporaries. The remark of the commentator *Migdal Oz* that 'everything in the chapter is based on principles derived from the sages and scattered through the Talmud' is wide of the mark. The truth of the matter is that Maimonides did not believe that the sages had an adequate knowledge of medicine, or that such knowledge could be obtained by the investigation of traditional texts; the Torah taught not the details of medical science, but rather that one should seek the best advice obtainable from whatever source it might come.

The Theological Approach

There is another trend, amply evident from the Bible onwards, in attitudes to healing. This third trend arises from the fundamental biblical concept that God is all-powerful, merciful and compassionate, and his providence extends to all his creatures. If this is so, then presumably individuals who are sick and suffer do so not by accident, but by God's design, whether on account of their sin or in some way to refine them. In this case, it is appropriate for us to pray to him, to seek his forgiveness, and if it is his will, he will heal us – 'for it is I, the Lord, who heal you' (Exodus 15:26). The Torah is the antidote to sickness; as the great Bible exegete Rashi (1040–1105) put it, commenting on that verse, '. . . the plain meaning is, that he has given us the Torah and the commandments so that we may be saved from them (*sc.* the diseases he inflicted on the Egyptians)'.

If it is not his will to heal us, then by utilising the art of medicine to heal ourselves are we not thwarting his will? If, for instance, God had 'designed' some individual with a defective kidney would we not be circumventing God's will by replacing it with a healthy one or by offering dialysis?

There have indeed been Jewish sects, including some Karaites,[16] who objected on religious grounds to the practice of medicine. Such an attitude is not without echoes amongst the mainstream Rabbanites, including Nahmanides (1194–1270), who held that God would protect from sickness any individual who served Him in complete faith, and that ideally the sick person should turn to repentance, not to doctors, even though the Torah granted 'permission for the doctor to heal'.[17] There are today to my knowledge, though I do not know whether they are documented, small orthodox groups who are reluctant to make use of mainstream medical expertise and, apart from prayer, rely either on 'alternative' therapies or on the regimens and specific remedies listed in the Talmud or mediaeval rabbinic sources. The justification for 'alternative' therapies is that they are considered, unlike mainstream medicine, to be in accordance with 'nature' and hence with spiritual principles.

The Talmud relates that Hezekiah, king of Judah, took six initiatives without consulting the sages;[18] *post factum* they approved of three but not of the others. Amongst those of which they did approve was his initiative in hiding away the *Sefer Refuot*, or 'book of cures'. Most commentators assume that the book listed the herbs which God, in his infinite wisdom, had created to cure each and every human malady; he hid the book, explains Rashi, 'because their heart was not humbled for the sick but they were healed immediately', that is, because the certainty of cure led people to ignore God.

Maimonides, to whom it was inconceivable that the sages should approve of the deliberate suppression of beneficial medical information or resources, rejects this explanation. In his opinion, the *Sefer Refuot* was a book containing cures forbidden by Torah, such as astrological talismans; to leave it around would have been positively dangerous; moeover, the 'cures' were worthless.[19]

The predominant Jewish view is indeed that endorsed by Maimonides, namely that the practice of medicine is not only permissible but virtuous. That the art of medicine is licit is inferred in the Talmud from the rules of compensation for injury. The law of Torah is that the malefactor must compensate the victim for pain, injury, shame, loss of earnings, and medical care; this implies that doctors are allowed to practise.[20]

But 'permission' is not enough. There is a *positive obligation* for those who are able to do so to use their skills and resources to heal the sick. Joseph Karo (1488–1575), author of the *Shulhan Arukh*, the most authoritative Jewish Code of Law, bluntly states, '. . . [to heal] is a positive obligation, tantamount to the saving of life, and one who avoids doing it sheds blood, even though there is someone else available to [effect the cure], since the patient does not respond equally to every doctor.' He goes on to formulate the principle that one may practice medicine only if duly authorised by a Jewish religious court.[21]

Even those unable to perform medical or nursing services are obliged to visit the sick and to pray for their welfare; and intercessions are made publicly in the Synagogue.[22]

David ben Shmuel haLevi (1586–1667) expressed theologically the relationship between 'permission' to heal and the 'obligation' to heal:

> True healing is through prayer, for healing is from heaven, as it is written, 'I have smitten, and I shall heal' (Deuteronomy 32:39). But not everyone is worthy of this [special divine intervention], hence it is necessary to achieve healing by natural means. He, blessed be He, agreed to this, and gave healing through natural cures; this is what is meant by 'He gave permission to heal'. Since human beings have got into this state [of having to rely on natural cures], doctors are obliged to effect cures [by natural means].[23]

By being subsumed within the *mitzvot*, or divine commandments, the practice of medicine becomes part of the spirituality of Judaism. Far from being an activity opposed to religion, it is an essential element within it. This is true even though the specific remedies used by the physician are not determined by the religious tradition itself, but by the science of medicine.

To the question, 'Does the physician play God?' we answer, yes. To aid the sick, it is our duty to 'play' – that is, imitate the ways of – God, to show mercy and kindness and to make our skills available to all in need.

Theodicy

We have seen that the physician, in practising his art, is a 'co-worker' with God in alleviating human suffering and misery. But if God is all-powerful, just and merciful, why does he allow humans to suffer and be miserable at all, other than when they clearly deserve it? Why do bad things happen to good people?

From the Bible onwards Jews have wrestled with this problem. The Reformist Jewish philosopher Hermann Cohen (1842–1918) outdid the traditionalists in making suffering a central issue in his religious system; suffering, according to Cohen, is the turning point at which religion emerges out of ethics.[24] Recent Jewish theologians have tended to focus their discussion of apparent divine injustice on the Holocaust, for it seems inconceivable that every one of the six million victims, including one million children, 'deserved' his or her fate.

Despite its almost total absence from the Hebrew scriptures, the belief in life after death is central to rabbinic teaching, whether expressed as bodily resurrection, eternal life of the spirit, or some combination of the two. Kabbalists, indirectly influenced by

Neoplatonist philosophy, adopted in addition the concept of reincarnation, though this was opposed by Saadia (*c*. 882–942)[25] and others and never achieved the status of a vital principle of faith.

Such beliefs simplify the theology of suffering, for (a) they diminish the significance of the vicissitudes of 'this world', and (b) they provide an opportunity for 'compensation' for the evils of this world in the next. The transmigration of souls easily explains the suffering of innocent children – either they are being punished now for sins committed in a previous incarnation, or else they will be compensated for their present sufferings in a later one.

God exercises providence in respect of individuals as well as in respect of Israel collectively. 'Collective providence' enables even the Holocaust to be rationalised; the destruction of a third of the Jewish people may be viewed as part of God's redemptive process, leading ultimately to Israel's restoration, whether or not in terms of the Land. But this leaves unanswered the question why each individual suffered. Maimonides denied that God extended Providence to individuals in the sub-lunar sphere other than to those whose spiritual excellence raised them above sub-lunar materiality, but most other Jewish theologians have strongly upheld the doctrine of universal individual providence, which is hard to reconcile with the observed facts of life.

Few have forgotten or completely repudiated the simple biblical explanation of suffering, including sickness, as the consequence of sin: '. . . if you listen to the voice of the Lord your God and do what is upright in his eyes . . . all the sickness which I set upon Egypt I will not set upon you, for I the Lord am your healer' (Exodus 15:26). But other concepts, both biblical and post-biblical, modify the picture.

The Talmud reflects on *yissurin shel ahava* ('sufferings of love') – 'those whom he loves the Lord chastises' (Proverbs 3:12) – which it sees as affording the suffering individual an opportunity for spiritual growth;[26] however, doubt is expressed as to whether suffering which distracts a person from Torah can be 'suffering of love'. Amos taught that it was precisely God's love for Israel that led Him to chastise them more than any other nation – 'For you alone have I cared among all the nations of the world; therefore will I punish you for all your iniquities' (Amos 3:2); suffering should thus be received as a token of God's special concern for Israel, or for the individual concerned.

Also familiar in Judaism are the concepts of redemptive suffering and of the vicarious atonement for sin. For instance, on

Numbers 20, 'Why is the death of Miriam juxtaposed to the law of the red heifer? To teach you that just as the red heifer atones (for sin) so does the death of the righteous atone (for sin)'.[27]

God is constantly present with those who suffer – 'Though I walk through a valley dark as death I fear no evil, for thou art with me' (Psalm 23:4), and 'I am with him in his distress' (Psalm 91:15). In line with this, on the collective level, is a graphic image found in rabbinic Midrash – God, or rather the *Shekhina* (divine presence), is 'in exile' with Israel.

God is sometimes said to 'hide his face', a thought expressed agonisingly in Psalm 44:24. Amongst the moderns, Eliezer Berkovitz is in accord with tradition when he not merely finds the hiddenness of God compatible with God's existence, but discovers God's actual presence within His silence. He argues that the Jewish response to the Holocaust should be modelled on Job's response to suffering, questioning God yet accepting his superior wisdom.[28]

Few today echo Maimonides's view of evil as *privatio boni*, the absence of good;[29] not only the Holocaust, but the 'ordinary' suffering of much of humanity, give too strong a strong sense of the reality of evil for such a doctrine to be credible.

The existence of evil is a central issue for kabbalists, who uphold the idea that ultimately all is from the Creator and therefore good. According to Isaac the Blind (1160–1235) the origin of what appears to us as evil lies in the dominance of the divine attribute, or emanation, of Justice, over that of Mercy. The Zohar (late thirteenth century) maintains that evil originates in the leftovers of previous, imperfect worlds which God destroyed; the *sitra ahara* ('other side') has ten *sefirot* (emanations) of its own, reflecting the direct emanations from God; good and evil are thus intermingled in our world, and it is our duty to separate them. Isaac Luria (1534–72) developed the concept of the *tzimtzum*, the concentration of the divine illumination in vessels not all of which were capable of containing it, and which therefore ruptured, causing the holy sparks to become associated with broken sherds and husks from which we must 'rescue' them by performing the commandments.

Richard Rubenstein is one of several non-orthodox Jewish theologians driven by reflection on the Holocaust to reject the traditional idea of God as the 'Lord of history'; God had simply failed to intervene to save his faithful.[30] 'Death of God' theologies have to be seen in a wider context, however; well before the Holocaust Jewish theologians such as Mordecai M. Kaplan were struggling to reinterpret the concept of God in the light of modern critical ideas.[31] A follower of Kaplan, the Jewish Reconstructionist theologian Harold Kushner, in his bestseller *When bad things happen to good people*, has explored the resulting attenuated view of God in the context of sickness and other forms of personal distress.[32]

Suffering brings redemption, whether for the individual, for Israel collectively, or for the world in its state of sin. Using imagery from the biblical *Song of Songs*, the late Joseph Dov Soloveitchik (1903–93), a leading Orthodox theologian, interpreted the revival of Jewish life after the Holocaust as a *tiqqun* ('restoration') which was the redemptive outcome of suffering: 'In the heart of the night of terror . . . a night of hiddenness . . . of doubts and apostasy . . . came a knock on the door, the knock of the beloved . . . Seven great reversals in Jewish life, seven miracles, commenced – political, military, cultural, theological, life – value, citizenship, and the new fertility of the land of Israel'.[33]

But how does the justification of the ways of God relate to the actual practice of medicine? The doctor's obligation to give treatment is not offset on the grounds that the patient has sinned and therefore deserves to suffer.[34] One only has to recall the example of Job's 'friends' to realise that it is not acceptable to harangue the patient for the sin which has caused him to suffer. The mediaeval codes nevertheless state that when visiting the sick you should create an opportunity for the patient to reflect whether he has undischarged debts or obligations; if he is seriously ill you should prompt him to confess and repent, at the same time 'reassuring' him that 'many have repented and not died'![35]

Whatever is appropriate for the doctor or the visitor to say or do, the patient may interpret suffering as a 'sign' prompting him or her to prayer and penitence, and may request and receive pastoral help in that undertaking. Most important, though, is the strength that comes from the faith that God is with the sufferer in his distress; 'One who visits the sick should not sit on the bed, nor [high up] on a chair, but sit [humbly] before him [respectfully] cloaked, for the *Shekhina* is above the head of the sick . . . the Holy One, blessed be he, sustains the sick'.[36]

How Questions in Medical Ethics are Decided

We must now examine some examples of how questions in medical ethics might be tackled by someone working within the Jewish tradition. Modern advances in the biological sciences and medical technology have generated economic, legal, and ethical questions, few of which were contemplated when the sources of Jewish law were formulated. To what extent can traditional *halakha* be extended to provide guidance in the contemporary situation? Further, is *halakha* the correct, or the only, available Jewish source on which to draw?

The topics selected are (a) Artificial Insemination by Donor and (b) Euthanasia. The choice of Euthanasia is obvious. A.I.D. has been chosen for three reasons:

1. Childlessness is regarded in most societies as an acute form of suffering. It is unlikely that anyone would attempt to justify A.I.D. other than as a method of relieving this form of suffering.
2. The discussion of A.I.D. illustrates the way a typical halakhic argument proceeds.
3. The discussion illustrates the divergent theological approaches of the main contemporary branches of Judaism.

Artificial Insemination by Donor (A.I.D.)

Halakha (Jewish law) faces three problems in considering the permissibility or otherwise of artificial insemination:

1. Is the child of a married woman who became pregnant from a man other than her husband, but without a normal act of intercourse, a *mamzer* (illegitimate)? Put another way, is the woman an adulteress?
2. Even if the woman's own husband was the donor, could the insemination take place when she is still *nidda* (technically in a state of menstruation, not having bathed in a *mikve* since her last period)?
3. Since masturbation is in other circumstances forbidden, how should sperm be obtained from the husband or donor?

Although artificial insemination appears to be a novel problem of the twentieth century, precedent was found in a Talmudic reference to the possibility of a virgin who had conceived 'in a bath place', that is, by accidentally absorbing sperm deposited there.[37] The case was much discussed in the Middle Ages; Simon ben Zemah Duran (1361–1444) reports that 'a number of non-Jews' as well as another rabbi had told him of virgins they knew of who had become pregnant in this manner.[38] Simon may have been unduly credulous, but even if the incidents were purely imaginary the legal precedents were set.

In the 1960s, when artificial insemination both by husband and by donor became widely available, Rabbi Moshe Feinstein (1895–1986) ruled that where there was no forbidden sexual act no adultery could be deemed to have taken place and therefore a child conceived in such a way would not be a *mamzer*.[39] Whilst not positively encouraging anyone to practise artificial insemination he argued that it was not actually forbidden.

Feinstein was bitterly attacked for his permissiveness by Rabbi Jacob Breisch (*Helqat Yaakov*), who castigated artificial insemination by a donor as abominable, forbidden, and disgusting, whilst conceding that the child could not be considered a mamzer nor its mother an adulteress, and that artificial insemination by the husband might be permitted. Breisch's opposition seems to have been based more on a sort of Jewish public relations concern than on a specific halakha to do with insemination; he felt that Jews should not appear more permissive in moral issues than Christians, and as the Catholic Church had condemned artificial insemination it would degrade Judaism if Jews were to be more lax. Feinstein rejected this argument out of hand, possibly reflecting a difference between American and European attitudes.

Joel Teitelbaum, the Hasidic rabbi of Satmar, and Feinstein's sharpest opponent, took the position that adultery was constituted by the deposition, by whatever means, of a man's sperm in a woman married to someone else. Feinstein had no difficulty in demonstrating the absence of halakhic support for such a position.[40]

Euthanasia

Three types of 'mercy killing' may be considered. Eugenic euthanasia, that is the killing of handicapped or 'socially undesirable' individuals, is in no way countenanced in Judaism. Debate centres on (a) active euthanasia, where a drug or other treatment is administered to hasten the patient's release from suffering, or (b) passive euthanasia, where therapy is withheld and the patient is allowed to die naturally.

An early rabbinic source unequivocally states:

> One who is dying is regarded as a living person in all respects . . . one may not bind his jaws, stop up his openings . . . move him . . . One may not close the eyes of the dying person. If anyone touches or moves them it is as if he shed blood, as Rabbi Meir said, 'This is like a flickering flame; as soon as anyone touches it, it goes out.' Likewise, if anyone closes the eyes of the dying it is as if he had taken his life.[41]

Judah the Pious of Regensburg (*c.* 1150–1217) ruled that if something, for instance the noise of chopping wood, is preventing 'the soul from departing', one may cease the activity in order to ease death.[42]

These two rulings establish the distinction between active and passive euthanasia, and much subsequent halakha hinges on refining and applying the distinction to contemporary situations. Active euthanasia is generally regarded as murder; passive euthanasia may sometimes be permitted. Physicians are urged to do their utmost to save and prolong life, even for a short time, and even if the patient is suffering great distress. Some authorities maintain that withdrawal of life-support is unlike 'removing the noise of chopping wood' referred to in the classical sources; life-support is positive therapy, whereas extraneous noise is simply an obstacle to death. Others are not so sure of the distinction.

Eliezer Yehuda Waldenburg (1912–), a leading Jerusalem *dayyan* (judge in a religious court), has permitted the use of narcotics and analgesics to relieve the pain of the dying even though these drugs might depress the activity of the respiratory system and hasten death, provided the intention of administering the drugs was solely to relieve pain. Moreover, one may not initiate artificial life-support for a patient who is incurably and irreversibly ill, though where artificial life-support apparatus has been connected it may not be disconnected until the patient is dead according to the criteria of halakha. To evade the harshness of the latter ruling Waldenburg made the novel suggestion that respirators be set with automatic time-clocks; since they would disconnect automatically after the set period, a positive decision would be required to continue their operation, and this would not be done unless there was now hope of cure.

The twelfth-century rabbi Jacob Tam seems to imply that it is permitted actively to take one's own life to avoid excessive torture, though it is unclear whether he meant this only in those circumstances where the suicide was primarily intended to save the individual from worse sin, that is, apostasy.[43] Byron L. Sherwin has cited this and similar rulings as a basis for reconsidering the case for active euthanasia; such arguments have made little headway amongst the Orthodox, though Conservative and Reform Jews have been more amenable.

Even though one may not take active, or in many cases even passive, measures to hasten the death of one who is suffering, many halakhists argue that it is permissible to pray for his/her release; the Talmud itself records, apparently with approval, that the maidservant of the great second-century sage, Judah ha-Nasi, when she saw his agony, prayed 'Those above (i.e. the angels) seek the master, and those below (i.e. the friends and disciples of Judah) seek him; may those above overcome those below'.[44] The nineteenth-century Turkish rabbi Hayyim Palaggi argued that this should only be done by persons who are not related to the sufferer; relatives might be improperly motivated.

Differences Amongst the Main Branches of Contemporary Judaism

Traditional Orthodox belief is that the Torah, being of divine authorship, is comprehensive, and that if we search diligently God will help us to find answers even to those problems that could not be spelled out explicitly in earlier times. Many thousands of responsa have now been published, therefore, by leading halakhists such as Feinstein in New York, and Eliezer Yehuda Waldenburg in Jerusalem, in the attempt to give firm practical guidance in this area.

Daniel H. Gordis[45] has argued that there is not only a measure of intellectual dishonesty in the programme of applying the classic halakhic approach to problems not envisaged by the rabbis, but also a risk of compromising the values they sought to inculcate. If, for instance, adultery is to be regarded as a precedent to forbid artificial insemination by a donor, one is not only making an unjustified extrapolation to the case under consideration, but also undermining the seriousness of adultery as a social issue, and undermining confidence in the halakhic process itself. In fact, claims Gordis, the real of objections of Rosner, Bleich and others to A.I.D. arise not from a genuine halakhic argument but from revulsion at the notion of a married woman being impregnated by another man's sperm; they are concerned, rightly, about issues of sexuality, parenthood, and the nature of marriage. 'But if these are the issues underlying our objection to A.I.D.' comments Gordis, 'we should say so clearly and discuss those issues on their own merits, rather than obscuring the salient halakhic issue by reference to secondary ones.' Gordis therefore favours using the resources of halakha not as a system of rules to be subjected to analysis, but as a stockpile to be scoured for its implicit concepts of humanness, of being made in the divine image; it is these concepts on which we should base our decisions in medical ethics.

Elliott Dorff,[46] focusing on issues at the end of life, writes 'This tension between continuity and change is probably most acutely felt in our day in the area of medical ethics'. He finds both the Orthodox and Reform resolutions of the tension unsatisfactory. The Orthodox are dominated by rules and precedents which they misapply or arbitrarily extrapolate because they do not allow sufficiently for the differences between the times in which the precedents were set and the radically different medical situation of our time; the Reform fail because their appeal to concepts such as 'covenantal responsibility' lacks the discipline of *halakha* and is ultimately indistinguishable from liberal secular ethics. His own preference, which he sees as that of Conservative Judaism in general, is for a three-stage approach. First, the Jewish conceptual and legal sources must be studied in their historical contexts. On this basis, one can identify the relevant differences between our own situation and that in which the texts were formulated. Then and only then can one apply the sources to the contemporary issue, using not only purely legal reasoning but 'theological deliberations concerning our nature as human beings created by, and in the image of, God'.[47]

I do not find Dorff's approach significantly different from the Orthodox one; few Orthodox rabbis would take issue with his three-stage approach of contextual study, historical evaluation, and application of principles, and by no means all commit the errors with which Dorff reproaches them collectively. But the fact is that it is not always easy to articulate the 'theological deliberations concerning our nature as human beings created by, and in the image of, God'. What, for instance, are we to make of the principle so frequently invoked by ex-Chief Rabbi (now Lord) Jakobovits, Fred Rosner and others, that 'every human life is of infinite worth'? Is there a clear source for such a principle within the *halakha*? It is certainly not stated in so many words in the Talmud. Daniel B. Sinclair has indeed commented on 'the apparent deviation of the *halakhah* from the [halakhic] principle of the supremacy of human life in areas such as treatment of the dying and foeticide'.[48] Sinclair doubts whether the theological concept of the 'sanctity of life' used by Bleich, Jakobovits, *et alia* is appropriate in Judaism, for in Judaism 'human life per se is not endowed with intrinsic holiness: rather, holiness is a state to be achieved by dint of sustained effort'.[49] He feels that the adoption of something like a 'holiness of life' principle has led Bleich *et alia* into serious conflict with regard to abortion of defective foetuses[50] and with regard to cases like that of Karen Ann Quinlan.[51]

Conclusion

A report to the central committee of the World Council of Churches in Moscow in July 1989 affirmed that health was not primarily medical. The causes of disease in the world were social, economic, political and spiritual, as well as bio-medical. Those in loving harmony with God and neighbour not only stay healthier but survive tragedy or suffering best and grow stronger in the process. As persons come to trust in God's unconditional love, they come together in a healing community.[52]

From a Jewish point of view this statement seems innocuous enough, provided one ignores its hidden agendas and innuendoes. Undoubtedly, traditional Jewish sources recognise that ill health stems from many causes, amongst them social, economic and spiritual as well as 'bio-medical'; one would have thought, indeed, that any adequately trained physician would agree. Living 'in loving harmony with God and neighbour' would likewise be endorsed by traditional Jews, and if translated to 'emotional stability' any good physician would regard it as a factor predisposing to good health; but I do not know of hard evidence that emotionally stable, socially adjusted Christians or Jews enjoy better health than emotionally stable, socially adjusted agnostics or atheists, nor can I envisage how such a claim could be substantiated.

As for the Jewish scene today, all three aspects of 'From Folk Medicine to Bioethics' – the popular, the scientific, the theological – remain with us, and they are often intertwined.

The folk medicine traditions of European Jews are very different from, say, those of North African or Iraqi Jewry; all have been influenced by the surrounding cultures even more than by Talmudic tradition, and are distinctively Jewish only in the wording of amulets and charms and in the associated forms of prayer. The 'healer' is a familiar figure in these societies.[53] Perhaps the most noted of all Jewish 'healers' was Israel ben Eliezer (1700–1760), the founder of Hasidism, generally known as the Baal Shem Tov, the 'good Baal Shem', from his reputation as an itinerant healer; the title *Baal Shem* (Hebrew בעל שם – 'master of the Name') was given to healers who were thought to achieve miraculous cures by writing or uttering letters of the divine names, as well as by dispensing herbal remedies. Many Hasidic leaders have emulated the founder's example as healers of the physical as well as spiritual maladies of their flock, indeed, they rarely distinguish between the two. Similar roles have been fulfilled by personalities, including rabbis, in 'oriental' Jewry.

This 'spiritual' healing tradition persists today; Hasidim routinely appeal to their 'Rebbe' to intercede with prayer or advice to overcome their ills, though often enough this is done side by side with recourse to the latest bio-medical techniques. The distrustful attitude it tends to breed towards more scientific therapies has joined forces recently with 'alternative medicine' and New Age ideas, a process which is part of the anti-rational, anti-Enlightenment backlash in contemporary religious circles.[54]

At the same time Orthodox Jews, especially from the non-Hasidic traditions, are engaged not only in the practice of 'scientific' medicine at all levels but in the serious discussion of bio-medical and bio-ethical issues, confident that guidance in these areas is to be found in the divinely revealed Torah; we cited above a sample of the thousands of published responsa. Hospitals such as Shaare Zedek in Jerusalem have allowed the halakhic rulings to put to the test; academic institutions such as Ben Gurion University in Beer Sheva have chairs in Jewish Medical Ethics; rabbinic organisations such as the Rabbinical Council of America issue regular updates on medical halakha; and books and articles on the ethics and halakha of medicine are authored by experts from all Jewish denominations.[55] In parts of Europe and in North America Jews take an active role in public discussion and the development of policy in medical ethics; some, at least, of the participants have sufficient knowledge and commitment to introduce the resources of their own tradition to the debate.

The function of theology in all this is to provide a framework within which the activity of healing, whether through folk or scientific methods, can be interpreted as a spiritual vocation. Even if the specific remedies used by the physician are not determined by the religious tradition itself, but by folklore or independent science, the art of healing is of the essence of the life of faith. It would be pretentious for a healer – say, a doctor routinely prescribing antibiotics to control an infection, or a surgeon routinely replacing a hip – to claim to be restoring the patient to a wholeness which incorporates not only physical healing but reconciliation with God and society. But without doubt the healer is playing a humble part within that process, and the divine art of healing is enhanced by the awareness of what is at stake in even the most routine procedures.

NOTES

Note: in these notes, BT = 'Babylonian Talmud'; JT = 'Jerusalem Talmud'. Unless otherwise specified, Talmudic references are to the Babylonian Talmud.

1. This and other references in similar format are to tractates of the Babylonian Talmud.
2. Maimonides *Mishneh Torah* Laws of Idolatry 11:16. He argues the case against astrology at great length in the *Letter to the Congregation of Marseilles*, stressing that astrology was not a Greek science, but part of the religion of Chaldeans, Egyptians and Canaanites.
3. *Biur ha-Gra* note 13 on *Shulhan Arukh Yore Deah* 179.
4. BT *Shabbat* 53a/b.
5. Preuss, Julius, *Biblical and Talmudic Medicine* tr. Fred Rosner. New York: Hebrew Publishing Company, 1978.
6. Mishna *Oholot* 1:8.
7. *Bekhorot* 7.
8. *Bekhorot* 6.
9. *Hullin* 3. For a translation of the relevant parts of Karo's *Shulhan Arukh* (Code of Law), together with a discussion of Talmudic anatomy in the light of the science of its day and the present time, see Levin, S.I. and Boyden, Edward A., *The Kosher Code of the Orthodox Jew*. New York: Hermon Press, 1969 (originally published in 1940 by the University of Minnesota). Boyden writes that 'although the Mishnaic portion of the Talmud, when redacted, was contemporary with Galen, and the commentaries of the Gemara were post – Galenic, the stage of development of Talmudic medicine is nearer that of the Hippocratic school . . .' (page vi).
10. Lieber, Elinor, 'Asaf's *Book of Medicines*: a Hebrew Encyclopedia of Greek and Jewish Medicine, possibly compiled in Byzantium on an Indian model', in *Dumbarton Oaks Papers* 38 (1984), 233–49. Lieber

herself (p. 238) maintains that the earliest certain reference to Asaph is *c.* 1200 in Kimhi's commentary on Hosea 14: 8. She thinks that parts of the *Book of Medicines* are a conflation of Greek and Jewish ideas, and makes out a strong case that the book presents a crude account of the circulation of the blood, anticipating Harvey by some centuries.

11. Lieber *loc. cit.* 244: 'While this shows many affinities with the Hippocratic Oath, it is not taken from it directly . . . From the literary point of view it constitutes a remarkable mosaic of Biblical phrases.'
12. 'Humours' would be the correct translation of *ruhot* in this context.
13. Richard Gottheil, in *The Jewish Encyclopedia* (1905 edition).
14. See Friedenwald, H., *The Jews and Medicine*. Baltimore: Johns Hopkins Press, 1944 vol. 1 page 333.
15. Maimonides *Mishneh Torah: Hilkhot Deot* 4, and in his medical works generally.
16. The Karaites, said to have been founded by Anan ben David in the eighth century, rejected rabbinic tradition and accepted only the written text of Torah as authentic revelation. The term 'Rabbanites' is used to distinguish mainstream Jewry from them.
17. Nahmanides, *Commentary* on Leviticus 26:1.11
18. There are versions of the story in BT *Berakhot* 1 Ob and *Pesahim* 56a and JT *Pesahim* 64a *Nedarim* 22b and *Sanhedrin* 5b.
19. Commentary on Mishna *Pesahim* end of chapter 4.
20. BT *Bava Qama* 85a, based on Exodus 21:19.
21. *Shulhan Arukh Yore Deah* 236:1.
22. Isserles note on *Shulhan Arukh Yore Deah* 235:10.
23. Taz, on *Shulhan Arukh Yore Deah* 236:1. Note that 'natural means' here refers to normal medical practice based on scientific method, at least as understood in the seventeenth century. David ben Shmuel roots his argument in a Talmudic discussion (BT *Berakhot* 60a) as to what prayers to say when letting blood.
24. Cohen, Hermann, *Religion of Reason out of the Sources of Judaism*, tr. Simon Kaplan. New York: Frederick Unger, 1972, p. 18. See also Leaman, Oliver, *Evil and Suffering in Jewish Philosophy*. Cambridge: Cambridge University Press, 1995.
25. Saadia Gaon, *The Book of Beliefs and Opinions* tr. Samuel Rosenblatt. New Haven: Yale University Press and London: Oxford University Press, 1948, book 6 section 8. Saadia was attacking Karaites rather than Kabbalists.
26. BT *Berakhot* 5; *Bava Metzia* 84b/85a.
27. BT *Mo'ed Qatan* 28a.
28. Berkovitz, E., *Faith After the Holocaust*. New York: Ktav, 1973. Compare BT *Hagiga* 5a: 'Whoever does not experience the hiddenness of God is not of them (*sc.* the elect)'. *See also* Laytner, Anson, *Arguing with God: A Jewish Tradition*. Northvale NJ and London: Jason Aronson Inc., 1990.
29. *Guide of the Perplexed* 1:1 0–12. Maimonides here adopts a Neoplatonic view, already espoused by Augustine and others.
30. Rubenstein, Richard, *After Auschwitz: history, theology and contemporary Judaism*. 2nd ed. Baltimore and London: Johns Hopkins University Press, 1992.

31. Kaplan, Modecai M. *Judaism as a Civilization: Towards a Reconstruction of American Jewish Life*. With an new Introductory Essay by Arnold Eisen. Philadelphia: Jewish Publication Society, 1994. (Original publication – New York: Macmillan, 1934.).
32. Kushner, Harold S., *When bad things happen to good people*. London and Sydney: Pan Books, 1982.
33. Soloveitchik, Joseph B., '*Kol Dodi Dofek*: It Is the Voice of My Beloved That Knocketh', in *Theological and Halakhic Relections on the Holocaust* ed. B.H. Rosenberg and F. Henman. Hoboken NJ: Ktav, 1992.
34. But how does the doctor allocate scarce resources if, for instance, there are two patients only one of whom can be treated? If one was thought to be afflicted on account of sin would priority be given to the other?
35. *Shulhan Arukh Yore Deah* 335:7 and 338:1.
36. BT *Shabbat* 12b.
37. BT *Hagiga* 14b/15a.
38. Responsa *Tashbatz* 263. Much relevant background information may be found in Cadden, Joan, *Meanings of sex difference in the Middle Ages* Cambridge: CUP, 1993.
39. Several responsa in *Iggerot Moshe*, for instance *Even ha-Ezer* 1:71, written in 1959.
40. For the material in this section see Rosner, Fred, and Bleich, David J., eds. *Jewish Bioethics*. New York: Hebrew Publishing Company, 1979; and Alfred S. Cohen, 'Artificial Insemination', in *Journal of Halakhah and Contemporary Society* 13 (1987) 43–59.
41. Tractate *Semahot* l; compare BT Shabbat 151b. This ruling is followed by all the major Codes.
42. *Sefer Hasidim*, #723.
43. Tosafot on BT *Avoda Zara* 18a.
44. BT *Ketubot* 104a.
45. Gordis, Daniel H., 'Wanted – The Ethical in Jewish Bio-Ethics', in *Judaism* 38,1 (Winter 1989) 28–40.
46. Dorff, Elliot N., 'A Methodology for Jewish Medical Ethics', in *Jewish Law Annual Association Studies* Vol. VI, ed. B.S. Jackson and S. M. Passamaneck, Atlanta, Georgia: Scholars Press, 1992, 35–57.
47. Dorffp. 46.
48. Sinclair, Daniel B., 'Law and Morality in Halakhic Bioethics', in *Jewish Law Association Studies* II, ed. B.S. Jackson, Atlanta: Scholars Press, 1986,143–163.
49. Footnote 2 on page 143.
50. Those diagnosed as having Tay-Sachs disease were a case in point; Chief Rabbi Jakobovits' ruling against abortion caused distress and controversy in Anglo-Jewry.
51. Quinlan's parents had requested her physicians to remove the mechanical respirator in order to let their daughter, who was comatose and without hope of recovery, die a natural death. The doctors refused, relying primarily on medical ethics, which they believed prohibited taking an action that might lead to the death of the patient. In 1976 lawyers for the Quinlan family argued successfully before the New Jersey Supreme Court that what was at stake was not medical ethics

but the legal rights of the individual patient to refuse medical treatment that was highly invasive and offered no chance for a cure. In the United States, the Quinlan rationale has been expanded to include the right of all mentally competent patients, whether terminally ill or comatose, to refuse any and all medical treatments.

52. Healing and Wholeness: the Churches' Role in Health. WCC/CMC, 1990.
53. Bleich, J. David, *Judaism and Healing*. New York: Ktav, Yeshivah University Press, 1989. Bleich is particularly interested in the halakhic aspects of the subject.
54. Beit-Hallahmi, Benjamin, *Despair and Deliverance: Private Salvation in Contemporary Israel*. Albany: SUNY Press, 1992.
55. In addition the the sources cited in previous footnotes, the following are helpful:

    Rosner, Fred, *Modern Medicine and Jewish Ethics* 2nd ed., Hoboken NJ: Ktav Publishing House with New York: Yeshivah University Press, 1991.

    Sinclair, Daniel B., *Tradition and the Biological Revolution: The Application of Jewish Law to the Treatment of the Critically Ill*. Edinburgh: Edinburgh University Press, 1989.

    See also the following journals:

    ASSIA (1970–) is published by the Falk-Shlesinger Institute for Medical Research at Sha'are Zedek Hospital, Jerusalem.

    The Regensburg Institute for the Advanced Study of Halakhah and Medical-Halakhic Problems (Jerusalem and Chicago) published its first volume, *Halakha u-Refuah*, edited by M. Hershler, in 1980.

    The Institute for Research in Medicine and Halakhah (Jerusalem) published its first volume, *Ha-Refuah l 'Or ha-Halakha*, edited by M. Stern, in 1980.

II

CHINESE HEALTH BELIEFS

Francesca Bray

The gentleman-scholar of imperial China was commonly said to be a Confucian in his office, a Taoist in his garden, and a Buddhist when contemplating death. Most of the other cases discussed in this volume concern religions which exhibit rather clear boundaries: they have supreme deities who created the world and who impose upon their faithful a set of well-defined beliefs and practices, including in most cases a prohibition on worshipping the gods of other religions. This was not the case in China.

The Chinese referred to what we might call their three main religions as the *san jiao*, three schools or doctrines, namely Confucianism, Taoism and Buddhism. Each primarily addressed a different facet of human existence, none had a supreme deity exacting exclusive allegiance, and on the whole they co-existed tolerably well.[1]

Confucianism, which derived from the ethical and political teachings of the fifth-century BC philosopher Confucius, was concerned with maintaining a productive and stable social order in which the family was the microcosm of the state, the human body the microcosm of the universe. People must work actively to reproduce the social order, fulfilling their proper roles in the interest of their family, their lineage, and good government – it was the duty of a man of talent to serve the state as an official. The fundamental virtue that underpinned the Confucian order was filial piety, the obligation to act respectfully towards one's parents and by extension towards any superior in the social hierarchy (its corollary, human-heartedness, required one to show consideration to those below one). Filiality was routinely enacted in the family rituals of ancestor worship (figure 1). The worst offence against filiality was the failure to provide a male heir to continue the line of ancestral worship.

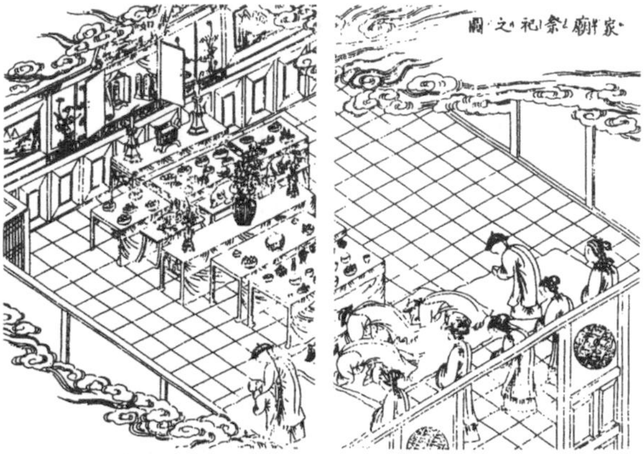

Figure 1: Celebration of an ancestral sacrifice. *Shinzoku kibun* [Recorded Accounts of Qing Customs], compiled by Nakagawa Tadahide (Nagasaki, 1800; facsimile ed, Taipei, Tali Press, 1983), 496–7. The sacrifice is performed by all the couples in the extended patrilineal family, each wife standing behind her husband, and also by the boys. The ancestral tablets can be seen arrayed in the alcove above the altar table, at the back of the room. This would be the central room of the house. The elaborate ordering of the dishes offered to the ancestral spirits varied according to local custom, and etiquette books or household encyclopaedias would often provide diagrams of the patterns that should be formed by the jars of wine and dishes of rice, meat, vegetables and fruit.

An easy-going eclecticism was characteristic of Chinese religious behaviour. But the Confucian doctrine had been officially adopted as the ideology of the state in the first century BC, and when Confucian philosophers or officials believed that this privilege was under threat they would campaign to control or eradicate their rivals. When Confucian philosophers or officials objected to Taoism and Buddhism, it was usually on the grounds that they offended against filiality and respect for the state. Taoist philosophy held that government was unnatural – a village was the largest community that could exist without the coercion and distortion inherent in any attempt at social regulation. During the two millennia of the imperial period (from the unification of the empire under the Qin dynasty in 221 BC to the fall of the Qing dynasty in 1911), Taoist cults led numerous rebellions against corrupt regimes. Even in times of peace, Taoist adepts were more concerned with their own longevity or immortality than with normal procreation, and the celibacy of Taoist monks and nuns was considered by Confucians to be a callous offence against their parents. A celibate clergy, whether Taoist or Buddhist, was considered disgraceful by

Confucians. Otherwise they deprecated Taoism mainly because they associated it with magic, sorcery and superstition.

From a strict Confucian perspective Buddhism too was anti-social, for it treated human desires and emotions, however well-regulated, as a source of suffering that bound individuals to the wheel of reincarnation. Only by renouncing human bonds could one hope to cast off desire and escape existence – Buddhism encouraged celibacy and celebrated neither births nor marriages. Between about AD 500 and 900 many rulers were devout Buddhists, and Confucian literati, afraid that their own doctrines might lose the hegemonic status they had enjoyed for centuries, led strenuous campaigns to convince successive emperors of the pernicious nature of the 'foreign' doctrine. After the establishment of the Song dynasty (960–1279) the hegemony of Confucianism was seldom in doubt; furthermore the majority of Chinese adherents to Buddhism, however pious, did not renounce the world until their procreative years were over and death began to loom in their thoughts. The forms of Mahayana Buddhism that emerged in China offered hope of salvation through piety and good deeds and were extremely popular among women and the elderly. Funerals, the one ritual over which Confucian and Buddhist doctrines competed for jurisdiction, were often a point of tension, for instance in the twelfth and thirteenth centuries when Confucians worried that ordinary people were turning to Buddhist-style funerals and wrote numerous tracts on how to turn the tide.

When asked for his views on the supernatural, Confucius declared that he did not care to speak of gods or ghosts, and Confucianism is in many respects a secular doctrine, whose moral imperatives are grounded in the requirements of social harmony, and which explains the nature of the universe and the workings of history in terms of a cosmology devoid of deities. But how, then, should we think of ancestor-worship? When the Jesuits attempted to convert the Chinese in the seventeenth century they decided to start with the educated elite, a number of whom who were happy to entertain their beliefs, but only on condition that they should not be asked to renounce their ancestral cult. The Jesuits tried – and failed – to convince their brethren in Rome that Confucianism was not a religion but a secular system of ethics, and that the mandarins should be allowed to continue their ancestral rites because they were not really worship, but rather a symbolic performance of social virtues. It is true that in Chinese philosophy the physical movements of ritual were considered indispensable steps in the inculcation of proper emotions, and this was certainly one important aspect of ancestral rituals. Nevertheless most Chinese did not regard the tablets on their altars as mere symbols of the lineage system of descent, but believed that the spirits of their immediate ancestors intervened actively in the affairs of their descendants.[2]

The Protestant missionaries who went to save Chinese souls in the nineteenth century took the opposite approach to the Jesuits and started at the grass roots. Working with the poor and uneducated, many of them hesitated to dignify the belief systems of their hoped-for flocks with the name of religion; they saw only rank and opportunistic superstition, an untidy multitude of gods, ghosts and ancestors holding sway over ignorant lives.[3] Nor was it only the lower orders who lit incense daily at the family shrine but saw no doctrinal contradiction in pasting up images of Bodhisattvas and Taoist deities beside the ancestral tablets. This eclecticism was possible because the *san jiao* represented not conflicting creeds but three philosophies of life, indicative of contrasting attitudes towards human relationships and politics as much as of differing visions of the sacred or the fate of the human soul.

Isolating a category of ideas or behaviour that is distinctly 'religious' is extremely difficult in the case of China, nor is it easy to draw clear boundaries between the cosmological, the divine and the supernatural. As far as ideas about health, sickness and suffering are concerned, lacking any belief in a supreme deity who was both omnipotent and benevolent, the Chinese were not faced with the dilemmas of theodicy discussed in other contributions to this volume. Moreover within a single *jiao* or doctrine, different explanations of sickness and suffering could be found. For a Taoist adept, illness might be inflicted by the celestial administration as a punishment for indulgence, or might stem from a failure in managing one's bodily energy. In either case the adept should be able to cure himself: the elimination of sickness and the enhancement of bodily vitality were indispensable steps in the cultivation of vital and spiritual energy that culminated in unification with the Tao or way, the flow of nature or primordial ruling principle. Within the framework of Confucian explanation, a child's sickness might be attributed to an internal imbalance triggered by exposure to cold, or to the anger of an ancestor. The first etiology required medical treatment, the second a rite to appease the angry ancestor;

most anxious mothers would try both. From a Buddhist perspective the child's sickness might be attributed to sinful behaviour in a previous life, but this did not prevent Buddhists from seeking medical treatment from physicians whose explanations of bodily process were based on a Taoist-Confucian cosmology of energetics.[4]

The central concept in this Chinese cosmology was *qi*[5], sometimes translated as breath, as *pneuma* or as cosmic or vital energy. *Qi* is the active and manifest force of Tao. The *qi* of the natural world transmutes, producing matter and dissolving it, building and transforming, following patterns described by the theories of *yin yang* and the five phases, *wu xing*, explained below. *Qi* was the breath and substance of life, the vital force that maintained the health of an individual, the well-being of the family and the prosperity of the dynasty. Whether in the language of medicine or of any of the other domains understood to affect sickness and health, *qi* was the basic term in which explanations of flourishing and decay were formulated. I have chosen to illustrate one fundamental dimension of Chinese health beliefs by discussing three common formulations of how *qi* impinged upon health and well-being, illustrating a complex intermeshing of categories that we might be tempted to separate into natural and religious. I shall take as my 'historical moment' the Lower Yangzi region in the seventeenth century (at the transition between the native Ming dynasty [1368–1644] and the Manchu Qing dynasty [1644–1911]), but in my conclusion I shall briefly discuss how this 'tradition' has transmuted into Chinese health beliefs in the late twentieth century.

The three perspectives on *qi* and its effects on human well-being that I discuss are: (i) *qi* in medical theory; (ii) *qi* and the practices of 'nourishing life', *yang sheng*; and (iii) *qi* in geomantic practice. All have ancient roots dating back two thousand years or more; by the seventeenth century not only could the theories be said to have stabilized, but also they were widely diffused among the general population, at least in the central Chinese provinces such as the prosperous and highly urbanized Lower Yangzi, whose cities were famous for their scholars, their physicians, and other experts in what one might call applied cosmology, including geomancers.[6] The region was also famous for its book trade, sustained by a flourishing market for household encyclopaedias, treatises on medicine, geomantic handbooks and philosophical excerpts. The level of information that I present here approximates what a seventeenth-century middle-class inhabitant of Suzhou, Hangzhou or Shanghai would have to hand in the various sections of a household encyclopaedia or in sundry handbooks on divination or on the maintenance of health in old age.[7]

Qi in medical theory

Medicine, *yi*, has been recognized as a specialized category of knowledge and practice in China for over two thousand years. Diviners and sorcerers healed the sick in early times, but by the early Han dynasty (206 BC–AD 220) the view emerges that the human body is a microcosm whose processes, normal and abnormal, are patterned by the universal characteristics of *qi, yin yang*, and the five phases, in specific ways determined by its physiology.[8]

The period from 400 BC to AD 300 saw an extraordinary flowering and cross-fertilization of schools of thought, and it makes little sense to try to separate out Taoist and Confucian contributions to the concepts that emerged in medicine. The original impulse to reflect upon and to work with the forces of nature was perhaps more characteristic of the early Taoists than of the early Confucians, yet Confucius was credited with editing the archaic *Book of Changes*,[9] which lays out the theory of *yin yang* transformations and their effects on human affairs for the purposes of divination. So far as medical thought is concerned, one might say that the Taoist approach was more concerned with the numinous, longevity and immortality, while the Confucian approach was more secular and concerned with the routine healing of bodily ills within a human life-span recognized as limited – by the Song dynasty the latter conception of the body and its life predominated in orthodox medicine.[10] Confucian physicians dealt with a mortal body, bounded like our own by the skin, whose disorders were explained without resort to the supernatural and were treated by the application to bodily *qi* of the cosmological principles of *yin yang* and Five Phase theory.

Primordial *qi* fills the cosmos; life comes from an accumulation of *qi* and death from its dissipation. A person must nurture the 'orthopathic' *qi* which regulates his bodily functions, preserving him in good health. But *qi* can also disrupt: 'pathogenic' external *qi* (such as cold, heat, damp or wind) triggers illness, pathogenic internal *qi* can be generated by immoderate appetites or emotions, and the nature of the pathogenic *qi* is what determines the illness's course.

One fundamental concept for analysing the patterning and distribution of *qi* is *yin yang*. To *yin* are attached a complex series of attributes which Westerners sometimes think of as polar opposites of the attributes of *yang*: female/male, dark/light, cold/hot, and so on. But these concepts are always relative. In any one phenomenon *yin* and *yang* are interrelated and changing cyclically: a baby's *qi* is more *yin* than an adult's, an old person's than a young person's, a woman's than the *qi* of a man of the same age. *Yin yang* structures patterns in space and time. *Yang* is more exterior, *yin* more interior. As pathogenic *qi* penetrates the outer *yang qi* which constitutes the defences of the body, it reaches the inner regions of *yin qi* on which the body depends for nourishment and growth, thus becoming more dangerous. A disorder like any natural process will go through active *yang* phases and latent *yin* phases: after a *yang* illness peaks it will enter a *yin* phase for which a different kind of treatment is required. *Yin yang* relations are fundamental, extremely complex, and can be understood at very different levels. As the famous physician Zhang Jiebin wrote in 1624: 'In diagnosis and therapy it is essential to consider *yin yang* first; it is the organizing principle of the medical art. If there is no error with regard to *yin* and *yang*, how can therapy be deficient?'[11]

The term *wu xing*, five phases, used regularly to be translated as 'five elements', but it does not correspond to Greek notion of elements at all: rather, the action of *qi* can be divided into distinct but interrelated categories. The five phases are Wood, Fire, Earth, Metal and Water. Each phase is characterized by a type of action or interaction; in a physiological context Wood denotes a phase of growth and of branching development, Fire a phase of rapid upward dispersal. Each phase is manifested in a characteristic colour, flavour, emotion, physiological system, bodily secretion, etc. The theory of how these phases and their manifestations interrelate is generally known in English as the theory of *systematic correspondence*: the five phases naturally give rise to each other in the order mentioned above (the order of 'mutual production'), and a sequence of 'mutual restraint' also occurs: Wood, Earth, Water, Fire, Metal. The normal physiological phases proceed according to the order of mutual production, while pathological processes are mostly transmitted through the sequence of mutual restraint.

Chinese medical theory was primarily interested in the processes of interaction and transformation that nourished and maintained

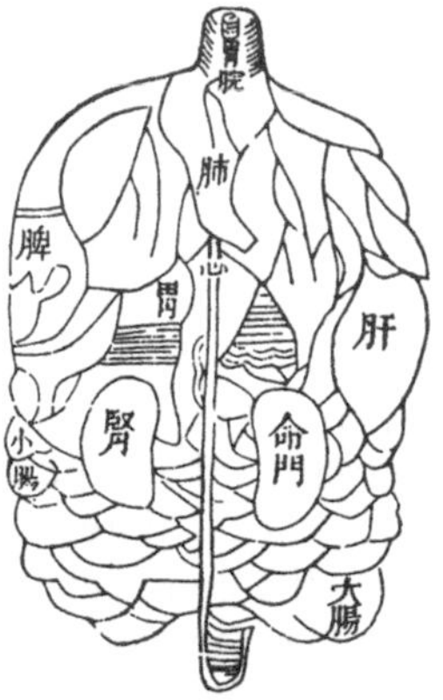

Figure 2: The organ systems of Chinese medicine. From the Ming treatise *Lingshu suwen jieyao* [Basic explanations of the Divine Pivot and Plain Questions] reproduced in Ilsa Veith, *The Yellow Emperor's Classic of Internal Medicine* (Berkeley: University of California Press), Figure 10. As well as the five organ systems, the throat, the stomach and the large and small intestine are shown.

the healthy body, and that also determined the transmission and evolution of disorders. The Chinese organs (Figure 2), Heart, Liver, Lungs, Spleen and Kidney, were not the anatomical entities of modern Western medicine. They were functional systems that connected different levels of the same type of physiological activity. To each of the inner, *yin* organs just named corresponded an outer, *yang* organ: small and large intestine, gallbladder, stomach and bladder. The teeth and hair belonged to the Kidney system, which regulated not only urination but also fertility. Nervousness and premature ejaculation were among the likely symptoms of a Kidney disorder; yellow sclerae, problems with muscles and sinews and outbreaks of anger were symptoms of a Liver disorder. Each system corresponded to one of the five phases, the Heart to Fire, the Spleen to Earth, the Lungs to Metal, the Kidneys to Water and the Liver to Wood, and the organ systems interacted with each other, absorbing food, producing energy, nourishing and building, lubricating and eliminating, in sequences determined by five-phase theory.

Qi in its various physiological manifestations circulated through the body, ensuring the function of the organ systems and maintaining a balance between *yin* and *yang* within them. The *qi* within the body took forms which in English are often referred to as *vital substances*, but which were processual as much as material. The

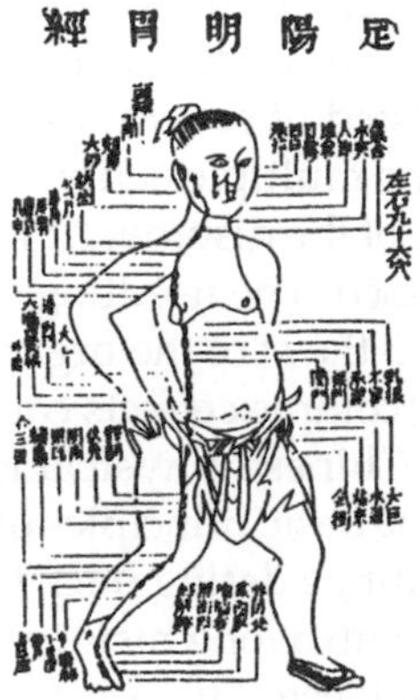

Figure 3: The 'bright yang' acupuncture tract of the stomach. From the same source, reproduced in Veith, *Yellow Emperor*, Figure 20. Forty-eight acupuncture points are shown.

yang component, simply called *qi*, was the non-material energetic *qi* that stimulated processes of transformation; one *yin* component of *qi*, called *xue*, blood, governed circulation, nourishment and growth. Another vital substance, often translated as 'essence', *jing*, encompassed both the nourishing forces and substances derived from food, and the reproductive forces and substances (including semen) necessary for procreation. The vital substances circulated through the body in regular cycles along the *circulation tracts* or *meridians* (*jing luo* or *jing mai*), connecting the elements of each of the inner and outer organ systems (Figure 3). These tracts included the anatomically identifiable blood vessels and the invisible tracts along which *qi* in its various manifestations circulated. Each organ system had its own pulse, which passed through the wrists at a different location or depth, and one of the principle techniques of diagnosis was a careful reading of the circulation of *qi* through the different pulses.

When a person fell sick, then, the deepest level of the problem was a dysfunction of *qi*. The physician observed the patient, elicited symptoms and made a careful reading of the pulses in order to diagnose both the type and the stage of the disorder. To restore the proper levels, balance and movement of *qi*, the physician would treat the patient with drug prescriptions and/or acupuncture. Some drugs acted directly on bodily *qi* or on its manifestations as blood or other fluids, building it up, stimulating its activity, breaking up stagnation; some shifted the balance between *yin* and *yang*, warming or dispersing heat; some acted on a particular organ system, each of which had its own role in the production of healthy *qi*. A prescription consisted of several drugs carefully dosed and combined to produce the multiple actions required by this particular patient at this stage of the disorder; it was adjusted or changed as the treatment progressed. The needling of an acupuncture point stimulated and regulated the *qi* of the organ system corresponding to that tract, so similarly complex effects could be produced.

For many centuries Chinese physicians have adhered to the image of the body and the basic principles of therapy contained in a canonical corpus of writings dating back to the Han dynasty. But China is a vast country with a long history, and not suprisingly the classical tradition was subjected to numerous different interpretations and challenges. The medical profession flourished as never before in the lower Yangzi cities of the seventeenth century, and we see a multitude of theoretical and therapeutic variants on the tradition in the writings of physicians competing to establish a reputation, to secure a clientele, or to meet the challenge of epidemics and of diseases endemic to the South (but unknown to the authors of the canonical texts, composed when the Northern plains were still the Chinese heartlands). Some believed the Heart system predominated in bodily processes, others were convinced it was the Spleen; some included ginseng in all their prescriptions, others swore by aconite. Acupuncture was considered by most respectable seventeenth-century physicians as a crude alternative to drug prescription, and it was left to quacks with a low-class clientele. Meanwhile the genteel public of the Lower Yangzi cities went in fear of *yin* depletion and clamoured for tonics and medicines to replenish *yin*, even though (the Suzhou physician Lu Maoxiu remarked darkly) they had not the slightest idea of what *yin* and *yang* were.[12]

Qi, alchemy and the nourishing of life

There was a ready market in the seventeenth century for works on *yang sheng*, literally 'the nourishing of life', which presented techniques for the cultivation of *qi* considered to prolong life and preserve health and vitality in old age. Some of the techniques included in *yang sheng* were shared with orthodox medical theory, including ideas about healthy nutrition and its role in producing beneficial *qi*. Others derived rather from a tradition of Taoist esoteric techniques (internal and external alchemy, *nei dan* and *wai dan*) originally intended to achieve immortality rather than longevity.

The goal of the medieval Taoist adept in search of immortality was not just to maintain his or her mortal body in normal health but to lighten and eventually discard it so that the immortal body could soar free into the empyrium and unite with the Tao.[13] Medicine attempted to restore the normal processes of *qi*, alchemy manipulated and reversed the normal courses of *qi* to purify it and prevent its loss. The immortality techniques of external alchemy consisted of the preparation and ingestion of alchemical elixirs containing gold and the rare and expensive mercury compound cinnabar (*dan*); these poisonous concoctions helped many noble or imperial adepts in medieval times to shuffle off their mortal coil. But although many experts considered that true immortality could only be obtained by the ingestion of gold, from the Tang dynasty (618–907) adepts more frequently chose techniques of internal alchemy that mobilized and cultivated primordial *qi* through the body's own resources, thus avoiding both the expense and the dangers of *wai dan*. The set of alternative techniques included refraining from the consumption of cereals, thus allowing one to absorb primordial *qi* effectively;[14] meditation and breathing techniques for absorbing primordial *qi*; and gymnastic exercises, *dao yin* ('guiding the *qi* and stretching the body'), meant to sustain long periods of meditation and facilitate *qi* absorption. These techniques permitted the adept to control *qi* in such a way as to cure any sickness they might develop – a good Taoist had no need of physicians, and *qi gong* techniques could also be used to channel *qi* so as to cure others who were sick. The gymnastic exercises also formed the basis of the various martial arts.[15]

As a person ages their vital *qi* becomes progressively less *yang* and more *yin*; alchemical techniques for nourishing life attempt to reverse this trend. The adept absorbs *qi* from the environment, which is why exercises and meditation are best performed at times of day (sunrise) or in places (on mountaintops, beside trees) where the *yang qi* of nature abounds. They are designed not to circulate the *qi* through the body according to the normal physiological patterns of medicine, but to concentrate and direct it through a body conceived of as a divinely inhabited landscape. While the natural direction of flow within the medical body is downwards, *nei dan* exercises reverse the flow of *qi*, 'driving the water uphill' (Figure 4,

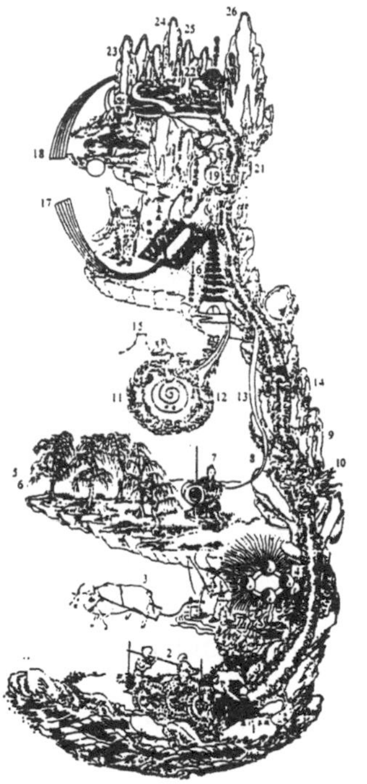

Figure 4: The body as a Taoist landscape. Despeux, *Immortelles*, Plate 5. 1: inversion of the water flow; 2: water-mill driven by yin and yang.

points 1 and 2) through the three 'cinnabar fields', from the lowest, just below the navel, where breath is transformed into essence, *jing*, through the median centre at the heart, where essence is transformed to spiritual energy, *shen*, and finally to the upper centre in the head, where spiritual energy reverts to the pure vacuity or blankness of the primordial Tao. In this spiritual processing of *qi*, the normal sequences of influence between the five organ systems are reversed.[16]

Techniques of alchemy and 'nourishing of life' are greatly concerned with *qi* in its fertile manifestation as essence, *jing* (which also denotes semen), and here again they turn the goals and techniques of medicine on their head. Seventeenth-century medical theory held that menstrual regularity was an essential prerequisite of female health and fertility, that both male and female procreative capacities depended on moderate but normal appetites and consumption, and that conception only took place if both partners reached orgasm simultaneously, mingling male and female

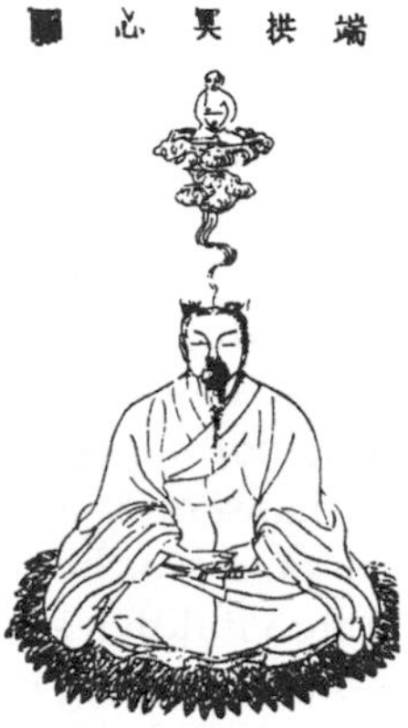

Figure 5: The *yang shen* emerges in meditation. From the sixteenth-century *Xingming guizhu* [Jade principles of innate nature and vital force], reproduced in Despeux, *Immortelles*, Plate 6.

essence.[17] The goal of inner alchemy, however, was not to engender living offspring, but to conceive a cinnabar embryo and give birth to an immortal child, the *yang* spirit, *yang shen* (Figure 5). In the 'reversing of the water' shown in Figure 4, water stands for the sexual organs and their powers, and the reversal of its flow for the channeling upwards of essence. This non-sexual form of procreation, in which men as well as women could give birth, required abstinence from sexual activity to avoid the dispersal of procreative *qi*, and the reversing of its normal flow – thus while menstrual regularity was a sign of health and fertility in a normal woman, a woman practising *yang sheng* techniques aimed for the cessation of the menses as an indispensable preliminary to more advanced techniques of nourishing inner life.[18]

An alternative to sexual abstinence, at least for men, was to reverse the emission of *yang* essence during sexual intercourse: refraining from orgasm and ejaculation, the man drove his semen back and upwards to the lower cinnabar field. The rejuvenating effects of this technique were still further enhanced by taking very young women as sexual partners, bringing them to orgasm and absorbing into one's own body the powerful primordial *qi* which they discharged in the form of female essence at the moment of climax.[19]

The commoner Confucian scholars who superseded the aristocracy as China's governing elite during the Song dynasty condemned many of the internal and external alchemical practices, and the goals they embodied, as immoral. Confucian orthodoxy insisted that immortality should be achieved not at the level of the individual but at that of the lineage: one became immortal through one's children; refraining from procreation was a serious offence against one's ancestors because it cut off the line. In a responsible and mature adult, sexual extravagance and sexual abstinence were equally to be condemned – the ingestion of cinnabar, like sleeping with bevies of virgins, was not approved and was confined to extravagant emperors or to Taoist nuns and monks[20] – but once one was past the age of procreation, it was both natural and desirable to wish to cultivate one's *yang* vitalities so as to live to a ripe and healthy old age. Treatises on nourishing life in which medical prescriptions for health mingled with alchemical techniques of *qi* control circulated widely in sixteenth- and seventeenth-century China, but for the general reader the goal was not immortality but longevity.

Qi in geomancy

Just as bodily *qi* could be regulated or directed to enhance individual health and vitality, so too the *qi* of the landscape could be manipulated to improve the well-being of its inhabitants. The Chinese science of siting, *dili* (the principles of the earth) or in more vulgar terms *fengshui* (wind and water), was used for the siting and design of graves and buildings. 'All human dwellings are at sites (*zhai*) . . . Sites are the foundations of human existence.'[21]

To summarize the principles of geomancy: a site for a house, pagoda, or grave was chosen at a favourable spot in the landscape, determined in part by orientation but also by the configuration and form of hills and streams, boulders and trees. As well as the site, the details of design (the arrangement of buildings within the compound, the height of roofs and gates) were all designed to channel cosmic *qi* for the benefit of the occupants and to exclude harmful influences. Since cosmic *qi* was constantly shifting according to seasonal and astral cycles, time was a factor that had also to be taken into account: a site was a locus in time as well as space, and a configuration that was inauspicious at one date might be auspicious at another. In order to relate a specific landscape to the cosmos the geomancer used a special compass in which some three dozen rings of symbols of *yin yang*, five phase and other systems of cosmological correspondence surrounded a needle 'vitalized by earth *qi*'. This enabled him to locate the arteries or tracts of the soil through which *qi* circulated; the seventeenth-century *Dili renzi xuzhi* [What everyone should know about geomancy] typically insists on the parallels between acupuncture and geomancy, and the shared techniques and terminology.[22]

Although geomancy was used for civic purposes to benefit a community (as in the construction of local administrative buildings, pagodas or temples) or even the whole empire (when imperial dwellings were concerned), the most frequent use of geomancy was in the siting of family houses and graves, in which cases it was used to direct auspicious *qi* for the benefit of the patrilineal family dwelling within the house, and the lineage to which it belonged. Geomantic techniques did not increase cosmic energy, they simply channelled it in new directions. Siting could therefore be a means of attracting fortune for one's own family at the expense of others, and was quite commonly used competitively: 'Let one man in a village build a fraction too high; let him build a window or a door which can be interpreted as a threat; and he has a struggle on his hands.'[23]

The well-being of a family depended on the health, fertility, happiness, wealth and wordly success of its members. At the core of this well-being was fertility: without healthy sons to continue the line it would become extinct; with numerous succcessful sons and grandsons, it would become glorious. The social body whose health was tended by the practices of geomancy included living family members, dead ancestors, and descendants not yet born. When a family bought land to build a new house, the geomancer's first task was to locate the ancestral altar, which was the heart of the house, its most auspicious place (Figure 6). If auspicious *qi* was successfully directed to the ancestral tablets on their altar then the rituals of ancestor worship would continue unbroken and the line would achieve immortality through descent (Figure 1).

While a family who could afford it would call in a professional geomancer to locate the altar, the carpenter was the cosmic expert who fine-tuned the geomantic details of the house (and who even decided on basic location and orientation for poor families who could not afford the services of a geomancer). The carpenter's main instrument for geomantic calculations was a wooden measure known as Lu Ban's foot-rule. Lu Ban was the patron saint of carpenters, and every carpenter's workshop had its own copy of the *Lu Ban jing* (Lu Ban's canon), containing computation and construc-

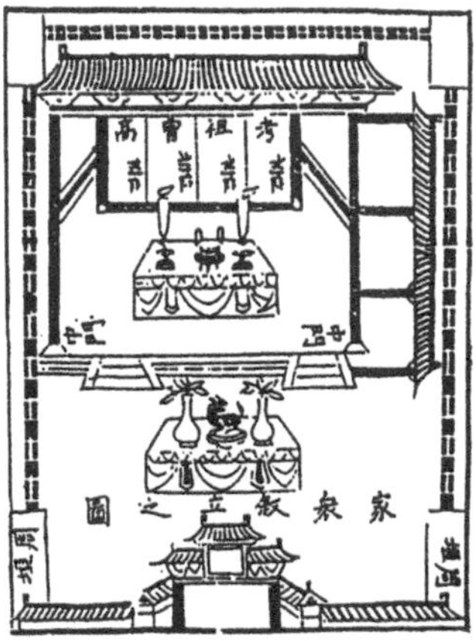

Figure 6: Family offering hall. From the 1602 edition of the *Zhuzi jiali* [Zhu Xi's *Family Instructions*], 7/78a, reproduced in Patricia B. Ebrey, *Chu Hsi's Family Rituals: a Twelfth-Century Chinese Manual for the Performance of Cappings, Weddings, Funerals, and Ancestral Rites* (Princeton: Princeton University Press), 7. Zhu Xi was probably the most influential of the Song dynasty philosophers who reformulated Confucianism into a new orthodoxy that lasted till the twentieth century. In this illustration the characters on the screen at the back of the offering hall indicate the genealogical order in which the tablets should be arranged.

tion techniques for buildings and articles of furniture as well as rhymed and illustrated rules of thumb for good and bad building configurations.[24]

In a family house the general configuration of roof heights and pitches was designed to capture and channel *qi* towards the altar. The relative height and length of main buildings and wings was important because it affected the relations between family members. The first section of the *Lu Ban jing* clearly illustrates the principles of ranking inherent in this sympathetic magic:

> A family temple is not like an ordinary house: whether or not sons or brothers will attain wisdom depends wholly on this place. Moreover the rear hall, main hall, corridors and triple gate may increase only gradually in height, since only then do sons and grandsons know their rank; and does not the younger aspire to the older's place. The builder must take careful notice of this.[25]

Roofs were not the only architectural features perceived as affecting the proper relations between kin. The *Lu Ban jing's* third section of illustrated rhymes on layout and siting contained precepts familiar

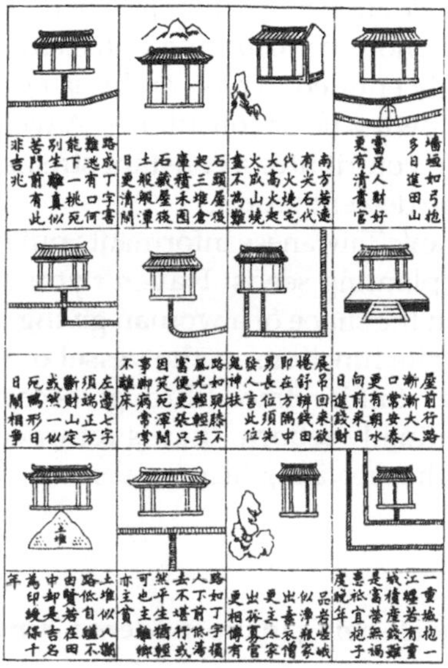

Figure 7: Lucky and unlucky building forms. Page of diagrams from the *Carpenter's Canon* depicting lucky and unlucky building forms; *Huitu Lu Ban jing* [The illustrated canon of Lu Ban], 1808, 3/14b–15a. This is a late Qing edition of the Ming text of the *Lu Ban jing*.

to everyone in seventeenth-century China through their reproduction in encyclopaedias and almanacs (Figure 7). As well as concerns about money, health, the number of sons and the virtue of daughters, these rhymes repeatedly refer to family harmony. In a house with two gates 'there will be no love between father and son', and 'young and old will put each other to shame'; pointed brackets over the roof bring continuous arguments; if the road in front of the house curves like an ox-tail, 'there will be division between father and son'.[26]

The family dwelling garnered and directed environmental *qi*, grave-siting affected the power of the ancestor's decaying bones which transmitted fertile *yang qi* to his living descendants. In medical theory the father endows his offspring with *yang qi* transmitted through his male essence in the form of semen at the moment of conception. This single, instantaneous contribution forms the child's spirit and intelligence, the immaterial aspects of his being, whereas the mother contributes his material, *yin* form which takes shape and grows as she feeds it first, during gestation, with her blood (the *yin* form of bodily *qi*), and then, after birth, with breast-milk which is a transformation of blood. A living man, then, makes one instantanous contribution to his child's existence; furthermore he is only entitled to pass on his *yang qi* through sexual congress with his own wife or concubines. A well-buried ancestor, on the other hand, contributes a constant stream of *yang qi* which fecundates a whole descent-group.

As one of Seaman's Taiwanese informants put it in 1983: 'To bury the bones is like planting seeds. Haven't you seen that Chinese graves are made in the shape of a woman giving birth?' As Seaman notes, 'The gravesite functions as the vessel of transformation in which the material stuff is refined [through decay] and from which the dead are eventually reborn, that is returned to the world as newborn infants, thus realizing in a social sense, at least, the goal of Taoist alchemy.'[27]

Qi, health and well-being in the modern Chinese world-view.

The preceding examples of *qi* and its relation to human health, reproduction and well-being illustrate the difficulty of disentangling the religious from the secular in Chinese cosmological reasoning. Medicine, alchemy and geomancy all applied to human affairs the basic logic of a natural philosophy concerning the Tao, *qi*, and its patterns of transformation. Confucianism, Taoism and Buddhism could all expound and apply this philosophy without reference to any deity; on the other hand between them the three doctrines could provide an array of ancestral spirits, celestial immortals, bodhisattvas, ghosts and demons, supernatural agents who rewarded and punished humans according to the different moral criteria of the three doctrines. Two points deserve emphasis. First, medicine, alchemy and geomancy were, in a sense, life sciences that applied the same natural principles, though in different ways and at different levels, to increase human well-being. Medicine was concerned with physical health while in alchemy bodily control was a step on the way to spiritual perfection; geomancy brought health, wealth and fertility to a family group rather than concentrating on the individual. All three, however, saw the essence of human well-being as health, fertility and immortality, attainable through the manipulation of cosmic *qi*. Second, then, medicine, alchemy and geomancy (to which we should add divination) are the 'life sciences' that evolved from the overarching 'astrobiological' conceptualization of human life typical of Chinese culture, not only in the imperial period, but still at the end of the twentieth century.[28]

After half a century of humiliation at the hands of the Western powers, Chinese radicals and reformers at the turn of the last century believed that it was essential to substitute science for the energy-sapping superstitions of traditional thought. After the fall of the Qing dynasty and the establishment of the Republic in 1911, the Nationalist government attempted to follow Japan's example and replace traditional Chinese medicine with Western medical science.[29] The other sciences of *qi*, geomancy, divination and alchemical gymnastics, were also frowned upon, but in fact the Nationalist government never had sufficient real control to suppress any of them; the traditions survived and evolved, whether among conservative scholars and nativists anxious to preserve the essence of Chinese philosophy, or among ordinary people untouched or unpersuaded by the virtues of Western modernity.

Many Nationalists had taken on muscular Christianity as part of the modern, progressive package offered by the West, but although they disapproved of China's old religions they had not eliminated them. With the establishment of the People's Republic of China in 1949, however, came a new regime of evangelical atheism and scientism under which Christian practices as well as the cults of the three doctrines became counter-revolutionary. Interestingly enough, though, the Chinese Communist Party could not dispense with *qi*. For one thing, despite the Marxist commitment to internationalism, the regime wanted to emphasize the Chineseness of modern China and its historical rootedness. Validating the traditional Chinese sciences was an important element in this strategy – hence the scientization of *qi* discussed below. Moreover, faced with the gigantic task of modernizing a poor and war-shattered country without support from abroad, the government realized that it would be necessary for China to 'stand on two legs', bringing in and developing whatever modern science, technology and expertise it could afford, but in the meantime capitalizing on indigenous resources wherever possible. The effects were particularly important in medicine. The socialist government naturally wanted to offer basic health care to the whole population, and this could not be achieved within a reasonable time-span unless the state integrated traditional medicine into its health services.[30]

Even after consolidating the development of a network of biomedical personnel and institutions the state has continued to encourage the parallel development of biomedicine and Chinese medicine. The public continues to favour the latter in many circumstances, particularly in cases of infertility, debility and complicated chronic ailments, where explanations in terms of *qi* easily trump the falterings of biomedicine. The Marxist government pushed for the extirpation of the 'superstitious' elements of Chinese medicine and encouraged what one might call the scientization of Chinese medical theory and practice – including the explanation, wherever possible, of Chinese medical concepts in the terms of Western science, the investigation of the pharmacological properties of Chinese materia medica, and the application of Chinese medical etiology and therapy to biomedically defined diseases like cancer. Although selective inclusions within the modernized Chinese medicine from the tradition of *yang sheng* and internal alchemy could be justified, the process of secularization generally required that medicine be distinguished and disembedded from the traditional web of complementary *qi*-manipulations, for instance geomancy and divination, where science found it difficult to justify the action of landscape or stellar conjunctions on the human body. The status of acupuncture benefited especially from the syncretism of Western science and Chinese cosmology. The acupuncture tracts or meridians are now systematically related to the nervous system; *qi* is measured and even explained in terms of electrical impulses in neurones or other cells; it is common to stimulate acupuncture needles with electric currents, or even to substitute laser beams. It is not as easy to translate the explanations of traditional disorder etiology or of drug therapy into the terms of biomedical science, but here too a cheerful syncretism is in evidence. At the end of the twentieth century Chinese medicine is in a flourishing state – it has not only withstood the challenge of biomedicine, but has drawn strength from it.

Despite the official efforts that have been made to tame *qi* by reducing it to the terms of Western science, it remains a powerful and potentially subversive force in Chinese society. Under the Maoist regime the population at large was expected to rise at dawn to practise *tai ji quan* and *qi gong*, mobilizing *qi*, that peculiarly Chinese form of energy, to strengthen their bodies and focus their minds in the service of the Revolution.[31] But mindful of *qi gong's* long history of rebellion as well as of its revolutionary potential, the state carefully controlled the schools of *qi gong* on offer, banning any which appeared to encourage subversive forms of expression.[32]

Now the population is ageing, the techniques of 'nourishing life' are in widespread demand, and since the New Economic Policies were introduced in 1979 the state has allowed private practices to offer what is essentially an uncontrolled range of health services. Control over religious practices has also relaxed and both *san jiao* and Christian cults are flourishing;[33] these include *qi gong* healing cults which are proliferating at a conspicuous rate. While science has been invoked rather successfully to justify the manipulations of *qi* in acupuncture, no satisfactory scientific explanation has been advanced for the esoterica of *qi gong* healing. Nevertheless, since it appears to work and since the theory of *qi* overlaps between indigenous medicine and *qi gong*, *qi gong* therapists are now to be found practising in Chinese hospitals. This does not worry the Chinese government, but *qi gong* healing cults are still regarded with considerable suspicion and go under constant threat of suppression. Meanwhile in private practice medical specialists can once again cross the boundaries into divination and other non-orthodox explanations of *qi*, for which there are large and enthusiastic clienteles, and under the new entrepreneurial economic order *fengshui* has become as popular in China as it is in Southern California.[34]

In contemporary Chinese society the astrobiological conceptualization of human life and well-being has taken on new life: far from being supplanted by Western science *qi* energy has acquired a new para-scientific aura, allowing it to be successfully harnessed to the new needs of a rapidly developing economy and society. Still today, in the minds of most Chinese, individual health and family well-being both depend on an efficient management of *qi*.

NOTES

1. As a good general introduction to the various schools of Chinese philosophical and religious thought, see William Theodore de Bary (ed), *Sources of Chinese Tradition* (New York: Columbia University Press, 1960). On the reworking of classic Confucian thought into neo-Confucian orthodoxy in the Song dynasty (960–1273) see Robert P. Hymes and Conrad Schirokauer (eds), *Ordering the World: Approaches to State and Society in Sung Dynasty China* (Berkeley: University of California Press, 1993). On Taoism see Anna Seidel and Holmes Welch, *Facets of Taoism* (New Haven: Yale University Press, 1979) and on

Buddhism, Erik Zürcher, *The Buddhist Conquest of China* (Leiden: Brill, 1972).

2. See the various papers in James L. Watson and Evelyn S. Rawski (eds), *Death Ritual in Late Imperial and Modern China* (Berkeley: University of California Press, 1988).
3. For a sympathetic account of this variety see J.J.M. De Groot, *The Religious System of China* (Leiden: E.J. Brill, 6 volumes, 1892–1910).
4. Buddhists shared with Confucians a sense of the moral obligation to relieve suffering. Although the first duty of an educated Confucian was to serve the state as an official, when this was not possible – and there were far more candidates for office than there were posts – an honourable alternative was to practise medicine: 'If you cannot become a good minister, then you may serve as a good physician', said the Song statesman Fan Chengda. If filiality led many Confucians to acquaint themselves with medicine (for a knowledge of medicine enabled one to take care of one's parents as they grew old and frail), human-heartedness encouraged them to treat non-family members, or to set up charity hospitals. During the Song dynasty the state trained physicians, set up hospitals and distributed free prescriptions during epidemics out of concern for the welfare of the common people (and in order to wean them from 'superstitious' and less politically sound alternatives). Buddhist charities also routinely offered medical services for the poor, and it seems that rivalry between the two may have driven their development. See for example Angela K.C. Leung, 'Organized medicine in Ming-Qing China: state and private medical institutions in the Lower Yangzi region', *Late Imperial China* 8, *1* (1987), 134–66.
5. Also spelled *ch'i* in the Wade-Giles romanization and *chhi* in the works of Joseph Needham; the Japanese form is *ki*.
6. A fourth and closely connected form of applied *qi* cosmology which I do not have space to include here was astrology and divination, which related individual fate to the movements of the heavens. On the everyday uses of divination in China see Richard J. Smith, *Fortune-Tellers and Philosophers: Divination in Traditional Chinese Society* (Boulder: Westview Press, 1991), and William A. Lessa, *Chinese Body Divination: its Forms. Affinities and Functions* (Los Angeles: United World, 1968).
7. On the culture of the seventeenth-century Lower Yangzi see, for example, Timothy Brook, *Praying for Power: Buddhism and the Formation of Gentry Society in Late-Ming China* (Cambridge, Mass.: Harvard University Press, 1993); David Johnson, Andrew J. Nathan and Evelyn S. Rawski (eds), *Popular Culture in Late Imperial China* (Berkeley: University of California Press, 1985); and Dorothy Ko, *Teachers of the Inner Chambers: Women and Culture in Seventeenth-Century China* (Stanford: Stanford University Press, 1994).
8. For a general historical survey of Chinese medicine see Paul Unschuld, *Medicine in China: A History of Ideas* (Berkeley: University of California Press, 1985). Ted Kaptchuk, a biomedical doctor who trained in Chinese medicine, offers a very accessible account of medical theory and technique in *The Web that has no Weaver: Understanding Chinese*

Medicine (New York: Congdon and Weed, 1983). Other useful but more detailed works include Manfred Porkert, *The Theoretical Foundations of Chinese Medicine* (Cambridge, Mass.: MIT Press, 1974), and Nathan Sivin, *Traditional Medicine in Contemporary China* (Ann Arbor: Center for Chinese Studies, University of Michigan, 1988). On acupuncture, see Lu Gwei-Djen and Joseph Needham, *Celestial Lancets: A History and Rationale of Acupuncture and Moxa* (Cambridge: Cambridge University Press, 1980).

9. The *Yijing* or *I-ching*, of which numerous translations exist, the best-known of which is still probably that by Richard Wilhelm.
10. As an example of the shift in emphasis, in the earliest *materia medica* drugs were classified into three categories: the upper class of drugs lightened the body and helped confer health and immortality, while the lower class were used as a response to the onset of disease. This Taoist classification was abandoned in Song and later *materia medica* for systems more directly based on the curative qualities of drugs, categorized according to a system of correspondences between *yin yang* and *wu xing*; see Paul Unschuld, *Medicine in China: a History of Pharmaceutics* (Berkeley: University of California Press, 1986). The great Tang physician Sun Simiao (581?–682), also an eminent Taoist and alchemist, was famous for having insisted that moderation (of appetites and emotions) was essential to avoid sickness. This view was later endorsed by Confucian physicians as an appeal for balance and for avoiding disruptions of *qi*, that is to say as a secular reasoning about the roots of disease. However Ute Engelhardt argues that Sun himself was probably influenced in his etiology by the teachings of the Taoist Celestial Masters, who considered that disease was primarily caused by moral trangression; Ute Engelhardt, '*Qi* for life: longevity in the Tang', in Livia Kohn (ed.), *Taoist Meditation and Longevity Techniques* (Ann Arbor: Center for Chinese Studies, University of Michigan, 1989), 294.
11. Sivin, *Traditional Medicine*, 62.
12. Yuan-ling Chao, 'Medicine and society in Late Imperial China: a study of physicians in Suzhou' (Los Angeles: unpublished Ph.D. dissertation, Department of History, UCLA, 1995), 39–40. See also Christopher Cullen, 'Patients and healers in Late Imperial China: evidence from the *Jinpingmei*', *History of Science* xxxi (1993), 99–150.
13. Although most immortals were male, women also figure in the biographies of adepts and immortals; see Catherine Despeux, *Immortelles de la Chine ancienne: Taoïsme et alchimie féminine* (Puiseaux: Pardès, 1990), including table p. 75. On Taoist internal and external alchemy more generally, see also Catherine Despeux, *La moelle du phénix rouge: santé et longue vie dans la Chine du XVIe siècle* (Paris, Guy Trédaniel, Editions de la Maisnie, 1988) Livia Kohn, *Taoist Meditation*; Joseph Needham, *Science and Civilisation in China*, vol. V.5, *Spagyrical Discovery and Invention. Physiological Alchemy* (Cambridge: Cambridge University Press, 1984); Kristofer Schipper, *The Taoist Body* (Berkeley: University of California Press, 1994); and Nathan Sivin, *Chinese Alchemy: Preliminary Studies* (Cambridge, Mass.: Harvard University Press, 1968).

14. Sima Chengzhen (647–735), the twelfth patriarch of the Highest Clarity school of Taoism, 'points out that when one begins to abstain from cereals and lives only on the absorption of *qi*, one first has to undergo a phase of weakening and decay. However, as soon as orthopathic *qi* becomes predominant in the body, all illnesses vanish. After nine years of further practice, one can rightfully be called a Realized One'; Engelhardt, '*Qi for life*', 273.
15. Chinese boxing (*tai ji quan*) and *qi gong* ('making *qi* work') evolved from the *daoyin* tradition.
16. See Despeux, *La moelle du phénix*, 44–8.
17. The Kidney system, which corresponds to the Water phase, regulates sexual activity and fertility and is responsible for the production of essence, *jing*, of which the male form is semen and the female the orgasmic secretions.
18. Just as men must avoid losing primordial *qi* through any emission of seminal essence, so women must perform exercises to achieve a gradual suppression of the menses, 'beheading the red dragon', and for female adepts as for men the culmination of self-cultivation is giving birth to the *yang shen* – not from the womb but from the head; Despeux, *Immortelles*, 243–68, 276–8.
19. On the contrast between Taoist and Confucian attitudes towards sex and procreation, see Charlotte Furth, 'Rethinking Van Gulik: sexuality and reproduction in traditional Chinese medicine', in Christina K. Gilmartin, Gail Hershatter, Lisa Rofel and Tyrene Whites (eds), *Engendering China: Women. Culture. and the State* (Cambridge, Mass.: Harvard University Press, 1994), 125–46. On female and male ideals of fertility, and on architectural and medical techniques for enhancing reproductive *qi*, see Francesca Bray, *Technology and Gender: Fabrics of Power in Late Imperial China* (Berkeley: University of California Press, 1997).
20. It appears that several Ming princes and emperors pursued immortality through *wai dan*, since alchemical apparatus was found in their tombs; Despeux, *Immortelles*, 73 n.8.
21. Steven J. Bennett, 'Patterns of the sky and earth: a Chinese science of applied cosmology', *Chinese Science* 3 (1978), 1–26; this quotation from the *Site Classic* is given on p. 2. A key work on geomancy is Stephan Feuchtwang, *An Anthropological Analysis of Chinese Geomancy* (Vientiane: Vithagna, 1974). The relations between geomantic and medical views of health and fertility are explored in a splendid article by Gary Seaman, 'Winds, waters, seeds and souls: folk concepts of physiology and etiology in Chinese geomancy', in Charles Leslie and Allan Young (eds), *Paths to Asian Medical Knowledge* (Berkeley: University of California Press, 1992), 74–97.
22. Seaman, 'Winds, waters', 79, 86.
23. Maurice Freedman, 'Geomancy', *Proceedings of the Royal Anthropological Institute 1968* (London, Royal Anthropological Institute, 1969), 14; Hugh Baker, *Chinese Family and Kinship* (London: Macmillan, 1979) gives a detailed account of a modern case of fighting with *fengshui* in Appendix II. Despite their a-social, selfish nature, because they

benefited family descent groups the principles of siting and orientation were not necessarily incompatible with Confucian values, indeed Song neo-Confucian philosophers developed cosmological systems which overlapped with geomancy in many respects; Feuchtwang, *Anthropological Analysis*, 16 f.

24. See Klaas Ruitenbeek, 'Craft and ritual in traditional Chinese carpentry', *Chinese Science* 7 (1986), 1–24; and Klaas Ruitenbeek, *Carpentry and Building in Late Imperial China: A Study of the Fifteenth-Century Carpenter's Manual Lu Ban Jing* (Leiden: E.J. Brill, 1993).
25. Ruitenbeek, *Lu Ban jing*, 197.
26. Ruitenbeek, *Lu Ban jing*, 278 f.
27. Seaman, 'Winds, waters', 87.
28. 'Astrobiological' is the term coined by Paul Wheatley, *The Pivot of the Four Quarters* (Chicago: Aldine, 1971), 414–19. For a concise account of the evolution of medicine in twentieth-century China see Francesca Bray, 'The Chinese experience', in J.V. Pickstone and Roger Cooter (eds), *The Encyclopaedia of Twentieth-Century Medicine* (London: Harwood, 1999).
29. See Margaret Lock, *East Asian Medicine in Urban Japan: Varieties of Medical Experience* (Berkeley: University of California Press, 1980) on the suppression and revival of traditional medicine in modern Japan.
30. On health policies in twentieth-century China see Judith Banister, *China's Changing Population* (Stanford: Stanford University Press, 1987); Ralph Croizier, *Traditional Medicine in Chinese Society: Science. Nationalism. and the Tensions of Cultural Change* (Cambridge, Mass.: Harvard University Press, 1968); and AnElissa Lucas, *Chinese medical modernization: comparative policy continuities. 1930s–1980s* (New York: Praeger, 1982).
31. The revolutionary anthem *The East is Red* likens Chairman Mao to the rising sun of the Revolution; by practising *tai ji quan* at dawn, the Chinese masses were not only absorbing the most powerful cosmic *qi*, they were also absorbing revolutionary loyalty and zeal.
32. Ute Eberhardt, 'Movement and tranquility in *qi gong*', unpublished paper presented at the 6th International Conference on the History of Chinese Science, Cambridge, 1990.
33. See for example Kenneth Dean, *Taoist Ritual and Popular Cults of Southeast China* (Princeton: Princeton University Press, 1993).
34. Judith Farquhar describes one small-town private physician who specializes in 'difficult diseases' which he diagnoses through a combination of systematic correspondence analysis and divination, another who combines her more conventional therapies with *qi gong* methods; 'Market magic: getting rich and getting personal in medicine after Mao', *American Ethnologist* 23, 2 (1996), 239–57.

MEDICINE AND MARTYRDOM: SOME DISCUSSIONS OF SUFFERING AND DIVINE JUSTICE IN EARLY ISLAMIC SOCIETY

Lawrence I. Conrad

The problem of suffering poses difficult questions within any society and at any time in history, in that the often indiscriminate scope of suffering, its apparent pointlessness and lack of recompense, the extremes of physical and emotional anguish it involves, and so forth, are universal concerns. Within monotheistic religion, however, the problem is particularly acute, since the existence of suffering in the world raises the question of how the one God can be characterized as just and merciful when the strict monotheistic insistence on His exclusive power and omnipotence tends to associate Him with responsibility for the miseries of the world.[1]

In the formative period of Islamic history in the seventh and eighth centuries this issue provoked detailed discussions, the particular character and urgency of which reflect several underlying factors that should be borne in mind. First, the Islamic efforts to come to terms with the problem of suffering were in an important sense more difficult than those posed to Judaism and Christianity in earlier times. Islam, for example, does not and never has proposed a broken God-man relationship requiring the healing ministrations of a redeemer figure, or locating the cause of human suffering in man's sinfulness.[2] Islam has also defined itself as the culmination of monotheistic religion in general. It views Judaism and Christianity as previous dispensations of the word of God, and indeed, as revealed by God and hence in origin identical to Islam; the present differences from Islam are attributed to distortions and errors introduced subsequently.[3] The self-image of Muslims from a very early point has thus been that of a community dedicated to the preservation of a pristine monotheism allowed to go astray by their predecessors, whose religions are simply distortions of Islam and now stand superseded. As the central doctrine of Islam is the omnipotence and unity of God, Islam has always taken a very strict position in any matter that might compromise this doctrine. The starting point for all Islamic discussions of suffering is therefore the fact of God's omnipotence and unity, and all solutions to problems posed by the fact of suffering are strictly bounded by a belief that God is the author, creator, and determining agent in all things, regardless of their character or consequences.

Second, early Islam's efforts to deal with the problem of suffering faced challenges not only from other monotheistic faiths, but also from its own past and from external opponents. In pre-Islamic Arabia, the trials and vicissitudes of human life were put down to 'fate' and the machinations of demons and spirits,[4] to which society responded with prophylactic and therapeutic magic of various kinds and a broad range of superstition and folklore.[5] After the rise of Islam this lore was of course opposed as diminishing the role of God as the author of all things, but the effort to limit the influence of pre-Islamic beliefs was hampered by the fact that the *jinn*, spirits very commonly blamed for misfortune, are mentioned in the Qur'ān and could therefore not be dismissed as fantasy. Even today, the belief that the *jinn* are responsible for afflictions and misfortunes of various kinds is extremely widespread in the Islamic world.[6]

Islam's defenders also had to cope with the very serious challenge of Manichaeism, an Iranian dualist religion that explained the course of events in the world in terms of the eternal conflict between opposing forces and essences – light vs. darkness, good vs. evil, and so forth. Manichaeism was not a popular religion at the grass-roots level in early Islamic times, but it did gain adherents among government functionaries and bureaucrats at the heart of the Islamic polity. In religious terms, its challenge was not just to Islam, but to monotheism in general, for challenges put to Muslims could as easily be aimed at Christians and Jews, and indeed, the other monotheistic faiths had long been involved in polemics with Manichaeism before the rise of Islam.[7]

Third, it is interesting to see how medical matters played a role in these discussions. The fact that this should have been the case is, on the face of it, distinctly unsurprising. But in the seventh and eighth centuries there was as yet no Arab-Islamic medical tradition, if by 'tradition' is meant a body of systematic knowledge with its own technical vocabulary discussed and taught by certain savants with the acknowledged credentials to do so. And even if specialized medical literature were to hand for this period, it is unlikely that it would be very informative on issues of concern to us here. It is in practical medical ethics, where doctor-patient relations are discussed, that we would expect to find the subject of suffering considered, but for the medieval Arab-Islamic tradition only one such work survives, and it does not discuss the matter.[8] Elsewhere the question of the suffering patient is hardly considered. As in other traditions, and as also in modern times, professional medical literature sought to explicate its field in a narrow sense, and raised the subject of the suffering patient in the same technical manner that all else was discussed. The authors of the medical compendia have much to say about pain, but only as a medical phenomenon to be categorised, classified, elucidated and confronted, and not as a dilemma at some other level. In his chapter on surgery, for example, al-Zahrāwī outlines the most horrific procedures in a completely detached and dispassionate fashion, and raises the subject of suffering only insofar as this is necessary to warn the surgeon about situations and procedures where he may anticipate some difficulty with his patient.[9]

The 'medical' material for early Islamic times is thus not medical in a professional sense, but rather comprises popular discussions in which broad religious and theological questions are raised by medical problems in society at large. For the seventh and eighth centuries, these problems revolved primarily, though not exclusively, around the great pandemic of plague that periodically ravaged the Near East between 541 and 749 AD.[10] The spectre of widespread and repeated loss of life, the demise of the faithful along with the unbelievers, and the apparent pointlessness of the pain and misery caused by these outbreaks, raised a stream of questions related to suffering. These were discussed and answered in a corpus of literature known as the *ḥadīth*, reports on the sayings and deeds of the Prophet Muḥammad and other respected early Muslims. It is in this material, and other related sources, that the relevant discussions are to be found.

In sum, then, larger questions posed by epidemic disease led Muslims in early Islamic times to embark on a broad-ranging discussion of issues pertaining to suffering. The range of possible solutions was defined and circumscribed by the fact that at the same time the same scholars were engaged in a crucial process of self-definition among Muslims, and a defense of their faith both from old traditional beliefs and from challenges from outside the Muslim community and from outside monotheistic religion.

But what exactly does it mean to investigate ideas of suffering and medicine in this formative period? To begin with, classical Arabic has no word that exactly conveys the notion of suffering. Related terminology certainly abounds, as in the words *waja'* ('pain'), *'adhāb* ('torment'), *muṣība* and *balā'* ('affliction', 'calamity'), *ḍarrā'* ('distress', 'adversity'), and *sharr* ('evil', 'iniquity', 'injury'). But to this the reply is surely that suffering has to do with its victim's reaction to adversity, and is not to be identified as the adversity itself. Suffering is not death, disease, hunger, privation, evil, or any other situation or cause of adversity *per se*. Rather, suffering is the emotional response to extreme adversity that one considers to be undeserved, unrequited, unexplained, or unrelieved, or some combination of these. The adversity can be more directly focused on someone else, or on a group or community with which one identifies. Thus, if one reads of a man returning to his home in al-Baṣra to find only his father and aged grandmother, who meet him in tears and tell him that all the rest of his family has been carried away in a recent epidemic,[11] the presence of a word for 'suffering' is not required to conclude that this is the emotion that the survivors feel. In fact, much of our information on such encounters was collected in plague and consolation treatises specifically compiled for the purpose of offering relief from suffering.[12]

The Qur'ānic Context

The religious context against which discussions of suffering and medicine took place can be investigated in a wide variety of sources. Unfortunately, however, almost all of these are from later times, and in important ways they retroject the thinking of their own day back into the period of Islamic origins. If we wish to know what sort of religious thinking there was in the time of Islam's infancy that would have been relevant to our concerns here, our main source must be the Qur'ān itself.[13]

As already intimated earlier, the Islamic scripture places its primary emphasis on the omnipotence of God. God is the Lord of all being;[14] to Him belong the East and the West, and whithersoever you turn, there is the face of God.[15] There is no god save He, and all that is in the heavens and the earth is His.[16] He is all-knowing: not a leaf falls but He knows it, and His knowledge is shared with no one.[17] His will carries all before it: no mercy He extends can be restrained, and no mercy he withholds can be secured.[18]

Though the Qur'ān does have a version of the Fall of Adam and Eve and their expulsion from the Garden of Eden,[19] God's relationship with man has not been fundamentally affected by this, for God subsequently forgave Adam, guided him anew, and revealed His word to him, recognizing that humanity can be unmindful.[20] When God decided to appoint a vice-regent to rule the earth in His name, he offered his covenant first to the heavens and the earth, but these shrank back in fear and declined; then He offered His covenant to man, who foolishly accepted.[21] Mankind is insolent and prides himself on what he thinks is his self-sufficiency;[22] he is fickle,[23] and having been granted all the earth and the good things in it, he shows little thanks.[24] But all of Adam's descendants nevertheless begin their lives in a state of righteousness and good terms with God: at the Creation, God summoned all the souls that would ever be born and asked them: 'Am I not your Lord?,' to which they answered: 'Yes, we so testify.'[25] This means that human beings are without exception Muslims at birth, though upbringing may subsequently result in them following another religion. The relationship between God and man, in other words, though fraught with inconstancy on man's part, is a relationship postulated in positive terms of opportunity and responsibility rather than a complete breakdown requiring restoration from without.[26] Indeed, the Qur'ān rejects the doctrine of intercession, though in later times it was to become very important. On the Day of Judgment, each individual will be held accountable for his or her own deeds; no one will be able to call on kinsmen or family members to plead for him with God.[27]

But what of suffering? How does the Qur'ān address the problem of upholding God as the author of all things when some of these things cause His creatures great torment and misery? Faced with the spectre, frequently mentioned in the Qur'ān, of the failure of previous peoples to maintain God's word unsullied and His message undiluted, the Islamic scripture opts firmly and unequivocally for divine omnipotence: 'No affliction befalls, except it be by the leave of God.'[28] God raises up and forgives whom He wills, and casts down and chastises whom He wills.[29] Some mistaken individuals are inclined to attribute all the good they enjoy to God, and all the adversity that befalls them to their enemies; they should be told, rather, that 'everything is from God.'[30] 'No affliction befalls in the earth or in yourselves, except that it be in a book (i.e. ordained) before We create it. That is easy for God.'[31]

The faithful are left in no doubt that just as God is capable of incomparable mercy, He can also deliver utter destruction. Various peoples, such as the Egyptians under Pharaoh, 'Ād, and Thamūd, were utterly destroyed by God, and those cast into Hell for their wicked deeds will remain there in torment forever. But other passages moderate this bleak picture with a message of hope:

> Did you suppose that you should enter Paradise without there had come upon you the like of those who passed away before you? They were afflicted by misery and hardship, and were so convulsed that the Messenger and those who believed in him said: 'When comes God's help?' Ah, but surely God's help is nigh.[32]

There may also be some consolation in the fact that all peoples suffer: does the believer not know that all towns to which prophets have been sent have endured affliction?;[33] does he think that he is the first ever to suffer injury?[34]

But what is the point of all this? If God's omnipotence is the first consideration, it is not the only one. If God is one, then His creation is also one and must operate in accordance to God's plan; and as God is not only omnipotent, but also munificent and merciful, this creation must work according to a plan that is discernibly God's and therefore, by definition, harmonious and beneficial for mankind. The Qur'ān repeatedly stresses this argument from design, and when doubters demand miracles, it often refers them to the marvels of God's creation, which clearly reflect God's harmonious and merciful plan.[35]

Suffering too is made a part of God's plan, in which it functions as a kind of test of faith. Most of mankind does not realise that afflictions have this function,[36] though scripture repeatedly insists on it. One particularly clear example is the following:

> Surely We will try you with something of fear and hunger, and diminution of goods and lives and fruits; yet give thou good tidings unto the patient who, when they are visited by an affliction, say: 'Surely we belong to God, and to Him we return;' upon those rest blessings and mercy from their Lord, and those – they are the truly guided.[37]

Elsewhere it is stated that every soul shall taste of death, and will be tried with evil and good for a testing. And in these and other passages the desired response is equally clear: a Muslim should be patient and trust in the mercy of God.

The doctrines elaborated in the Qur'ān were reinforced by numerous examples of pious and righteous men who managed to live their lives in accordance with them. The archetypical example of this is of course Muḥammad himself, whose early career in Mecca, where he was reviled and threatened by all but a minority of the community, is depicted in terms of patient fortitude in the face of adversity – in essence, actualizing the tenets of faith as articulated in the scriptures entrusted to him by God.[38] But he was not the first to have done so. As in the Judeo-Christian tradition, the Qur'ān presents the suffering Job as a model for the believer to emulate:

> And Job – when he called unto his Lord, 'Behold, affliction has visited me, and Thou art the most merciful of the merciful.' So We answered him, and removed the affliction that was upon him, and We gave his people, and the like of them with them, mercy from Us, and a reminder to those who serve.[39]

Elsewhere the same themes of exemplification and remembrance are likewise stressed:

> Remember also Our servant Job; when he called to his Lord, 'Behold, Satan has visited me with weariness and chastisement' 'Stamp thy foot! This is a laving-place cool, and a drink.' And We gave to him his family, and the like of them with them, as a mercy from us, and a reminder unto men possessed of minds; and, 'Take in thy hand a bundle of rushes, and strike therewith, and do not fail in thy oath.' Surely We found him a steadfast man. How excellent a servant he was! He was a penitent.[40]

The example of Abraham is similarly deployed as a model of how the Muslim should react to situations of adversity. Referring to the uselessness of idol-worship, Abraham is made to argue as follows:

> They are an enemy to me, except the Lord of all Being who created me, and Himself guides me, and Himself gives me to eat and drink, and, whenever I am sick, heals me, who makes me to die, then gives me life, and who I am eager shall forgive me my offence on the Day of Doom.[41]

In later discussions the role of such *exempla* is made very prominent. Stories about them were collected into didactic compilations,[42] and entire biographical dictionaries were dedicated to their exemplary lives.[43]

Challenges to the Islamic Position

Even without the challenge posed by epidemic disease, there were serious obstacles in the way of the Qur'ānic approach to suffering outlined above. First, there was a marked tendency for old traditional views to continue after the rise of Islam, even if they posed major contradictions to the tenets of the new faith. Ancient Near Eastern medical folklore was a case in point. Throughout the region, it was generally believed that the *jinn* and other spirit forces of various kinds were responsible for illness and especially epidemics. The *jinn* were considered to be material beings of the physical world; they were visible to human beings and related with them in various ways. One could negotiate with the *jinn*, gain benefits from them, and defeat them, and some individuals even claimed to be married to a *jinnī* or to be the child of a *jinnī*. Many kinds of illness and misfortune were ascribed to the activities of the *jinn*; and continuing a belief already attested in ancient Greece, Canaan, and Babylonia,[44] it was considered that epidemics were caused by the *jinn*, who spread the disease from one victim to another with jabs of poisoned weapons.[45] Such lore has proven extremely tenacious in the region; as recently as 1947, Egyptian peasants tried to protect themselves from a cholera epidemic by snapping the air with wooden scissors to frighten away the *jinn*,[46] and practical manuals on how to protect oneself from them or drive them out of one's house, or away from one's wife and children, find a ready market to this very day.[47] Nor were the *jinn* alone in the medical pantheon. Contagion, for example, was regarded as a malevolent living willing entity.[48]

To combat these spirit forces, people quite naturally resorted to the supernatural. Incantations were worn as amulets to protect an individual, or were written into magic bowls and kept in the house to protect the premises from spirit intruders. Other types of amulets provided alternative forms of protection: animal teeth were worn to ward off spirits afraid of being bitten, bells or bits of jingling metal were considered to make sounds obnoxious to the *jinn*, and amulets containing menstrual rags or bones of the dead were believed to disgust spirits and thus also keep them at arm's length.[49] Though quaint or ridiculous-looking from an outsider's perspective, such systems of belief did possess their own internal logic. Someone with a fever-blister, for example, would carry a sieve around his village on his head asking for donations of scraps of food, which would then be tossed in front of a dog to be eaten.[50] Here the idea was one of transference; the spirit responsible for the blister would be attracted to the food in the sieve, and thus would be killed and eaten by the dog when the sieve's contents were thrown on the ground. A caliph offered a cup of water by a leper at the roadside, we are told, drank the water for fear of contracting leprosy[51]. The story is surely apocryphal, but the point is the prophylactic measure brought to bear. To refuse the cup of the leper would be to reject the hospitality of a wretched subject with nothing else to offer; this insult would surely be noticed by the spirit of 'contagion', whose attention would thus be drawn to the caliph and lead to his infection despite his precautions.

The fact that the *jinn* were acknowledged in the Qur'ān guaranteed that beliefs in the role of such spirits would be extremely difficult to counter.[52] And indeed, for quite some time it seems not to have been noticed that there was a problem, since there was even a tradition from the Prophet Muḥammad stating that the plague was caused by the *jinn* or by spirits motivated by one's enemies.[53] Nevertheless, opposition did eventually arise, on the grounds that attribution of events to spirits implied that events could occur independent of the will of God, and thus detracted from His omnipotence.[54]

The other challenge was external, and came, as noted above, from Manichaeism.[55] The polemic between the two sides is difficult to trace, since the Manichaeans lost and their literature was largely destroyed in its original form; for the Islamic period, what we now know about their arguments is limited to quotations cited by Muslims in order to refute them.[56] Citations attributed to the early 'Abbāsid litterateur and caliphal adviser 'Abd Allāh ibn al-Muqaffa' (d. *ca*. 140/757) and refuted in a treatise against him by the Zaydī *imām* al-Qāsim ibn Ibrāhām (d. 246/860) are especially important for present concerns. Here Ibn al-Muqaffa' is said to have argued against the omnipotence, justice and mercy of God by pointing out that His creatures turn against Him, revile Him with impunity, and kill His prophets and apostles, while God causes His creatures to fall ill and torments them with the diseases He has unleashed upon them, so that His Creation is reduced to complete ruin.[57] The anonymous author of the *Dalā'il wa-l-i'tibār* attributed to al-Jāḥiẓ speaks along similar lines and specifically attributes to the Manichaeans the belief that loathsome adversities and calamities could not afflict mankind if the universe followed the will of a merciful clement God, a denial that the order of nature reflects the will and purpose of God, and indeed, a denial that there is any meaningful order to nature at all.[58] In order to mount a systematic defense of the faith from such attacks, he marshals a wealth of examples with which he can demonstrate or argue for the physical world as the manifestation of a perfect divine plan. But the discussions began at a time when the plague was recurring all across the Near East, and it was the plague that served as the exemplary vehicle for the Islamic position in general.

Traditions on the Plague

The Islamic response to the challenge of plague is presented primarily in the form of traditions attributed to the Prophet Muḥammad, and to Muslims through the ages these sayings and deeds have been regarded as authentic reports on what Muḥammad actually said and did. In some cases this may be so, though the sources available to us do not allow us to trace traditions much earlier than the mid-first century, i.e. at least two generations after the Prophet's death in 632.[59] In the main, however, it is clear that the corpus cannot all be from Muḥammad, since parts of it routinely contradict other parts, or are clearly derivative from some earlier formulation of the same problem. That is, what has survived to us is a continuum of discussion that took place from the seventh to the ninth centuries, with the Prophet cited in order to give one's position sufficient authority to stand against that of a rival, who has also cited the Prophet for his point of view.[60] Non-Muslims were quick to point out what was going on,[61] but Muslims as well acknowledged it; the great traditionist al-Bukhārī (d. 256/870), for example, conceded that in his critique of traditions for inclusion in his own *ḥadīth* compilation, he was able to accept as authentic only a tiny minority of the traditions known in his day.[62] Modern scholarship questions the vast majority of even this small corpus.[63]

An early stage of the debate, one that I have discussed elsewhere, denounced contagion as false, not because Muslims denied the transmissibility of disease, but because contagion had been conceived of as a living willing force within the animistic pantheon of ancient Arabia, and thus, as we see once again, had to be denied as a diminution of God's omnipotence.[64] But if there is no 'contagion', and if the spirit world has no power to afflict mankind with epidemic disease, then how does epidemic disease arise? The answer of the early thinkers is to drive home the point that had been motivating the earlier discussions all along: epidemic disease – and here the plague is the archetype usually evoked – is an affliction visited upon man by God. The earliest arguments along these lines seem to be those in which the Prophet or one of his Companions makes the point that God has inflicted pestilence upon other peoples in the past: epidemic disease is a chastisement (*rijz, 'adhāb*) sent by God upon 'a group of the Israelites', 'those who were before you', 'the righteous who were before you', 'certain communities which have gone before you', or even just 'a group'.[65] These discrepancies in identification of the group in question are in themselves revealing: the point is clearly not whom in particular God chose to chastise, but rather the workings of divine will in general in times of adversity.

The favoured example of this, commonly cited in *ḥadīth* compendia, Qur'ān commentaries, and plague treatises, is the story of Ezekiel. In a tale reminiscent of the Biblical story of this prophet and the valley of dry bones,[66] the Islamic version is largely exegesis of Sūrat al-Baqara (2), vv 243–44:

> Hast thou not regarded those who went forth from their habitations in thousands, fearful of death? God said to them: 'Die!' Then He gave them life. Truly God is bounteous to the people, but most of the people are not thankful.[67]

The explanation given for this verse is that a certain people suffered an epidemic of plague from which some fled while others did not. Those who stayed were devastated by the pestilence, while those who had left remained safe. So the next time an epidemic struck, all of them fled; but before they reached the haven where they expected to be safe, God's angels struck them all dead in one fell swoop. Later, the prophet Ezekiel passed by the place where their bones lay (variants have it that he was of this people and had gone out in search of them), and as a token of mercy God allowed him to recall them to life.[68]

The Old Testament version is clearly a metaphor prophesying the restoration of the kingdom of the Israelites (pestilence has nothing to do with this and does not appear in the account), but in the

Islamic version the tale teaches the lesson that ancient peoples too discovered that as epidemic disease comes at the bidding of God, flight from it is futile and a sign of weak faith. Just as God smites the Muslims with epidemic disease, so also in past times he has smitten other favoured peoples and righteous persons. This is, of course, very similar to one of the Qur'ān's replies to the question of why mankind suffers in the first place. It also strikes an implicitly positive note, again similar to what we have seen in the Qur'ān, in that it suggests that such affliction is not a sign of implacable divine wrath or impending universal destruction, as well may have seemed to be the case during many of the severe plague epidemics of Umayyad times, or from accounts of these outbreaks.

But if epidemic disease is a manifestation of the activity of God and comes as a matter of divine decree, then is there any point to efforts to avoid epidemics, and indeed, are not such acts defiance of the will of God? The answer here is essentially that flight is indeed futile and calls one's faith into question. Many reports in *ḥadīth*, Qur'ānic exegesis, and history stress this, and a favoured motif, one that stresses the absurdity of attempts to escape, is that of a man fleeing on his donkey, as if a dumb animal will save him from God's decree.[69]

This stage of the discussion has yet to encounter the crucial question of how a merciful and benevolent God could send upon man a scourge which kills the righteous with the wicked, the faithful Muslim with the unbeliever: how can it be that God allows the righteous to suffer along with the wicked? As we have seen above, it is precisely this challenge that was thrown back at the Muslims by the Manichaeans. The basic problem of why man is allowed to suffer from delibitating and painful illness had already been addressed in a tradition stating that 'every illness has its cure', or more to the point, 'God has sent down no illness without also sending down a cure for it', the sole exception being death itself.[70] While perhaps sufficient for addressing single or individual cases of suffering and death, this was inadequate as an explanation during outbreaks of plague, when entire families were destroyed, neighborhoods could lose the majority of their populations, and whole villages could be snuffed out.[71] Clearly God had not sent down a cure for bubonic plague.

This problem is addressed in a new set of traditions in the *ḥadīth* literature: the plague, or *ṭā'ūn*, is an affliction which God visits upon whomsoever He wills, but while it is a painful chastisement for the unbeliever, it is a martyrdom for the Muslim.[72] A believer who perishes of the plague or, by analogy, certain other diseases, will not have to wait for the balance of his good and evil deeds to be reckoned on the Day of Judgment, but will be granted immediate admission into Paradise.[73] Lists of categories of martyrdom quickly came into circulation, but since the plague victim appears far more frequently than any other category, it seems likely that the challenge of pandemic plague was the starting point for these lists, and indeed, for this entire line of discussion.[74] Its earliest expression is probably its simple assertion. In a tradition of the Baṣran scholar 'Āṣim ibn Sulaymān al-Aḥwal (d. 142/760), the famous Companion Anas ibn Mālik inquires about the cause of someone's death; when told that he died of the plague, Anas responds: 'The Apostle of God said: '"The plague is a martyrdom for every Muslim."'[75] This is then developed into other traditions in which it is asserted that the plague victim will enjoy status as a martyr equal to that of a slain warrior in God's cause, that if a Muslim remains in his home and does not flee from an epidemic his steadfast faith will gain him a martyr's reward should he be stricken, and that while the plague is a martyrdom for the Muslim it is a painful chastisement for the unbeliever.[76]

Here we can see the argument proceeding on from the consideration of the omnipotence of God to the issue of His justice. That is, to propose that epidemics come from God secures the case (where epidemic disease is concerned) for His all-encompassing dominion; but in Umayyad times the plague was of greatest severity in the towns, where Arab Muslims were concentrated. The ensuing slaughter of believers during these epidemics would thus now call into question any argument for God's justice. A solution is thus found in the proposition that while death in an epidemic simply hastens the unbelieving on their way to Hellfire, it is an act of divine mercy for Muslims, who will as a result proceed directly to Paradise regardless of the measure of their earthly deeds.

It is interesting to find that these discussions of martyrdom make little reference to the explicit remarks on the subject in the Qur'ān. In one passage in the Islamic scripture, the principle of martyrdom as a status awarded to slain warriors is established:

> If you are slain or die in God's way, forgiveness and mercy from God are a better thing than that you amass; surely if you die or are slain, it is unto God you shall be mustered.[77]

Elsewhere it is more explicitly stated that this status involves admission to Paradise:

> And those who are slain in the way of God, He will not send their works astray. He will guide them, and dispose their minds aright, and he will admit them to Paradise, that He has made known to them.[78]

Finally, in a third passage we find that this admission is immediate:

> Count not those who were slain in God's way as dead, but rather living with their Lord, by Him provided, rejoicing in the bounty that God has given them, and joyful in those who remain behind and have not joined them, because no fear shall be upon them, neither shall they sorrow, joyful in blessing and bounty from God, and that God leaves not to waste the wage of the believers.[79]

These verses confirm that God does not fail to recompense those who risk their lives by fighting for His cause, and then are killed. The question here is one of earned reward. But the lists of martyrs concern people who die of plague, in childbirth, in a fire, in a collapsed house, by drowning and so forth: i.e. not individuals who have knowingly put their lives at risk and thereby have earned a reward, but rather the righteous and suddenly overwhelmed innocent who would have expected a better fate at the hands of God. The problem here is God's justice and mercy, and again one sees the crucial importance of the underlying issue under consideration in determining how a topic will be discussed, where the argument will lead, and what evidence will be brought to bear. In the martyr lists, knowledge of the category of 'martyr' is simply presumed; the object is to assert that consideration for God's justice and mercy, and for the validity of the argument from design, requires that the category be extended into new areas.[80]

Wensinck long ago argued that the Islamic doctrine of martyrdom parallels that of eastern Christianity so closely that the former can be said to derive from the latter.[81] While this clearly seems to be the case in some respects, in others the Islamic formulation of the idea marked a radical departure from earlier Judeo-Christian tradition. In the latter, epidemics were often regarded as God's punishment for sin[82] and certainly no merit accrued to an individual by virtue of falling victim to an epidemic.[83] As the doctrine of original sin meant that all mankind is inherently sinful, the problem posed to Christian thinkers by the suffering of the believer was less acute, in that the possibility of an utterly innocent victim was less prominent.[84] Islam also broke with its monotheist predecessors in asserting that martyrs proceed to Paradise in their physical bodies. This was later brought into line with the Christian position, i.e. that only the martyrs' souls gain immediate felicity, while their bodies must await the Judgment Day in their graves;[85] but the Qur'ānic passages cited above clearly presuppose an immediate physical mustering to Paradise, and early references to Muslim martyrs make it clear that in earliest Islamic times the faithful were not troubled by this proposition.[86] The early Islamic view also excluded intercession by martyrs,[87] while earlier Christian thought had accepted this possibility.[88] Early Muslims can thus be said to have taken up the general view of martyrdom that prevailed in the seventh-century Near East, but quickly adapted it to suit the differing doctrines and priorities of their own community.

The Elite vs. the Masses in Medicine and Martyrdom

It would be a grave error to suppose that it was only in *ḥadīth* that the debate over the medical aspects of suffering were pursued. Medical topoi and metaphors were in fact commonly used to illustrate the arguments of theologians and philosophers in discussions of theodicy,[89] in which human suffering is often characterised in terms of loathsome medication, painful or distasteful therapies, the agony, indignity or disfigurement of a long illness, and undeserved death from disease. The author of the ps-Jāḥiẓian *Al-Dalā'il wa-l-i'tibār*, for example, uses medical examples to argue that suffering does not disprove the argument from design. To the challenge that a merciful Creator God solicitous of the welfare of mankind would not allow or cause certain of his creatures to lose some of their faculties, he replies that this teaches them discipline, serves as a lesson to others, and invites them to bear up patiently and await God's rewards in Paradise.[90] To the Manichaeans' argument that the outbreak of epidemics demonstrates that the world is not the work of a merciful clement Creator, he replies that without God such disasters might well become permanent and engulf the whole world, as opposed to remaining temporary afflictions limited to certain places. Comparing the sceptics to children who object to bitter medicine, he argues that the life of ease encourages arrogance and profligacy, while adversity reminds man of his duties to others and to God. To the objection that epidemics sweep away the good with the wicked, he retorts that calamities remind the good of God's blessings in better times past, while chastising the wicked and encouraging them to repent.[91] It is perhaps significant to find that the anonymous author of this treatise does not argue that victims of epidemics are martyrs; i.e. his position is more characteristic of Christian rather than Muslim views, and thus suggests that we have to do here with a Christian rather than a Muslim author.

Al-Qāsim ibn Ibrāhīm's scathing refutation of Manichaean criticisms of Islam and monotheism in general offer an insight into how Muslim thinkers responded to the challenge. The Zaydī Imām turns immediately to the argument from design, asserting that all aspects of human character and physiology, down to the smallest details, are the handiwork of God, who endows man with what he needs for protection from spiritual and physical harm. Ibn al-Muqaffa''s claims are the sort of thing one hears from cunning jailbirds, crude storytellers, and lunatics, and people should beware of taking seriously any of his claims that God gratuitously afflicts His creatures with deafness or blindness, forces them into disobedience, obstructs them in their faith, or causes them illness and torment for no reason or cause. Citing the examples of Job and Abraham, which we have seen already in the Qur'ān, he argues that God responds to supplications and enlightens with His guidance. It is from God that a sufferer ought to seek relief; when affliction ends it is God who has raised it, and if a victim dies it is God who will restore him to life.[92]

The great theologian al-Ghazālī (d. 505/1111) is an especially valuable example of the use of medical metaphors and motifs among Muslim thinkers. In his magnum opus, the *Revival of the Religious Sciences*, he tells a story in which Jesus passes by a blind leprous cripple and exclaims: 'Praise be to God for sparing me from that with which he has afflicted so much of mankind.' Jesus asks the leper from what affliction he has been spared, and the man replies that at least he is better off than those who have no knowledge of God.[93] Elsewhere al-Ghazālī uses a medical metaphor to argue that suffering is often misunderstood. A mother, for example, might not want to have her small son cupped, while the father insists on the procedure despite the discomfort and fear involved for the child. A dull-witted critic will say that the mother has shown compassion for her son, but the sagacious observer will recognise that as cupping is good for the boy, the father is displaying consummate compassion, while the mother is an enemy in disguise.[94]

If intellectually appealing to the elite, these formulations opened the way to endless counterarguments and tangential developments at a level beyond the comprehension of non-specialists,[95] and in any case they did not offer the sort of response that the ordinary believer found either engaging or fulfilling. While agreeing that the tenets of Islam could and should be defended, the man in the street was more concerned with issues of immediate and personal relevance to himself, his family, and his community: Why do I suffer? How can my people deserve such affliction? Can it be that God really does not care what happens to His faithful?

In its response to such basic questions the doctrine of martyrdom was simplicity itself. Drawing a stark dichotomy between those who believe and seek to follow God's will on the one hand, and mortal sinners and unbelievers on the other, it promises victims from the former immediate admission to the joys and gratifications of Paradise while assuring them that sinners and infidels are simply being hurried on their way to Hellfire. God's omnipotence and authorship of all that is are upheld while at the same time His boundless mercy and absolute justice are similarly sustained. The focal point for the doctrine was the case of the plague victim, of which there were endless examples through the first 130 years of Islamic history, when the early discussions were taking place. But this example quickly led to the extension of the category, and that it was regarded as paradigmatic and not exclusive to the questions posed by the plague is clear from the many other kinds of martyrs that join it in the martyr lists: victims of pleurisy or dysentery (neither of which could have been precisely identified), drowning, fires or collapsed buildings (i.e. earthquakes?), those killed in defense of their property or family or fighting injustice, women who die in childbirth or as virgins, those who die in foreign countries or in accidents 'in God's cause', and so forth.[96] In the face of overwhelming suffering and disaster, then, the assurance of personal salvation remains unblemished.

The appeal of these and similar formulations can be seen in their staying power through the history of Islam. During the great fourteenth-century Black Death and the plague epidemics that followed it, the arguments and doctrines articulated in early Islamic times were as prominent as they had been in the days of their origins,[97] and even today the medieval Arabic plague treatises are published with a more didactic and hortatory rather than historical agenda in mind.[98] Discussions of medical ethics refer heavily to *ḥadīth*, law, and Qur'ānic exegesis,[99] and publications of the traditions of the Prophet pertaining to medicine are undertaken with devotional and practical use in mind.[100] No less so now than in the early centuries of Islam, the overarching concern continues to be that if adversity and suffering are to be confronted, this must proceed in acknowledgement that no human catastrophe can call into question the omnipotence and all-embracing will of God, or place in doubt His justice, mercy, and solicitude for the welfare of mankind.

NOTES

1. For discussions of suffering in Islamic contexts, see John Bowker, *Problems of Suffering in the Religions of the World* (Cambridge, 1970), pp. 99–136; W. Montgomery Watt, 'Suffering in Sunnite Islam', *Studia Islamica* 50 (1979), pp. 5–19.
2. E.E. Elder, 'The Development of the Muslim Doctrine of Sins and their Forgiveness', *Moslem World* 29 (1939), pp. 178–88; Georges C. Anawati, 'La notion de "péché originel" existe-t-elle dans l'Islam?', *Studia Islamica* 31 (1970), pp. 29–40; Fedwa Malti-Douglas, 'Faces of Sin: Corporal Geographies in Contemporary Islamist Discourse', in Jane Marie Law, ed., *Religious Reflections on the Human Body* (Bloomington and Indianapolis, 1995), pp. 36–45.
3. J.-M. Gaudeul and R. Casper, 'Textes de la tradition musulmane concernant le *taḥrīf* (falsification) des écritures', *Islamochristiana* 6 (1980), pp. 61–104.
4. Werner Caskel, *Das Schicksal in der altarabischen Poesie* (Leipzig, 1926); Helmer Ringgren, *Studies in Arabian Fatalism* (Uppsala, 1955); Toufic Fahd, 'Anges, démons et djinns en Islam', in *Génies, anges et démons*, Sources orientales VIII (Paris, 1971), pp. 153–214.
5. See, for example, Ibn Abī Sarḥ (wr. 274/887–88), *Kitāb al-rumūz*, ed. S.M. Ḥusayn in *Maiallat al-majma' al-'ilmī al-'arabī bi-Dimashg* 11 (1931), pp. 641–55; trans. James A. Bellamy in *Journal of the American Oriental Society* 81 (1961), pp. 224–46; Ibn Abī l-Ḥadīd (d. 656/1258), *Sharḥ nahj al-balāgha*, ed. Muḥammad Abū l-Faḍl Ibrāhīm (Cairo, 1959–64), XIX, 382–429. Cf. also Julius Wellhausen, *Reste arabischen Heidentums*, 2nd ed. (Berlin, 1897), pp. 159–67.
6. There is a vast and thriving popular literature on how to detect and defeat the machinations of the *jinn*. The authors are primarily religious authorities and their books are published by the presses of such major religious establishments as al-Azhar in Cairo. See below, n. 47.
7. See below, n. 56.

8. Martin Levey, 'Medical Ethics of Medieval Islam, with Special Reference to al-Ruhāwī's *Practical Ethics of the Physician*', in *Transactions of the American Philosophical Society*, New Series, 57.3 (1967), pp. 1–100. The primary theme of this work is the behaviour the physician should display in order to safeguard and promote the status of the profession.
9. Al-Zahrāwī (Albucasis), *On Surgery and Instruments*, ed. and trans. M.S. Spink and G.L. Lewis (London, 1973), e.g. pp. 4–5, 10–11, 118–27, 166–67, 242–43, 576–77.
10. See Josiah C. Russell, 'That Earlier Plague', *Demography* 5 (1968), pp. 174–84; Jean-Noël Biraben and Jacques Le Goff, 'La peste dans le Haut Moyen Age', *Annales* 24 (1969), pp. 1484–1510; Michael W. Dols, 'Plague in Early Islamic History', *Journal of the American Oriental Society* 94 (1974), pp. 371–83; Pauline Allen, 'The Justinianic Plague', *Byzantion* 44 (1979), pp. 5–20; Lawrence I. Conrad, 'The Plague in the Early Medieval Near East', Ph.D. dissertation: Princeton University, 1981; *idem*, 'Die Pest und ihr soziales Umfeld im Nahen Osten des frühen Mittelalters', *Der Islam* 73 (1996), 81–112. On Syria in particular, see Lawrence I. Conrad, 'The Plague in Bilād al-Shām in Pre-Islamic Times', in Muḥammad 'Adnān al-Bakhīt and Muḥammad 'Aṣfūr, eds., *Proceedings of the Symposium on Bilād al-Shām During the Byzantine Period* (Amman, 1986), II, 143–63; *idem*, 'Epidemic Disease in Central Syria in the Late Sixth Century: Some New Insights from the Verse of Ḥassān ibn Thābit', *Byzantine and Modern Greek Studies* 18 (1994), pp. 12–58.
11. Al-Mubarrad (d. 285/898), *Kitāb al-ta'āzī wa-l-marāthī*, ed. Muḥammad al-Dībājī (Damascus, 1396/1976), p. 211.
12. Michael W. Dols, *The Black Death in the Middle East* (Princeton, 1977), pp. 320–35; Lawrence I. Conrad, 'Arabic Plague Chronologies and Treatises: Social and Historical Factors in the Formation of a Literary Genre', *Studia Islamica* 54 (1981), pp. 51–93; Avner Gil'adi, *Children of Islam: Concepts of Childhood in Medieval Muslim Society* (Oxford, 1992), pp. 69–100; Muḥammad 'Alī al-Bār, *Mā rawāhu l-wā'ūn fī akhbār al-ṭā'ūn li-l-imām Jalāl al-Dīn al-Suyūṭī* (Damascus, 1418/1997), pp. 75–99.
13. It has been argued by John Wansbrough that the Qur'ān in fact did not reach the complete state in which we have it today for several centuries after the death of Muḥammad; see his *Qur'ānic Studies* (London, 1977). But this thesis has now been decisively refuted by Fred M. Donner in his *Narratives of Islamic Origins: the Beginnings of Islamic Historical Writing* (Princeton, 1998), pp. 35–63 , which demonstrates that the text available today is a work that originated in the time of the Prophet himself.
14. Sūrat al-Fātiḥa (1), v. 1; trans. A.J. Arberry, *The Koran Interpreted* (London , 1955), p. 1.
15. Sūrat al-Baqara (2), v. 109; = Arberry, p. 14.
16. Sūrat al-Baqara (2), v. 256; = Arberry, p. 37.
17. Sūrat al-An'ām (6), v. 58; Sūrat al-Anbiyā' (21), v. 4 ; = Arberry, pp. 127, 323.

18. Sūrat Fāṭir (35), v. 2; = Arberry, p. 444.
19. Sūrat al-Baqara (2), vv. 33–36; Sūrat al-A'rāf (7), vv. 18–24; Sūrat Ṭāhā (20), vv. 114–24; = Arberry, pp. 5–6, 144–45, 319–20.
20. Sūrat al-Baqara (2), vv. 35–37; = Arberry, p. 6.
21. Sūrat al-Aḥzāb (33), v. 73; = Arberry, p. 435.
22. Sūrat al-'Alaq (96), vv. 6–8; = Arberry, p. 651.
23. Sūrat Ṭāhā (20), v. 114; = Arberry, p. 319.
24. Sūrat al-A'rāf (7), v. 9; = Arberry, p. 143.
25. Sūrat al-A'rāf (7), v. 171; = Arberry, p. 164.
26. Cf. Tilman Nagel, *Der Koran. Einführung-Texte-Erläuterungen* (Munich, 1983), p. 253.
27. Sūrat al-An'ām (6), vv. 70, 164; Sūrat al-Najm (53), vv. 36–41; Sūrat 'Abasa (80), vv. 33–36; = Arberry, pp. 129, 142, 552, 631.
28. Sūrat al-Taghābun (64), v. 11; = Arberry, p. 588.
29. Sūrat Āl 'Imrān (3), vv. 25, 124; = Arberry, pp. 48, 61.
30. Sūrat al-Nisā' (4), vv. 78–79; = Arberry, pp. 83–84.
31. Sūrat al-Ḥadīd (57), v. 22; = Arberry, p. 567.
32. Sūrat al-Baqara (2), v. 214; = Arberry, p. 29.
33. Sūrat al-A'rāf (7), vv. 94–96; = Arberry, p. 155.
34. Sūrat Āl 'Imrān (3), vv. 137–48; = Arberry, pp. 62–63.
35. The clearest example of this is Sūrat al-Raḥmān (55), vv. 1–78; = Arberry, pp. 557–59.
36. Sūrat al-Zumar (39), v. 49; = Arberry, p. 477.
37. Sūrat al-Baqara (2), vv. 155–57; = Arberry, p. 20.
38. See, for example, Ibn Hishām (d. 218/833), *Sīrat Rasūl Allāh*, ed. Ferdinand Wüstenfeld (Göttingen, 1858-60), I. 1, 155–323; trans. Alfred Guillaume, *The Life of Muhammad* (Oxford, 1955), pp. 111–218.
39. Sūrat al-Anbiyā' (21), vv. 83–84; = Arberry, p. 330.
40. Sūrat Ṣād (38), vv. 41–47; = Arberry, p. 467.
41. Sūrat al-Shu'arā' (26), vv. 78–82; = Arberry, p. 374.
42. See D. Sidersky, *Les origines des légendes musulmanes dans le Coran et dans les vies des prophètes* (Paris, 1933); Tilman Nagel, *Die Qiṣaṣ al-anbiyā'. Ein Beitrag zur arabischen Literaturgeschichte* (Bonn, 1967); Raif Georges Khoury, *Wahb b. Munabbih* (Wiesbaden, 1972); *idem, Les légendes prophétiques dans l'Islam depuis le Ier jusqu'au IIIe siècle de l'Hégire* (Wiesbaden, 1978).
43. Cf., for example, Abū Nu'aym al-Iṣbahānī (d. 430/1038), *Ḥilyat al-awliyā' wa-ṭabaqāt al-aṣfiyā'* (Cairo, 1354/1935), where ten volumes of this material are compiled.
44. See Iliad I.43–67; and in the Old Testament, Deuteronomy 32:23–4; Job 5:7; Psalms 76:4, 78:48. Cf. also A. Caquot, 'Sur quelques démons de l'Ancien Testament (Reshep, Qeteb, Deber)', *Semitica* 6 (1956), pp. 55, 57–59, 61; Francesco Vattioni, 'Il dio Resheph', *Annali dell'Istituto orientale di Napoli*, Nuova Serie, 15 (1965), pp. 67–68; William J. Fulco, *The Canaanite God Reshep* (New Haven, 1976), pp. 12–13, 24–25, 27, 37, 50, 56–62, 69–70.
45. Lawrence I. Conrad, 'Epidemic Disease in Formal and Popular Thought in Early Islamic Society', in Terence Ranger and Paul Slack,

eds., *Epidemics and Ideas: Essays on the Historical Perception of Pestilence* (Cambridge, 1992), pp. 82–85.

46. Nancy Elizabeth Gallagher, *Egypt's Other Wars: Epidemics and the Politics of Public Health* (Syracuse, 1990), pp. 120–21.
47. From this vast literature two examples may be cited: Abū Bakr Jābir al-Jazā'irī, *Wiqāyat al-insān min al-jinn wa-l-shayṭān* (Cairo, 1988); Sa'īd Jār 'Alī al-Badawī, *Kayfīyat ikhrāj al-jān min jism al-insān* (Cairo, 1992). This sort of lore is not limited to Muslims. See, for example, Nessim Henry Henein and Thierry Bianquis, eds. and trans., *La magie par les Psalms* (Cairo, 1975), a text used by Copts in Egypt.
48. See n. 51 below.
49. Many such amulets and talismans are discussed in Ibn Abī Sarḥ, *Kitāb al-rumūz*, pp. 641–55; trans. Bellamy, pp. 224–46; Ibn Abī l-Ḥadīd, *Sharḥ nahj al-balāgha*, XIX, 382–429. Cf. Dietrich Brandenburg, *Medizin und Magie. Heilkunde und Geheimlehre des islamischen Zeitalters* (Berlin, 1975). Extant pieces are studied in Ludvik Kalus, *Catalogue of Islamic Seals and Talismans* (Oxford, 1986); Peter W. Schienerl, *Schmuck und Amulett in Antike und Islam* (Aachen, 1988). On Aramaic spells, amulets, and magic bowls, see the two works by Joseph Naveh and Shaul Shaked: *Amulets and Magic Bowls: Aramaic Incantations of Late Antiquity*, 2nd ed. (Jerusalem, 1987); *Magic Spells and Formulae: Aramaic Incantations of Late Antiquity* (Jerusalem, 1993).
50. Ibn Abī Sarḥ, *Kitāb al-rumūz*, p. 647; = trans. Bellamy, p. 237.
51. Ibn Sa'd (d. 230/844), *Kitāb al-ṭabaqāt al-kabīr*, ed. Eduard Sachau *et al.* (Leiden, 1904–40), IV. 1, 86–87.
52. See, for example, Sūrat al-An'ām (6), vv. 100, 128, 130; Sūrat al-Isrā' (17), v. 88; Sūrat al-Kahf (18), v. 50; Sūrat Saba' (34), v. 12; Sūrat al-Ṣāfāt (37), v. 158; Sūrat al-Aḥqāf (46), v. 29; Sūrat al-Raḥmān (55), vv. 15, 33, 39, 56, 74; Sūrat al-Jinn (72), vv. 1, 5–6; Sūrat al-Nās (114), vv. 1–6; = Arberry, pp. 133, 136–37, 284, 294, 438, 462, 525, 557–59, 611, 669.
53. See, for example, Aḥmad ibn Ḥanbal (d. 242/855), *Musnad* (Cairo, A.H. 1311), IV, 395, 413; al-Jāḥiẓ (d. 255/868), *Kitāb al-ḥayawān*, ed. 'Abd al-Salām Muḥammad Hārūn, 2nd ed. (Cairo, 1385–89/1965–69), I, 351; VI, 220; Ibn Qutayba (d. 276/889), *'Uyūn al-akhbār*, ed. Aḥmad Zakī al-'Adawī (Cairo, 1343–48/1925–30), II, 114.
54. Conrad, 'Epidemic Disease', pp. 86–87.
55. On the history of Manichaeism, see Samuel N.C. Lieu, *Manichaeism in the Late Roman Empire and Medieval China*, 2nd ed. (Tübingen, 1992).
56. See H.A.R. Gibb, 'The Social Significance of the Shu'ūbīya', in *Studia orientalia Ioanni Pedersen setuagenario A.D. VII Id. Nov. anno MCMLIII a collegis discipulis amicis* (Copenhagen, 1953), pp. 105–14; reprinted in his *Studies on the Civilization of Islam*, ed. Stanford J. Shaw and William R. Polk (Boston, 1962), pp. 62–73; Johann Fück, *Arabische Kultur und Islam im Mittelalter. Ausgewählte Schriften* (Weimar, 1981), pp. 258–71.
57. Al-Qāsim ibn Ibrāhīm, *Al-Radd 'alā al-zindīq al-la'īn Ibn al-Muqaffa'*, ed. Michelangelo Guidi in his *La lotta tra l'Islām e il manicheismo, un libro di Ibn al-Muqaffa' contro il Corano confutato da al-Qāsim b. Ibrāhīm* (Rome, 1927), pp. 17–24 (lemmata).

58. Ps-Jāḥiẓ, *Al-Dalā'il wa-l-itibār*, trans. M.A.S. Abdel Haleem as *Chance or Creation? God's Design in the Universe* (London, 1995), pp. 90, 114–15, 124. There is unfortunately no good edition of this important book, which exists in two recensions, one a simplified revision of the other. Wim Raven in Frankfurt has collected all of the known manuscripts and is preparing a critical edition of the original text, and Abdel Haleem announces a forthcoming edition in the translation above, which is based on the simplified revision. Abdel Haleem also seems to uphold the traditional attribution of this work to al-Jāḥiẓ (in his translation he promises a full discussion in his forthcoming edition), but the book is not written in a Jāḥiẓian style and the argument for authorship by a Christian Arab who knew Greek seems preferable. See H.A.R. Gibb, 'The Argument from Design: a Mu'tazilite Treatise Attributed to al-Jāḥiẓ', in Samuel Löwinger and Joseph Somogyi, eds, *Ignace Goldziher Memorial Volume*, I (Budapest, 1948), pp. 150–62; Hans Daiber, *Das theologisch-philosophische System des Mu'ammar ibn 'Abbād as-Sulamī* (Beirut, 1975), pp. 159–60.
59. See Harald Motzki, *Die Anfänge der islamischen Jurisprudenz. Ihre Entwicklung in Mekka bis zur Mitte des 2./8. Jahrhundert* (Stuttgart, 1991), where it is argued that much early and perhaps authentically Prophetic material can indeed be recovered from the later collections of *ḥadīth*.
60. The case for this interpretation of the evidence is argued in detail in my 'Epidemic Disease', pp. 78–82.
61. J.-B. Chabot, ed., *Incerti auctoris chronicon anonymum pseudo-Dionysianum vulgo dicto* (Paris, 1927–33), II, 149–50; Qusṭā ibn Lūqā (d. *ca.* 300/912), *Kitāb al-i'dā'*, ed. and trans. Hartmut Fähndrich, *Abhandlung über die Ansteckung von Qusṭā ibn Lūqā* (Stuttgart, 1987), p. 12 nos. 4–5.
62. Al-Khaṭīb al-Baghdādī (d. 463/1071), *Ta'rīkh Baghdād* (Cairo, 1349/1931), II, 8, 14, quoting al-Bukhārī as stating that he compiled his collection from an original corpus of 600,000 traditions. The final text of his collection, eliminating repetitions, contains only 2,602 traditions. One must allow for exaggerations in the figure of 600,000, the fact that this would have included many traditions differing only in their chains of transmitters (from which al-Bukhārī would have selected the most authoritative), and the presence in the corpus of traditions not attested all the way back to Muḥammad and thus less attractive to al-Bukhārī. Still, it seems clear that within only two and a half centuries after the time of the Prophet, Muslim scholars were finding that very little of what was being attributed to him could actually be authenticated according to the critical standards of the day.
63. See Joseph Schacht, *The Origins of Muhammadan Jurisprudence* (Oxford, 1950); G.H.A. Juynboll, *Muslim Tradition: Studies in Chronology Provenance and Authorship of Early Ḥadīth* (Cambridge, 1983); *idem, Studies on the Origins and Uses of Islamic Ḥadīth* (Aldershot, 1996).

64. Conrad, 'Epidemic Disease', p. 88; *idem*, 'Discussions on Contagion in Medieval Islamic Society', in Lawrence I. Conrad and Dominik Wujastyk, eds., *Conceptions of Contagion: Perspectives from Pre-Modern Societies* (London, 1999), forthcoming.
65. See, for example, Mālik ibn Anas (d. 179/795), *Al-Muwaṭṭa'*, ed. Muḥammad Fu'ād 'Abd al-Bāqī (Cairo, 1370/1951), II, 896, *Jāmi'* no. 23; 'Abd al-Razzāq al-Ṣan'ānī (d. 211/827), *Muṣannaf*, ed. Ḥabīb al-Raḥmān al-A'ẓamī (Beirut, 1390–92/1970–72), XI, 146; Ibn Sa'd, III. 2, 124; Aḥmad ibn Ḥanbal, *Musnad*, I, 173, 176–77, 182, 196; V, 202, 207–208, 209, 213, 240; al-Bukhārī, *Al-Jāmi' al-ṣaḥīḥ*, ed. Ludolf Krehl and T.W. Juynboll (Leiden, 1862–1908), II, 377, *Anbiyā'* no. 54; IV, 344, *Ḥiyal* no. 13; Muslim (d. 261/874), *Ṣaḥīḥ*, ed. Muḥammad Fu'ād 'Abd al-Bāqī (Cairo, 1375–76/1955–56), IV, 1737–40, *Salām* nos. 92–97; Ibn Ḥibbān al-Bustī (d. 354/965), *Ṣaḥīḥ*, in the recension of 'Alī ibn Balbān al-Fārisī (d. 739/1339), *Al-Iḥsān bi-tartīb Ṣaḥīḥ Ibn Ḥibbān*, ed. Kamāl Yūsuf al-Ḥūt (Beirut, 1407/1987), IV, 264–65, 266, nos. 2941, 2943.
66. Ezekiel 37:1–14.
67. Arberry, pp. 34–35.
68. See Conrad, 'Arabic Plague Chronologies and Treatises', pp. 77–79, for a translation of the story from an important plague treatise.
69. Conrad, 'Epidemic Disease', pp. 92–94.
70. See, for example, the materials collected in A.J. Wensinck, *Concordance et indices de la tradition musulmane* (Leiden, 1936–88), II, 156–57.
71. See Conrad, 'Die Pest und ihr soziales Umfeld', pp. 90–92, 97–98.
72. Cf. the brief discussion of plague martyrs in Etan Kohlberg, 'Medieval Muslim Views on Martyrdom', *Mededelingen der Koninklijke Nederlandse Akademie van Wetenschappen* 60 (1997), pp. 301–302.
73. On the early Islamic conception of Paradise, see Josef Horovitz, 'Das Koranische Paradies', *Scripta universitatis atque Bibliothecae Hierosolymitanarum (Orientalia et Judaica)* 1.6 (1923), pp. 1–16; Jane Idleman Smith and Yvonne Yazbeck Haddad, *The Islamic Understanding of Death and Resurrection* (Albany, 1981), 87–91.
74. See Wensinck, *Concordance*, III, 198–202.
75. E.g. Aḥmad ibn Ḥanbal, *Musnad*, III, 150, 220, 223, 258, 265–66; al-Bukhārī, *Ṣaḥīḥ*, II, 209, *Jihād* no. 30; IV, 60, *Ṭibb* no. 30; Muslim, *Ṣaḥīḥ*, III, 1522, *Imāra* no. 166.
76. E.g. Aḥmad ibn Ḥanbal, *Musnad*, IV, 128, 128–29, 185; V, 81; al-Bukhārī, *Ṣaḥīḥ*, IV, 60-61, *Ṭibb* no. 30.
77. Sūrat Āl 'Imrān (3), vv. 157–58; = Arberry, p. 65.
78. Sūrat Muḥammad (47), vv. 4–5; = Arberry, p. 526.
79. Sūrat Āl 'Imrān (3), vv. 169–71; = Arberry, pp. 66–67.
80. Cf. Kohlberg, 'Medieval Muslim Views on Martyrdom', pp. 300–303.
81. A.J. Wensinck, 'The Oriental Doctrine of the Martyrs', *Mededeelingen der Koninklijke Akademie van Wetenschappen, Afdeeling Letterkunde*, 53 (1921), pp. 147–74.
82. Cf. Exodus 11:1; Leviticus 26:21; Numbers 11:33, 14:37, 16:47; Deuteronomy 28:59; Joshua 22:17; I Samuel 6:4; and Lawrence I.

Conrad, 'The Biblical Tradition for the Plague of the Philistines', *Journal of the American Oriental Society* 104 (1984), pp. 281–87.

83. See, for example, Cyprian (wr. A.D. 252), *De mortalitate* xvi-xvii; ed. M. Simonetti in *Sancti Cypriani episcopi opera*, II (Turnhout, 1976; *Corpus christianorum, Series Latina*, IIIA), pp. 25–26, where he refers to Christians' fear that death in the epidemic raging at the time would *deprive* them of martyrdom; i.e. death of illness would prevent them from dying for their faith in Roman persecutions.
84. See again Cyprian, *De mortalitate* viii; ed. Simonetti, pp. 20–21. To queries about why the righteous die with the sinners, the faithful with the pagans, he replies that all share a common origin and the bond of mortal human flesh. An epidemic destroys all in the same way that a shipwreck (a favoured motif in this text) claims the lives of all the passengers. It is only in the Hereafter that the Christians will receive their reward.
85. See Wensinck, 'Oriental Doctrine of the Martyrs', pp. 149, 157. The shift in the Islamic positon may have been a reaction to the fact that on occasion the graves of individuals considered to have been martyrs were opened and the bodies discovered within; for some stories of such incidents, cf. Kohlberg, 'Medieval Muslim Views on Martyrdom', pp. 292–93.
86. See, for example, al-Ṭabarī (d. 310/923), *Ta'rīkh al-rusul wa-l-mulūk*, ed. M.J. de Goeje *et al.* (Leiden, 1879–1901), II, 710, where the martyred al-Ḥusayn is called 'lord of the youth of Paradise'; *ibid.*, II, 1515, where a mortally wounded warrior beseeches God to grant him Paradise when he meets Him that evening, instead of preparing the traditional Arab guest meal (*qirā*) for him. Such accounts make sense only if the milieu in which they arose conceived of martyrs as entering Paradise in their physical bodies. Cf. also Kohlberg, 'Medieval Muslim Views on Martyrdom', pp. 290–92. The same attitude can still be found among the modern bedouins; see William Gifford Palgrave, *Narrative of a Year's Journey throuqh Central and Eastern Arabia 1862–1863* (London and Cambridge, 1866), I, 32–33; Jibrail S. Jabbur, *The Bedouins and the Desert: Aspects of Nomadic Life in the Arab East*, trans. Lawrence I. Conrad, ed. Suhayl J. Jabbur and Lawrence I. Conrad (Albany, 1995), pp. 377–80.
87. See above, n. 27.
88. Wensinck, 'Oriental Doctrine of the Martyrs', p. 164.
89. See Eric L. Ormsby, *Theodicy in Islamic Thought: the Dispute over al-Ghazālī's 'Best of All Possible Worlds'* (Princeton, 1984).
90. Ps.-Jāḥiẓ, *Al-Dalā'il wa-l-i'tibār*, trans. Abdel Haleem, pp. 81–82.
91. *Ibid.*, pp. 113–18.
92. Al-Qāsim ibn Ibrāhīm, *Radd*, pp. 22–24; trans. Guidi, *La lotta tra l'Islām e il manicheismo*, pp. 52–54.
93. Al-Ghazālī, *Iḥyā' 'ulūm al-dīn* (Cairo, 1334/1916), IV, 298–99.
94. Al-Ghazālī, *Al-Maqṣad al-asnā fī sharḥ ma'ānī asmā' Allāh al-ḥusnā*, ed. Fadlou A. Shehadeh (Beirut, 1971), pp. 68–69.
95. E.g. could God have created a universe better than the present one? Is God, by virtue of His divinity, required to do what is best (*al-aṣlaḥ*) for mankind?

96. Wensinck, *Concordance*, III, 198–202.
97. Jacqueline Sublet, 'La peste prise aux rêts de la jurisprudence: le traité d'Ibn Ḥağar al-'Asqalānī sur la peste', *Studia Islamica* 33 (1971), pp. 141–49; Dols, *The Black Death in the Middle East*, pp. 109–21.
98. See, for example, Abū Ibrāhīm Kaylānī Muḥammad Khalīfa's edition of Ibn Ḥajar al-'Asqalānī (d. 852/1449), *Badhl al-mā'ūn fī faḍl al-ṭā'ūn* (Cairo, 1413/1993), p. 3, where the editor indicates the relevance of his book for modern times, when God has repeatedly been obliged to chastise mankind for 'disregarding His religion and violating His laws'.
99. Muḥammad 'Abd al-Jawād Muḥammad, *Buḥuth fī l-sharī'a al-islāmīya wa-l-qānūn fī l-ṭibb al-islāmī* (Alexandria, 1991); Vardit Rispler-Chaim, *Islamic Medical Ethics in the Twentieth Century* (Leiden, 1993).
100. See, for example, Muḥammad Sa'īd Suyūṭī, *Mu'jizāt fī l-ṭibb li-l-nabī al-'arabī Muḥammad* (Beirut, 1984); al-Sayyid Jumaylī, *I'jāz al-ṭibb al-nabawī* (Beirut, 1986); Muḥammad 'Alī al-Bār, *Hal hunā ṭibb nabawī?* (Jedda, 1409/1989); Fu'ād Ḥusayn Muzannir, *Tibb al-nabī al-muṣṭafā fīmā ikhtāra wa-iṣṭafā* (Beirut, 1989); Mukhtār Sālim, *Al-Ibdā'āt al-ṭibbīya li-rasūl al-insānīya* (Beirut, 1995). On the copyright page of his *Natural Healing with the Medicine of the Prophet, from the Book of the Provisions of the Hereafter by Imam Ibn Qayyim al-Jawziyya* (Philadelphia, 1993), Muhammad Al-Akili has the following disclaimer: 'Note to the reader: The medical knowledge contained in this book is intended solely for the information and study of qualified physicians. The section on Physician's Liability in this book governs a disclaimer by the translator and the publisher of this book. Therefore, the use of any medical information contained in this publication, and if applicable, must be administered solely by a qualified medical practitioner, or *ḥakīm*, and at his or her discretion'.

APPEASING THE SPIRITS: HEALING STRATEGIES IN POSTWAR SOUTHERN MOZAMBIQUE[1]

Alcinda Manuel Honwana

Introduction

Healing systems are both cultural and social systems which articulate ill health as a cultural idiom and establish a systematic relationship between beliefs about causation of illness, the experience of symptoms, decisions concerning treatment and evaluations of therapeutic outcomes.[2] This chapter discusses healing strategies adopted by war affected population in Southern Mozambique. It examines the role played by cultural beliefs and practices in people's health-seeking decisions and healing strategies to overcome distress and illness. Spiritual agencies such as the ancestral spirits, the malevolent spirits and the spirits of those killed during the war are believed to be central in the process of causation and healing of ill-health. Thus, 'appeasing the spirits' becomes a mechanism of social healing and reconciliation, of redressing the wrongs of the past and of rebuilding life after war.

The present study emphasises the importance of cultural notions and understandings of diagnosis and healing and of distress and trauma since the ways people express, embody and give meaning to their afflictions are generally tied to a specific cultural context. In this perspective, biomedical and psychotherapeutic notions of distress and trauma constitute cultural constructs and may often not be effective in contexts where cultural beliefs and world views are different. The biomedical approach to healing war trauma should, thus, be regarded as only one of the several ways of dealing with post-war healing in Africa since there are other ways of understanding health and healing in post-conflict situations which are culturally specific. Further, the chapter suggests that, alongside biomedical and psychotherapeutic interventions, it is fundamental to take into account and use local healing and conflict resolution mechanisms and involve the family, traditional healers, religious congregations and other community-based support groups. In rural communities, at times of personal and wider societal crisis these 'institutions' are the essential means through which healing and order can be re-established.

Initial research was undertaken in 1992–3 in southern Mozambique in the periphery of Maputo (Dhlavela, Zona Verde and Khongoloti), and in two rural districts (Boane and Manhiça). Further research was conducted in 1995 in Gaza (Chokwe, Xibuto and Manjacaze). The research focus included both those who were directly and indirectly affected by the war. I interviewed traditional healers, diviners, spirit mediums; traditional chiefs and *régulos;*[3] war-affected people – refugees, displaced people, kidnapped children, ex-soldiers; as well as many other civilians.

Cultural Basis of Health, Illness and Healing

The dominant paradigms shaping aid policies and interventions in African conflicts have been informed by Western biomedical notions of health, illness and healing. Western definitions and understandings of diagnosis and healing, and of distress and trauma, have been applied to societies that possess very different ontologies and social and cultural patterns. Such notions and understandings cannot be effectively applied across cultures since the ways in which people express, embody and give meaning to that distress are tied to a specific cultural context. Geertz[4] has defined culture as a 'pattern of meaning' that shapes human experiences and provides a framework of understandings and beliefs which underpin people's life actions. Therefore, culture plays an important role in social and emotional well-being since the ways in which people manage their afflictions are at least in part built on cultural perceptions.[5]

In Western biomedical tradition, and according to Descarts' legacy, body and mind are perceived to be distinguishable and separate entities. The implication is that in these circumstances the causes of ill health are located either in the body or in the mind, but never in both. Also, dominant Western psychotherapeutic models locate the causes of psychosocial distress within the individual and devise responses which are primarily based on individual therapy. Recovery is achieved through helping the individual 'come to terms' with the traumatic experience, and healing is held in private individual sessions aimed at 'talking out', externalising feelings and afflictions on a one-to-one basis, or through drug therapy. These approaches have been successful in the Euro-American contexts because these methods are rooted in local ancient religious traditions (such as the institution of the confessional);[6] and the fact that modern psychological therapy became part of the popular consciousness and is a form of 'common sense'.

However, in contexts (such as the Mozambican) particularly those which are closer to traditional religious and healing practices, other forms of 'common sense' routes to understanding and healing psychological trauma may exist.[7] Boyden and Gibbs' work on Cambodia has shown that individual therapy conducted by a biomedical expert was often ineffective because it did not account for the place that ancestral spirits, malevolent spirits and other forces have in the causation and healing processes, and it undermined the role of the family and the community in providing support and care. Marrato's[8] study of a war-affected population in Mozambique, also shows how recalling the traumatic experience through verbal externalisation was not part of the process of 'coming to terms' with it. She points out that people perform healing rituals which do not necessarily involve verbal expression of the affliction.

Indeed, in societies which possess a holistic cosmological model, the Cartesian dichotomy does not apply because mind and body are perceived to be integrated. Beliefs in the powers of spiritual agencies are directly linked to bodily afflictions and other misfortunes. In this context health and illness acquire a particular significance which differs from the biomedical tradition. While it is true that the biomedical and psychotherapeutic practices have a lot to offer, they constitute only one of several ways of dealing with distress and trauma in the African context. Apart from not embracing local African traditions and world views, Western psychotherapeutic interventions are expensive and limited in the numbers they can reach.

Local Notions of Health, Illness and Healing

In Southern Mozambique people perceived health as being a natural state for all human beings. So, to be unhealthy denotes abnormality, showing that somewhere something is out of its normal place, that harmony is jeopardised. Health in this context is, therefore, approached in terms of a life process rather than just in terms of a bodily process and in this sense it acquires a broader dimension in comparison to Western concepts. Thus, health is defined by the harmonious relationships between human beings and the environment (their surroundings), between them and the spiritual world and amongst themselves within the environment. Rather than being narrowly defined realms, the social (the spirits and the living) and natural world are united within a larger cosmological universe.[9]

Thus, rain should fall at its ordinary time, crops should grow, people should not fall sick and children should not die. If this harmonious state fails to come about, it is perceived as the result of intervention of malevolent spirits controlled by the *valoyi* (witches and sorcerers) or a sanction of the ancestral spirits for incorrect behaviour or of other spiritual forces.[10] Therefore, if the relationships between human beings and their ancestral spirits, between them and the environment and amongst themselves are balanced health ensues. However, if they are disrupted in any way, the well-being of the community is jeopardised. Thus, there is a complex set of rules and practices which govern the maintenance of fecundity (of the land and of women) and general well-being of the communities.

Ill health[11] is, therefore, considered to be primarily a social phenomenon which establishes an alteration in the normal course of the individual's life. Traditional healing has thus a holistic approach combining both the social and the physical dimensions of the malady in order to treat the person as a whole. Here there is an overall integration between body and mind. The social imbalance in a patient's life is generally reflected in the physical body, and both dimensions are equally taken into consideration to restore the patient's health. The corollary is that healing is achieved through a double strategy: divination, which deals with the social causes of the patients affliction; and the physical healing which addresses the suppression of the bodily symptoms.

Moreover, the individual is never treated as a singular entity but rather as part of a community. During the divination seance the diviner always looks at the state of the patient's social relationships in the community (relationships with the living and with the spiritual world) to achieve a diagnosis. The diviner-patient dialogue, developed during the consultation, represents a reciprocal learning process in which, as Jackson[12] puts it, a process of transference and counter-transference of information occurs and brings them together. Thus, in this context the relationship between practitioner and patient is very close and enhances the cultural bonds between them. In this regard traditional healing can be extremely effective to heal trauma and other social disorders caused by war.

These notions of health and healing also entail that both the living world and that of the spirits (supernatural) play a role in the process of causation and healing of ill health. In fact, health practitioners commonly known as *tinyanga* or *nyanga* (singular) are generally possessed by spirits, or function under spiritual inspiration. There are several types of *tinyanga* as they can be herbalists, diviners or spirit-mediums. People take recourse to the spirits, through the *tinyanga*, for several reasons: to cure illness, to seek protection from the hazards of life, to discover the causes of a death in the family, or even to discover why domestic animals are dying and agricultural production is not going well. Above all, people seek the powers of the ancestral world to find out the reasons beyond such events and how to restore balance into their lives.

Spiritual Agencies' Role on Health and Healing

The ancestral spirits constitute part of everyday life action. It is believed that when an individual dies and the body is buried, his/her spirit remains as the effective manifestation of his/her power and personality. Thus, death does not constitute the end of an individual's existence, but rather marks the transition to a new dimension of life. Spirits of the dead take possession of a person's body and operate through him/her, exercising a powerful influence over the living.[13]

The supreme being, *Xikwembu* or *Nkulukumba*, the Creator, constitutes a remote divinity which does not have a direct relationship with the community.[14] People relate directly to the ancestral spirits with whom they share a combined existence, and interact in everyday life action. Thus, the ancestral spirits are believed to be real entities whose action interferes with the life of human beings in society. They are the ones who protect and guide the communities. They promote fertility of the land and of women, good agricultural production, good hunting and good relations among members of the group. They also protect them against misfortune, disease, ecological dangers and evil, namely witchcraft and sorcery. In short, the spirits care for the well-being of the communities. However, the ancestral spirits can also withdraw their protection and create a state of vulnerability to misfortune and evil intentions, or even cause maladies to show their displeasure or anger with their descendants. They are believed to protect and give health and wealth to those who respect social norms, and to punish those who are anti-social, who act against the norms, who disrespect social order. Ill health can also be caused by the intervention of malevolent spirits manipulated by witches and sorcerers, or by the spirits of bitterness, those of individuals wrongfully killed or not properly buried.

Communities venerate and worship the ancestral spirits through special rituals to propitiate them. *Ku pahla* is a verb which means 'to venerate' or 'to honour' the ancestral spirits. *Ku pahla* is a permanent way of paying respect to one's ancestors, and it is performed in multiple occasions such as: the birth of a child, before harvesting, during a meal, before a long trip and the like. The performance of *ku pahla* gives individuals and groups a sense of security and stability which they need to carry on with their lives. It is this permanent liaison between the living and the dead that gives meaning to the existence of both the spirits and the community. Another way of establishing contact with the spirits is through possessed *tinyanga* who are the intermediaries between the living world and that of the ancestral spirits.

Post-War Healing and the Spirits of the Dead

The use of traditional religious beliefs and practices during the war was widespread in the southern region. Both the military and the civilian population made recourse to traditional healers, diviners and spirit mediums. This is not particular to Mozambique, in other contexts such as in Zimbabwe similar phenomena occurred.[15] In the post-war period these religious beliefs in the powers of the spirits do not disappear as people believe that the spirits of dead soldiers and civilians will haunt and kill them. This phenomenon is known as *Mpfhukwa*. *Mpfhukwa* are the spirits of the soldiers and civilians killed during the war who did not have a proper burial with all the rituals aimed at placing them in their proper positions in the world of the spirits. Thus, their souls are unsettled; they are spirits of bitterness. It is believed that these spirits have the capacity to afflict, provoke maladies and even kill those who killed or mistreated them in life. This revenge is also extended to the family of the killer, who have to pay for their relatives behaviour in the war. The *Mpfhukwa* spirits may also be nasty to passers-by, especially to those who cross their path.

Mpfhukwa is particularly important after a war, when soldiers and civilians are not appropriately buried. Some of my elder informants recalled that after the *Nguni* wars in southern Mozambique in the nineteenth century,[16] the spirits of the *Nguni* and *Ndau* warriors killed in the southern region away from their homes afflicted and killed local *Tsonga* families. The *Ndau* spirits are reported to have been the most dangerous ones. Most informants believe that the *Ndau* spirits are very powerful and that the *Mpfhukwa* phenomenon is originally *Ndau*. Apparently, the capacity to become a *Mpfhukwa* is acquired through the powers of a plant called *mvuco*. And in the traditions of the *Ndau* every individual has to drink the solution made from this plant just a few weeks after his/her birth. The solution is believed to make the individual stronger, and once dead to resuscitate for vengeance.

The war between the government and RENAMO (Mozambique National Resistance) also had a strong *Ndau* component as the support base of RENAMO was mainly *Ndau* (although it has changed in the last years of the war). Also, since there has been a greater interpenetration between the *Tsonga*, the *Nguni* and the *Ndau* the secret of *Mpfhukwa* is no longer exclusively *Ndau*. For that reason many people fear that the re-emergence of *Mpfhukwa* spirits will be greater and stronger than in the past. Many informants were unanimous in saying that rituals for appeasing these spirits must be performed in the places where battles happened and people died. These rituals are vital to calm their souls and place them in their proper positions in the spiritual world. These rituals are generally performed by the *tinyanga*, the ones who have the capacity to capture and exorcise or appease these spirits.

Appeasing the Mpfhukwa Spirits

Fabião Sitoe from Manhiça shared a very interesting case with me. He said that in April 1993 the *tinyanga* of the locality of Munguine in Manhiça were asked to perform a ritual in the road that links the locality of Munguine to the village Manhiça. The ritual was needed because as soon as it got dark nobody could use this road to get to the Manhiça. The *Mpfhukwa* spirit of a RENAMO commander killed nearby was afflicting passers-by. Local people reported that as they approached the place they felt something beating them or heard voices sending them back or became blind and could not see their way to Manhiça.

Sitoe continued saying that the *tinyanga* performed *ku femba* (to catch the spirit). Then the spirit said who he was and that he wanted money, *capulanas* (local pieces of fabric) and to be accompanied to his home in Ndauland. The local population agreed to contribute with money to give the spirit and buy the *capulanas*. A week later the spirit was caught again and tied with the pieces of fabric and the money and was buried far away from the locality. Sitoe said that the *tinyanga* also placed some medicine in the money and fabric to prevent the return of the spirit. According to the local people since then no more problems occurred in that road. People believe that these rituals are necessary to bring back peace and order impaired by the war.

Another example of *Mpfhukwa* is one which was widely discussed by the media in Mozambique in mid 1996. During the war in the district of Govuro a battalion of *Maconde*[17] soldiers killed Laquene Nguluve, ex-*régulo* of Vuca. According to Carvalho's[18] reports the killing of the *Ndau régulo* happened ten years ago when the soldiers suspected that he was supporting RENAMO in the war against the government. In 1996 that battalion started to suffer the retaliation of the *régulo* Nguluve's spirit. In two months six members of that battalion died in strange circumstances, and the commander who ordered the killing is suffering from a serious mental breakdown (he is said to wander naked in the streets of Beira – the provincial capital). Members of the battalion and their relatives took recourse to local diviners for help. Divination has revealed that the spirit of the dead *régulo* wants revenge and is asking for the life of a *Maconde* child to be taken with the same gun used to kill him. The *Maconde* apologised and pleaded with the spirit to accept as a settlement three goats, a bottle of brandy and a virgin maconde girl to take care of the hut of the spirit. Apparently the spirit has rejected that offer and people fear he will continue to afflict and kill the soldiers of the battalion until his demands are met. Interviewed by a journalist the current traditional chief of Vuca, brother of the deceased stated that:

> . . . our spirits (the *Ndau*) are stronger than the *Maconde* spirits . . . the spirit of my brother knows what he wants. I asked him to save the (*Maconde*) boy and accept their offerings but he refused, saying that he will finish that group who killed him unjustly.

The matter has become of public concern and local authorities in the Govuro district (the government, the Association of Traditional Healers and the Association of War Veterans) were involved in trying to mediate the conflict but so far with no success. While the first case seems to have been successful in appeasing the spirit, the second appears to be more problematic. The very fact that the spirit wants the death of an innocent child also complicates the matter. This illustrates the complexities of these problems some of which might be easily resolved and others might not. The *tinyanga's* role is precisely to try and mediate these complex situations by establishing the liaison between the living and the dead.

Pollution, Cleansing and Purification

The notion of social pollution is thus an important factor in the context of southern Mozambican post-war healing. In the rural communities most people believe that individuals are potentially exposed to pollution in their contacts with other social groups and environments. Those who migrate across group boundaries, such as migrant workers are particularly exposed to social contamination. This kind of contamination comes from being victims of witchcraft and sorcery, by picking up unknown spirits, or by being more vulnerable to illness in an unknown environment. Ecological conditions too may be a source of pollution.[19]

Social pollution may also arise from being in contact with death and bloodshed. Thus, individuals who have been in a war, who killed or saw people being killed are believed to be polluted by death and other atrocities of war. They are the vehicles through which *Mpfhukwa* spirits might enter the community as referred to above. After a war when soldiers and refugees return home, when war affected children return to their families, they are believed to be potential contaminators of the social body. The *Mpfhukwa* (spirits of the dead) that haunt them can disrupt life in their families. Thus the cleansing process is seen as one of the fundamental conditions for the reintegration of these individuals into society.[20]

In this post-war period many families perform cleansing rituals to purify and protect their relatives from the atrocities of the war. This is more predominant in the countryside where family solidarity, age hierarchies and traditional religious beliefs and practices still have a considerable influence in people's health-seeking decisions and strategies. In urban and semi-urban settings, where people are exposed to other ways of solving their afflictions, some practice these traditional rituals, others do not and others might combine a series of therapeutic strategies. Religious and political alliances also determine people's decisions concerning treatment alternatives. The rituals which are described next are, in a way, what most participants from rural areas considered to be the ideal way of dealing with these afflictions in a rural context.

The healing process, rather than being an individual session for 'talking out' the afflictions on a one-to-one basis, is constituted of several ritualistic procedures. These rituals bring together a series of symbolic meanings aimed at cutting the links with the past, at cleansing and reintegrating the afflicted into the community. While modern psychotherapeutic practices emphasise verbal exteriorisation of the affliction, here the past is locked away. Recalling the past would mean to open a door for malevolent forces to intervene. The cleansing process and the idea of closing the way to malevolent spirits is tied to the notion of social pollution. According to most informants this kind of treatment is essential to cleanse the individual and help release traumatic experiences. The treatment does not finish with the ritual, which only represents the beginning of the healing process. Next I will discuss two cases in which a boy and a soldier were submitted to cleansing rituals as part of after-war healing.

The first one is that of nine-year-old Paulo Mongo. Paulo was kidnapped by RENAMO soldiers in an attack on his village and was taken to the RENAMO military base of Chinhanguanine where he stayed about eight months. Paulo managed to escape from the camp weeks before he was due to start military training. When the child finally arrived home he was taken to the *ndomba* (the house of the spirits) to be presented to the ancestral spirits of the Mongo family. The child's grandfather addressed the spirits informing them that his grandchild had returned home. The grandfather also thanked the spirits for their protection as Paulo was able to return alive. A few days after his arrival Paulo was submitted to a ritual of purification in which many members of his family participated. His father described it to me:

> . . . we took him to the bush (about 2 km away from our house). There we built a small hut covered with dry grass in which we put the child, dressed in the dirty clothes he came back with from the RENAMO camp. Inside the hut the child was undressed. Then we set fire to the hut and Paulo was helped out by an adult relative. The hut, the clothes, and everything else that the child brought from the camp, were burned in the fire.

After that Paulo had to inhale the smoke of some herbal remedies as well as be bathed with water treated with medicine. These treatments were meant to cleanse his body internally and externally. Finally, small incisions were opened on the child's body and were filled with a paste made of various powders. This practice is called *ku thlavela* and it is aimed at giving him strength and protection against evil.

The second case is that of Titos, son of one of my key informants. Titos' mother said that protection and cleansing rituals for soldiers are essential to avoid the danger of being caught by the *Mpfhukwa* spirits as discussed above. She explained that some people tend to neglect traditional rituals and completely embrace biomedicine, but from her own experience, certain things have to be done 'in our own way' (traditional way). Ana (Titos' mother) said that when Titos had gone to join the colonial army in the 60s she had performed a protective ritual for him. The ritual was performed at home and she, as a *nyanga*, treated her son with a series of herbal remedies aimed at protecting him against the dangers of the war. First he was 'vaccinated' (*ku thlavela*) by having small incisions made on his body and filled with a medical paste obtained from a blend of different plants. This 'vaccination' was aimed at making him courageous and strong to fight a war. Then Titos had to drink a solution made from several remedies and bathe himself with water mixed with medicine. After that she took him into the *ndomba* and informed the spirits of the family that he was going to fight the war and asked them to protect him. She then prepared him a talisman (*nhlulo*) which he had to carry around the waist for the duration of his military service.

She also mentioned that when Titos came home after fighting the colonial war he went through a purification ritual. His clothes were burned outside his home, then he inhaled the smoke of a remedy called *mbasso* (a paste resulting from the combination of different plants and vegetable oils) which was blended with some dry grass from the hut in which Titos was supposed to sleep that night. Then he had to bathe himself with water treated with a remedy called *hlambu* (a powder made with the leaves and roots of different plants). After his bath he was taken to the family *ndomba* (the hut of the spirits) where he was welcomed and blessed by the ancestral spirits.

These cases demonstrate that both Paulo and Titos' afflictions were collective ones, which involved directly not only his relatives (grandfather and father in Paulo's case; and mother in Titos' case) but also the spirits, who are considered to be part of the family (spirits were asked to protect them and bring them back home alive; both Paulo and Titos were taken to the hut of the spirits to be welcomed by them). They were believed to be home alive due to spiritual protection and so the spirits had to be thanked for their role. Spirits, in this context have an active role in guiding and protecting their living relatives against the dangers and hazards of life and in restoring health and harmony. So, the process of overcoming an unhealthy state transcends the individual and involves the community (living and dead). This collective participation becomes fundamental in the sense that one polluted individual can contaminate the social body, the *Mpfhukwa* also harm family relatives and passers-by. Therefore, healing the polluted individual is also healing the whole community.

Verbal articulation of the experiences which brought about the unhealthy state is not a feature in these rituals. Instead the experiences of the past are suppressed as we have seen in both cases in the burning the hut and the clothes and by cleansing the bodies with water treated with special medicines. In the case of Titos, adult men are expected to become soldiers so, a protective ritual was performed before he joined the army. This did not happen to Paulo who was kidnapped and was about to become a soldier, had he not managed to escape. Thus, Paulo was much more vulnerable than Titos, not only for being a child but also for not having protection. Similarly to the soldiers, and as some informants stated, migrant workers who go to work in the South African mines are also submitted to protective rituals, for they are going to face a different social and cultural environment and are believed to be exposed to social pollution.

Venerating the Ancestral Spirits

Mhamba is a propitiatory ritual which is performed to honour the ancestors. Through *timhamba* (plural) communities venerate (*ku pahla*) the ancestral spirits. Junod gives the following definition of *mhamba*: *Mhamba* is the object, the act or the person used to establish the link between the ancestral spirits and their descendants.[21] I would suggest that a *mhamba* is a ritual and therefore, a set of beliefs and practices that unite together the members of a community to pay respect to their ancestral spirits. The *mhamba* is not just the object, the isolated act or the person but rather the combination of all this. It has action, dynamism and a profound symbolic value which is intelligible for the members of that community.

Mhamba rituals take place at dawn. First, an animal is sacrificed. In times of peace and prosperity the most common sacrificial beast was an ox but today with the widespread poverty caused by the war a goat or even a chicken might do. The animal is killed by piercing its neck with an assegai. The animal's blood has to be spread all over the ritual place – the *gandzelo* or the family cemetery. The meat is then prepared into a meal to be offered to the spirits and also consumed by the members of the family. The person who presides over the ritual, generally the senior individual of the family, speaks to the ancestors. He invokes the names of all the family's deceased ancestors starting usually with the *hahani* or *kosezana* (the elder sister of the paternal grandfather) unless the spirits have indicated differently. After that, the officiant informs the ancestral spirits about the state of the family, thanks them for their protection and guidance, and asks them to continue to look after the family. Other members of the family are allowed to express their feelings to the ancestors at this moment.

Having done that, the participants can have a small portion of the remaining sacrificial meal. Everyone must eat that meal. The children are the first to eat and they have the front legs of the ox because these are *mpakama* (the ramifications, the arms of the family). The *vakonwana* (the sons-in-law) eat the back legs, the best meat of the animal as a sign of respect and consideration, for they have paid the *lobolo* (bridewealth) to the family. The *nkosikhazi* (the daughters-in-law) have the *nhlana* (the rump) for they are the ones who reproduce the group and nurse the children, taking them on their backs. The remaining parts are consumed by the other participants. In addition to the sacrificial meal, more food and drinks are available to the members of the family to celebrate the occasion. At the end of the meal and throughout the day, drums are played and people sing and dance. It is a festive occasion for the whole family united by their ancestral spirits.

Timhamba rituals entail collective healing and re-establishment of balance. The bloody sacrifice which characterises these rituals also emphasises reciprocity towards the ancestral spirits to whom the individual owes his possessions. The purpose of the *timhamba* is both the communication and the communion with the dead. Communication which comes through addressing them verbally to seek protection, healing and guidance – as the headman or the person in charge of the ritual addresses the spirits any other person of the group can do so if he/she wishes. Communion which is achieved through sharing the same sacrificial beast in a meal which is consumed by both the spirits and the living.

In returning to their communities after the war the first rituals to be performed by the population are the *timhamba*, to venerate the ancestral spirits buried in the family land or symbolised by the *gandzelo* (the tree of the ancestral shades). These rituals, also known as *ku pahla* are aimed at restoring the liaison between the individuals and their ancestors who were abandoned during the war, and receiving the guidance and the protection of the spirits to rebuild their lives. I can recall some of the conversations that I had with refugees and displaced people who were preparing to return to their places of origin, which they were forced to leave because of the war.[22] They were unanimous in stating that the first thing they would do on arriving at home would be to organise a big *mhamba* for their ancestors who remained unattended in their land. Some had been back home after the cease fire just to check and prepare the conditions for the return of the whole family. And even in that short stay they performed *ku pahla* to honour the dead. Xitoquiso who left his home in Mukodwene in 1987 after being tortured by RENAMO soldiers said that in January 1993 he went to Mukodwene:

> I went to see the place and give it a good clean. Next June (in two months time) I will return but this time to make a *mhamba*. I will go with my family and I will take everything for the

> ceremony: goats, chicken, maize meal etc. We are going to present ourselves to our ancestors and thank them for their protection because most of us managed to survive the war. We will move back home for good probably at the end of the year as we want to make sure that the war is really over.

Another informant, Damião from Xibondzane in Manjacaze is a demobilised government soldier who brought his family (mother, brothers and sisters) to live with him in Massaka due to the escalation of RENAMO attacks in Xibondzane. He said they would not rush to go back as he wanted to see what would happen after the elections, saying that:

> I have heard about what happened in Angola, so I would rather wait here. Nevertheless, we will go home for visits and prepare the fields. Also the elders in the family are organising a *mhamba* for next month. *Timhamba* are a tradition in our family, my grandfather had always organised *ku pahla* ceremonies.

Carlos Matxane a refugee from Xibuto said that he wanted to take his family home as soon as possible. However, he will stay in town because he has got a good job which he prefers to keep. He also mentioned that in August he and his relatives are going to Xibuto (his home land) to perform a big *mhamba* for their ancestors. They are going to call the *nyanga* of the family (who he knows has survived the war and is back in the village) to officiate the ritual.

From the accounts of these participants[23] one can see how central the ancestral spirits are to people's lives. The first thing they do, even before returning for good, is to re-establish the relationship with the dead ancestors, a relationship which has been impaired by the war. Despite the fact that some people do forget about venerating the ancestral spirits when everything in their lives goes well, and may not perform a *mhamba* for years, in a moment of affliction or crisis many seek for the help of the spirits. This is very common in the urban and semi-urban environments, especially when the modern institutions do not provide adequate answers to their problems.

Conclusion

This paper has demonstrated that in southern Mozambique, beliefs about the power of spiritual agencies in the lives of individuals and groups are strongly embedded in everyday action. It is by means of spiritual powers that people make sense of themselves and can restore meaning and a sense of balance to their lives. In this context, spiritual agencies form an integral part of the wider system of meanings in rural communities. Yet, although spiritual entities can be a stabilising factor in social relations, they are by no means a static regulator of human endeavour and identity. On the contrary, it is precisely their capacity for allowing individual and collective changes of identity that explains much of its ontological force and persistence. Through rituals involving spiritual power, individuals and groups are able to regain their identity and be reaccepted into society.

The paper has also discussed peoples' perceptions and understandings of the post-war healing and the role of social pollution and the *Mpfhukwa* spirits in the causation of ill health. 'Appeasing the spirits' thus, becomes a fundamental strategy for redressing the past and rebuilding health and well-being in the communities. The purification and protective rituals were aimed at liberating the individual from pollution and restoring his/her identity as a member of the group. Polluted individuals are temporarily excluded by going through a period of separation in which they do not belong to the social body and cannot enjoy social interaction. Only after compliance with all ritual prescriptions are they reincorporated into society.

These healing and protective rituals do not involve verbal exteriorisation of the experience. Healing is achieved through non-verbal symbolic procedures which are understood by those participating in it. That is why clothes and other objects symbolising the past had to be burnt to impress on the individual and the group a complete rupture with that experience and the beginning of a new life. Recounting and remembering the traumatic experience would be like opening a door for the harmful spirits to penetrate the communities.

The examination of local healing strategies demonstrates that biomedicine and psychotherapy are but among many ways of understanding and healing distress and trauma. Considering that the majority of the Mozambican population affected by the war is rural, a combination of several healing approaches seems to be necessary in order to take into account patient's world views and systems of meaning. This paper has suggested that the role of traditional healing systems in this regard cannot be ignored and should not be antagonised as has happened in the past.[24] Traditional practitioners and elderly family members are already creating their space in this process of healing the social wounds of war. They are not waiting for the government to bring the psychologists and other medical practitioners to solve their problems. They are using the means available to them to restore peace and stability in their communities.

NOTES

1. A similar version of this chapter was published in 1997 by *Peace and Conflict: The Journal of Peace Psychology*, 3(3), 293–305, Lawrence Erlbaum Associates, Inc.
2. Arthur Kleinman, *Patients and Healers in the Context of Culture*, (Berkeley: University of California Press, 1980).
3. *Régulos* were African traditional chiefs appointed by Portuguese colonial administration. They were not necessarily the traditional chiefs of the areas as the colonial administration appointed those who were more docile to them.
4. Clifford Geertz, *The Interpretation of Cultures*, (New York: Basic Books).
5. See Joan Boyden and Sara Gibbs, 'Vulnerability and Resilience: Perceptions and Responses to Psychological Distress in Cambodia' (Oxford: INTRAC, 1996).
6. Andy Dawes, 'Helping, Coping and Cultural Healing', *Recovery and Cooperation on Violence. Education and Rehabilitation of Young People*, (1996), Vol.1 no.5.
7. Dawes, 'Helping, Coping and Cultural Healing'.
8. Josefa Marrato, 'Superando os Efeitos Sociais da Guerra em Moçambique: Mecanismos e Estratégias Locais', Paper presented to the 4th congress of Lusophone Social Sciences, Rio, September, (1996).
9. See also Carolyn Nordstrom, 'Estudos sobre Medicina Tradicional-Zambezia'. Maputo: Ministério da Saúde, (1991).
10. Keith Rennie,'Christianity, Colonialism and the Origins of Nationalism among the Ndau of Southern Rhodesia 1890–1935', (1973), D.Phil. Thesis in History. Northwestern University, Evanston, Illinois.
11. The use of terms such as ill health and malady is intended to avoid the disease/illness dichotomy used in Cecil Helman, *Culture. Health and Illness*. (London: Wright, 1984). Such a dichotomy appears to be irrelevant in this context.
12. Michael Jackson, 'An Approach to Kuranko Divination', *Human Relations* (1978) 31 (2).
13. For more information on spirit possession in southern Mozambique see Alcinda Honwana, 'Spiritual Agency and Self-Renewal in Southern Mozambique' (1996), Ph.D. Thesis in Social Anthropology, University of London, SOAS.
14. C. Fuller, 'An Ethnohistoric Study of Continuity and Change in Gwambe Culture', (1955), D.Phil. Thesis in Anthropology, Northwestern University, Evanston Illinois.

15. For more information on traditional religion and war in Mozambique see Christian Geffray, *La Cause des Armes au Mozambique: Anthopologie d'une Guerre Civile*, (Paris: Credu-Karthala, 1990); Alex Vines, *Renamo: Terrorism in Mozambique*. (London: Centre for Southern African Studies, University of York and Indiana University Press, 1991); Otto Roesch, 'Renamo and the Peasantry in Southern Mozambique: A View from Gaza Province', *Canadian Journal of African Studies*, (1992), vol. 26, 3, 462–84; Kenneth Wilson, 'Cults of Violence and Counter-Violence in Mozambique', *Journal of Southern Africa Studies*, (1992), Vol.18, 3; Honwana, 'Spiritual Agency and Self-Renwal in Southern Mozambique'. In relation to Zimbabwe, see Terence Ranger, *Peasant Consciousness and Guerilla War in Zimbabwe*, (London: James Currey, 1985); David Lan, *Guns and Rain: Guerrillas and Spirit Mediums in Zimbabwe* (London: James Currey, 1985); Pamela Reynolds, 'Children of Tribulation: The need to heal and the means to heal war trauma', *Africa*, (1990), 60:1–38.
16. In the nineteenth century the *Nguni* broke from the *Zulu* state of Shaka and migrated towards Mozambique, conquering and dominating the peoples they encountered in their way. During this process they subjugated the *Ndau* (a group from central Mozambique) and forced them down south as slaves in the *Nguni* state of Gaza which they established in the southern region after dominating the *Tsonga*. For more information see Rennie, 'Christianity, Colonialism and the Origins of Nationalism; Gerard Liesegang,'Notes on the Internal Structure of the Gaza Kingdom of Southern Mozambique, 1840–1895', in J.B. Peires (ed.) *Before and After Shaka*, (Grahamstown: Institute of Social Economic Research, Rhodes University, 1981), 179–208; Antonio Rita-Ferreira, *Fixação Portuguesa e História Pré-colonial de Moçambique*, (Lisboa: Junta de Investigações Científicas do Ultramar, 1982).
17. *Maconde* is a social group from northern Mozambique. This group had a very strong representation in the armed forces throughout the country (both during the liberation war and in the post-independence government).
18. R. Carvalho, 'Filho por filho', *Mediafax*, (1996), 26 June, Maputo.
19. Harriet Ngubane, *Body and Mind in Zulu Medicine*. (London: Academic Press, 1977). Ngubane presents a very interesting analysis of social pollution among the Zulu.
20. For more information see Alcinda Honwana and Enny Pannizo, 'Evaluation of the Children and War Project', (1995), Consultancy Report for Save the Children USA in Mozambique.
21. Henrique Junod, *The Life of a South African Tribe*. Vol. 2, (London: Macmillan, 1927), 382.
22. See Alcinda Honwana, 'Instituições Religiosas Tradicionais e a Reintegração Social dos Grupos Vulneráveis', (1993), Consultancy Report for the Suisse Cooperation for Development in Mozambique.
23. These interviews were conducted in April 1993 in the villages of Massaka I and II, district of Boane, and in the village of Munguine in the district of Manhiça.

24. The colonial and post-colonial governments both repressed traditional beliefs and practices. For the former tradition was an hindrance to Christian conversion and to 'civilisation'; and for the latter it was regarded as mere superstitions which were locking people in the past and impairing change and development.

MISCARRIAGES OF JUSTICE: DEMONIC VENGEANCE IN CLASSICAL INDIAN MEDICINE

Dominik Wujastyk

Some people say pregnant women smell sweet, like a melon, and that is why they attract evil spirits.[1]

Introduction

In the classical tradition of Indian medicine, called *āyurveda* in Sanskrit, disease is seen as being caused by several agencies, including the supernatural. The question of disease etiology in *āyurveda* is of great interest, and is far from simple. One of the central etiological ideas in *āyurveda* is the 'crime against wisdom' (*prajñāparādha*), the idea that we fall ill through – to put it at its mildest – lapses of judgement. At its strongest, the idea proposed in the ancient medical compendia is that the immutable law of *karma* punishes us with disease for past abrogations of our integrity.[2] In the present essay I shall discuss some of the issues surrounding demonic possession viewed as medical punishment. There is a great deal about this topic in the classical treatises on *āyurveda*, and it is treated by both ancient and medieval authors as an important part of the classical tradition of medicine.

Given what the Sanskrit medical texts say about demonic possession, this essay inevitably becomes a meditation on the historically persistent and all too human tendency to add the weight of criticism, guilt and moral condemnation to the burden of natural suffering through illness or disease.

Amongst the most painful and difficult of all human conditions is the sickness or death of a child, whether before, during, or after childbirth. And while this is of course a shared pain for everyone around the child, the earlier in the process the disaster occurs, the more intimately the event involves the child's mother in particular.

It might seem, therefore, inhumanly harsh to make the mother the focus of special judgement and condemnation, and yet this is what we see again and again. Voices of sympathy or support are rare in the medical literature. More usual is the depiction of the woman as having caused her own disaster by laying herself open to demonic attack.

Carl Sagan, the late Cornell astronomer and space scientist, entitled one of his last books *The Demon-Haunted World*. This title he took from one of the earliest of Indian scriptures, the *Īśā Upaniṣad*, a short and deeply spiritual tract from the first millennium BC, still very popular in India today, which uses this phrase to describe the hell into which bad people are cast. Sagan's subtitle explains the purpose of the book: *Science as a Candle in the Dark*. His book is a splendidly enthusiastic and enjoyable tirade against all kinds of pseudo-science, unreason, and 'demonolatry.'[3] In Sagan's view, it is only Science – taken in the contemporary sense – that can provide the light by which we may travel the path of reason. Whether or not we agree with Sagan, his book is a deeply felt and passionate argument for values that few of us would openly deny, even as we avoid walking under ladders or treading on the cracks in the pavement.

As part of his characterization of pseudo-science, Sagan cited a striking passage in which Leon Trotsky described Germany on the eve of the Hitler takeover.

> Not only in peasant homes, but also in city skyscrapers, there lives alongside the twentieth century the thirteenth. A hundred million people use electricity and still believe in the magic powers of signs and exorcisms . . . Movie stars go to mediums. Aviators who pilot miraculous mechanisms created by man's genius wear amulets on their sweaters. What inexhaustible reserves they possess of darkness, ignorance, and savagery![4]

There is probably no country in the world today to which this characterization could not be applied, to a greater or lesser extent. The rise of unreason in its various guises is not to be taken lightly, and whatever our view of the details of Sagan's arguments, we do well to think seriously of some of the darker consequences of dogmatism and superstition, from which science is not immune either, of course.

All this can certainly be applied to India, whose *fin-de-siècle* population is approaching one billion, over seventy per cent of which still lives in villages. In this *real* India, people live by ideas and practices which have been changed little by the advent of dish-washers and personal computers in middle-class homes. Perhaps antibiotics have made a difference even at the grass roots, although when I was living in an Indian village in 1995, I learned, after the fact, of a man who died nearby from an infected wound in his leg which could have been treated easily with antibiotics. And the prevalence of cholera today in some areas shows that the germ-theory of disease transmission through contaminated water is still not as widely appreciated at the practical level as one might expect as we approach the dawn of the twenty-first century.

In the present essay I wish to address the question of what women in ancient India were told was happening when they had miscarriages, or when their children fell sick, how the voices of authority in their societies explained these personal tragedies. And in this matter, as the research of many ethnologists and social anthropologists has shown, the beliefs of the thirteenth century have not disappeared, but are living happily alongside the twentieth century.[5]

Demons and miscarriage in the Veda

An Indian preoccupation with demons as the cause of miscarriage is in fact considerably older than the thirteenth century, and can be traced back to the very earliest corpus of Indo-Aryan religious material. From the late second millennium BC, we have the following hymn of the *Ṛgveda* (10.162) in which the fire-god Agni is invoked in a prayer to help the suppliant drive away the incubus who brings disease to a woman's unborn child:[6]

> 4. The one who spreads apart your two thighs, who lies between the married pair, who licks the inside of your womb – we will drive him away from here.
> 5. The one who by changing into your brother, or your husband, or your lover lies with you, who wishes to kill your offspring – we will drive him away from here.
> 6. The one who bewitches you with sleep or darkness and lies with you – we will drive him away from here.

The theme of demonic attack causing miscarriage also occurs frequently in the *Atharvaveda*.[7] Hymn 2.25, for example, is a charm employing the plant *pṛṣṇiparṇī* against a flesh-eating demon called Kaṇva who is particularly known as a devourer of embryos.[8]

However, in neither of these sources is this theme elaborated, nor is it related especially to issues of responsibility. For that, we turn to the specialist literature of ancient Indian medicine.

Demons in Sanskrit medical literature

Like so many important works in ancient Indian literature, the basic medical literature springs into history without prelude, like Athena from the head of Zeus. These texts, which are of encyclopaedic length and style, probably began to be shaped from the time of the Buddha, and reached their present form in the early centuries of our era.[9] Already in their earliest form, they divide medical science into eight canonical sections, one of which is 'Bhūtavidyā' or the science of spirits. The next division is 'Kaumārabhṛtya' or the nurturing of children. In practice, this eightfold division of medicine is not followed closely in the arrangement of most medical textbooks, and these two subjects in particular are commonly dealt with as a single topic, since children and mothers are seen as being the people most vulnerable to demonic influence.

Suśruta

The last book of Suśruta's *Compendium*, one of the original Indian medical encyclopaedias, contains a series of chapters on the demons of disease. These chapters are thought to be a later addition to the main text, but nevertheless they probably date from the early first millennium AD, and contain much material that was in still earlier circulation.

Suśruta describes nine demons. They are called – in Saṇskrit – '*graha's*, that is 'grabbers', 'graspers,' 'seizers'. The same word, *graha*, is also used in astral literature to mean a planet, because of the planetary influence on the mundane world, and there are also nine planets in traditional Indian astrology. This parallelism of terminology has led to confusion in the past, and attempts to interpret the medical material with astrological implications. But we can be certain that in the early Sanskrit medical literature no astrological connection with planets plays a part. Medical *grahas* are demons pure and simple.

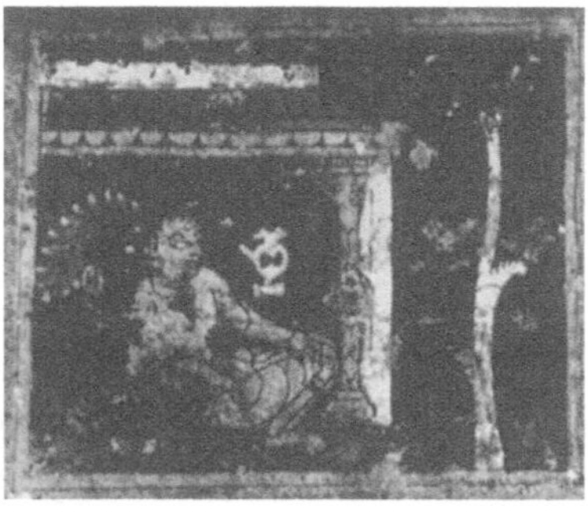

Fig. 1

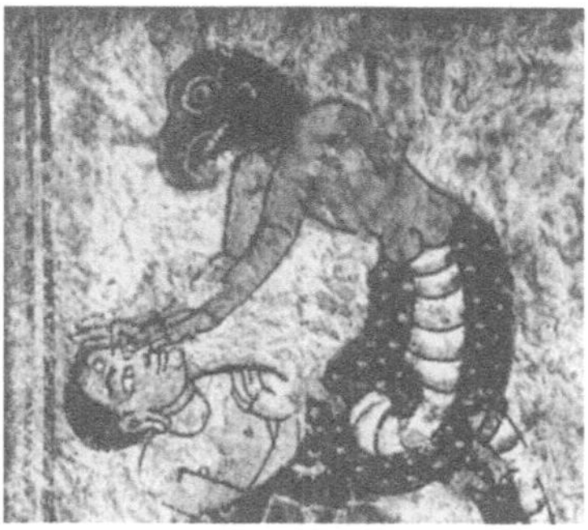

Fig. 2

Figure 1: A particularly sinister image of the demon king Skanda (also called 'Kumāra'), Wellcome Institute MS Indic α 1936, f. 16r (courtesy of the Governors of the Wellcome Trust). *Figure 2:* Śakuni as bird-serpent attacks a victim's eye, from Wellcome Institute MS Indic α 1937, f. 2v (courtesy of the Governors of the Wellcome Trust).

The texts describing the demons are very vivid, and it is therefore perhaps not surprising that from an early period there has existed in India a tradition of illustrating such demonic figures. The library of the Wellcome Institute for the History of Medicine includes three Nepalese Sanskrit manuscripts which contain miniature paintings showing some of Suśruta's demons in graphic detail. Although these vivid and frightening images deserve fuller treatment for their importance in the history of Indian miniature painting, they are included here to exemplify the emotional impact which these images evoke today, and must have evoked for the patients to whom they were shown in pre-modern times.[10]

Suśruta calls the nine demons by the following names:[11] Skanda (Fig. 1), Skandāpasmāra (epileptic Skanda), Śakunī (Fig. 2), Revatī (Fig. 6), Pūtanā (Fig. 3), Andhapūtanā, Śītapūtanā, Mukhamaṇḍikā (Fig. 4), and Naigameṣa.

Immediately after listing these demons, Suśruta introduces the moral dimension, which we shall see again and again. These demons, says Suśruta, attack children whose mothers or nurses have not behaved properly. If a mother or nurse has not followed Suśruta's earlier advice, or has not kept the child properly clean, or in a state of ritual grace, then these demons will attack and torment the child. This is Medical Justice: disease as retribution.

Suśruta gives detailed descriptions of the symptoms of each kind of demonic attack. For example, when attacked by Mukhamaṇḍikā (Fig. 4), the child is pale and distended, frightened, has a huge

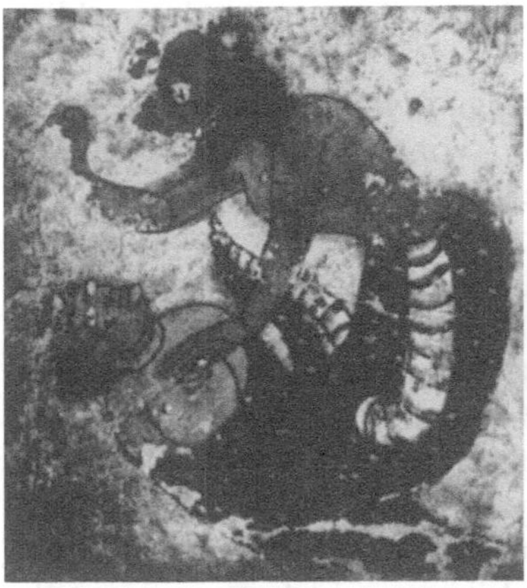

Fig. 3

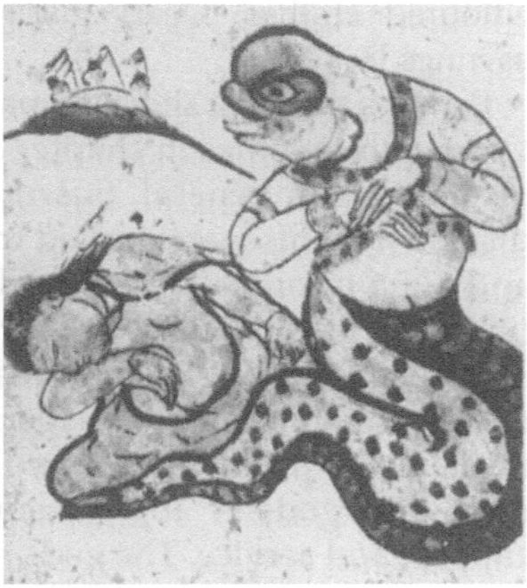

Fig. 4

Figure 3: Pūtanā, 'Stinking Lady,' from Wellcome Institute MS Indic α 1937, f. 11r (courtesy of the Governors of the Wellcome Trust). *Figure 4:* Mukhamaṇḍikā, from Wellcome Institute MS Indic β 1409, f. 7r (courtesy of the Governors of the Wellcome Trust).

appetite, develops a net-like tracing of veins on the belly, and smells of urine.

The general treatment for such a demonic seizure is to anoint the child with rancid butter, to put mustard seeds on the floor and burn a mustard oil lamp in the room, and to perform fire offerings and prayers to various gods, including Skanda (Fig. 1), who is called the lord of the nine demons. In later chapters, more detailed treatments are described. These are more medically-oriented, and include the application of several herbal balms and fumigations.

Or take the example of the demoness Revatī, 'Lady Opulence,' about whom we shall in due course learn much more (Fig. 6). When she attacks, the child turns yellowish-brown, with a blood-red face. The child gets an inflamed mouth, feels bruised all over, and constantly rubs his or her nose and ears. The affected child must be sprinkled with a herbal decoction, anointed with a medicated oil, and given daily doses of medicated ghee. The child must wear a protective amulet, and the physician should perform certain rituals to propitiate Lady Opulence. Her fearsome appearance is described in terms which are very similar to those of Kāśyapa's *Compendium*, a text which will be examined in more detail below. She has a dark complexion, is dressed in multicoloured clothes, wears garlands of flowers, and sparkling earrings.[12]

Perhaps the most shocking passage in this section of Suśruta's *Compendium* comes in chapter 37, when the author discourses on demons in general. Suśruta first describes how the nine disease demons were created from the gods Agni, Śiva, Kṛttikā and Umā in order to be guardians for the newly-born Guha (Skanda). Skanda, who is described as the leader of the armies of heaven, then asks the great god Śiva how his guardian disease-demons might be expected to support themselves. Śiva explains the process whereby the three-fold world of animals, men, and gods is able to survive only through reciprocal support and service. The gods provide weather, especially rain, to support men and animals, while men in turn support the gods by offering worship and prayer. But what happens if this system breaks down? Then people do not worship the gods. Priests (*brāhmaṇas*), guests, and gurus do not get treated with the proper deference and hospitality. Beggars get no alms from people like this.

Śiva then gives his terrible judgement on this rupture of the fabric of mutual-dependence: these are the people upon whom the disease demons may prey. Śiva puts this very strongly: he urges the demons to attack such people without the slightest compunction or mercy. And if the parents of the sick children begin, in their desperation, to worship the demons, then it only proves the tactic was justified, and this worship provides support and subsistence for the demons.

And this, Suśruta concludes, is ultimately why the demons came into existence and started to attack the children of bad people.[13]

It could not be made more clear that disease is the direct result of moral turpitude. And the great god Śiva himself has sanctioned the demons of disease mercilessly to attack the children of bad parents.[14]

The *Kumāratantra* of Rāvaṇa

It is impossible to address the topic of demons in pre-modern India without referring to perhaps the most well-known demon text of all, the *Rāvaṇa-Kumāratantra*. It dates from a period over a millennium later than the ancient material in Suśruta's famous

Compendium, yet is is still a very old text. It is a short Sanskrit work on female demons who attack children at particular times of the day, month, or year. The twelve female demons, or 'little mothers' (*mātṛkās*), are not identical to nine demons of Suśruta, but several are the same. They are Nandā (happy lady), Sunandā (very happy lady), Pūtanā (stinker), Mukhamaṇḍitikā (Fig. 4), Kaṭapūtanā (stinker), Śakunikā (omen bird lady, Fig. 2), Śuṣkarevatī (dry lady opulence), Āryakā (Her Ladyship), Sūtikā (Birthing lady), Nirṛtā (Decay), Pilipicchikā (Fig. 5), and Kāmukā (Lover lady).

The *Kumāratantra* is known from individual manuscripts, but also as a text embedded within longer medical works. It forms a section in the eleventh-century *Cikitsāsārasaṃgraha* by the distinguished commentator Cakrapāṇidatta. It is also present as a section within Trimallabhaṭṭa's eighteenth-century *Yogataraṅgiṇī* But we only get an idea of the true influence of this little work when we realize that translations and reworkings appeared all over the Middle and Far East: translations of the *Kumāratantra* can be found in Tamil, Tibetan, Chinese, Cambodian, and even in Arabic.[15]

As an example of the tenor of the work, let us examine what the text says about the demoness Pilipicchikā (Fig. 5):[16]

> Signs:
>
> On the eleventh day, month, or year, the little mother called Pilipicchikā takes possession. Then, immediately upon being possessed, a fever arises, food is rejected, the gaze is turned upwards, the limbs thrash, and there is vomiting.

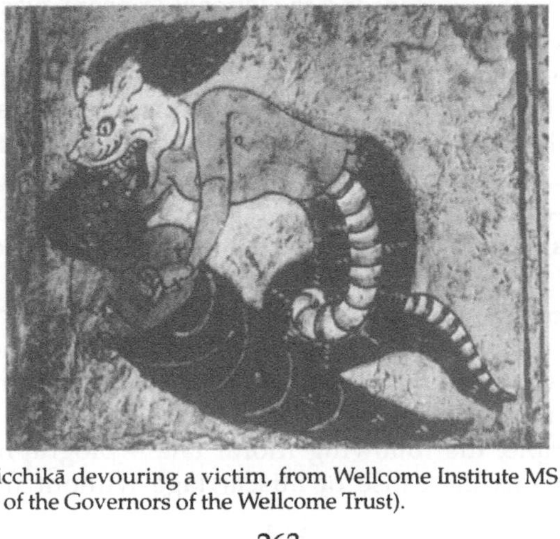

Figure 5: Pilipicchikā devouring a victim, from Wellcome Institute MS Indic α 1937, f. 7v (courtesy of the Governors of the Wellcome Trust).

Medicine:

An image should be made out of rice-flour with its face painted red with red sandalwood paste, and should be sprinkled with milk. A tribute offering should be made to the east with yellow flowers, perfume, betel leaves, seven yellow pennants, seven lamps, eight cakes, eight buns, eight sweet bread rolls, fish, meat, and wine. A bath should be taken in still water, and there should be a fumigation with bael leaves, myrrh, cow's horn, a cast-off snakeskin, and melted butter. This should be accompanied by the incantation 'Oṃ bow to Rāvaṇa, please release so-and-so from the disease. Release.' This should be done for three days. On the fourth day one should give food to priests. Then the child will become himself again.

This is how a good result is obtained.

Haunted women and the ripening of deeds

That such ideas were widespread in early India is confirmed – if confirmation were necessary – by the testimony of early foreign vistors to India. The Greek philosopher Apollonius of Tyana is reported by his biographer Philostratus (fl.ca. AD 170) to have travelled through Asia to India in the early part of the first century AD.

Apollonius described how, during his stay in India, the spirit of a dead man had haunted his widow. Iarchus, the Hindu king with whom Apollonius was in audience, 'drew a letter out of his bosom and gave it to the woman; and the letter, it appears, was addressed to the ghost and contained threats of an alarming kind.'[17]

The more specific idea that women are not merely subject to hauntings, but are guilty for their own miscarriages is also clear from popular Indian texts in other genres, such as the *Vṛddha-karmavipāka*, the 'Great Ripening of Deeds.' This text, available in an eighteenth-century manuscript,[18] consists of thousands of micro-biographies which explain the difficulties in ordinary people's lives in terms of the fruition of past *karma*. It is the level of detail that makes the text interesting: it describes short episodes of personal defeat and disaster in the lives of individuals, together with an account of what they did in previous lives to bring the present retribution down upon their heads.

For example, the following moral tale – biography number 1793 – explains the cause of miscarriage without reference to demons, yet it highlights the fact that the mother is personally responsible for the disaster:[19]

> Once upon a time, in a previous incarnation, a woman wanted to make her unborn baby thrive, so she ate some chicken's eggs. Then, in her present life, she was born into a mixed caste, and was very greedy. She was rich in money and grain, because of her previous good deeds. But because of the previous bad deed of eating an egg, she could not maintain a pregnancy.

The text continues to explain that by performing the correct propitiation of priests (*brāhmaṇas*), and performing rituals (*pūjās*), she was able to restore her fertility and became the mother of many sons.

The *Compendium* of Kāśyapa

Let us turn now to a text which has so far escaped general notice in this context, the ompendium ascribed to Kāśyapa. This work has not before been translated into any European language, and its contents have not been generally integrated into studies of ancient Indian medicine.[20] Therefore, I shall dwell on this work in slightly more detail.

Kāśyapa's *Compendium* survives only in two fragmentary Sanskrit manuscripts. As such, it is amongst the group of important āyurvedic texts that have barely reached the twentieth century.[21]

The first of the manuscripts of Kāśyapa's *Compendium* was discovered by the great Bengali scholar Haraprasād Śāstrī in Kathmandu in 1898. This Nepalese manuscript consisted of only thirty-eight palm leaves, and covered just a fraction of the text. Subsequent scholars have been unable to find this manuscript again, but before it disappeared it was copied out by hand and photographed by the French scholar Palmyr Cordier. He deposited these copies in the Bibliothèque National in Paris.[22]

The second manuscript of the text came into the hands of the learned pandit Hemarāja Śarman some time before 1938, although we do not know from where. His manuscript consisted of palm leaves numbered 29–264, with many gaps. He published the text based on this manuscript, and included a photograph of five leaves in his introduction. Pandit Hemarāja judged his manuscript to be between 700 and 800 years old.

The following discussion is based on Pandit Hemarāja's edition.[23]

The date of Kāśyapa's Compendium

A short text called *Kāśyaparṣiproktastrīcikitsāsūtra*, or 'The Sūtra of Women's Medicine Declared by the Sage Kāśyapa,' though lost in Sanskrit, has been discovered in a Chinese translation as part of the Chinese Buddhist Tripiṭaka. It appears to be one of the lost chapters of Kāśyapa's *Compendium*. The Chinese translation was done by the Buddhist monk Dharmadeva (or Dharmabhadra), who travelled to China in AD 973, and remained there for almost thirty years, until his death in AD 1001.[24]

Based on this and other evidence, the composition of the Sanskrit text may tentatively be pushed back to about the seventh century, though parts may have been extracted from or modelled on earlier texts. There are some extremely archaic words and usages in the *Revatīkalpa* chapter, which we shall look at in more detail, usages which one normally associates with the *Brāhmaṇas* and *Upaniṣads* of the first millennium BC. While it is impossible to be certain, I suspect that this is not a deliberate attempt to write something old-fashioned, but rather a genuine survival of extremely ancient material perhaps from before the beginning of the Common Era.

Revatī, Lady Opulence the demoness child-killer

A full chapter in Kāśyapa's *Compendium* is devoted to the demoness Revatī (Fig. 6), who is described in the following vivid terms:

> She is extremely violent, full of life-force, and she looks horrifying. She is feral, with her folded wings, diamond-hard beak, talons, teeth, and fangs. Her eyes burn like gems, and her great wings are many-splendoured. At her throat she wears sparkling gold and jewels, and she wears assorted flowers, perfumes, clothes, and she carries a club, all ablaze. She has a fine crown and wears anklets, necklaces, shell-bracelets, armbands, earrings, and bells. She is decorated with pennant, umbrella, firebrand, and a garland of clouds flashing with lightning.

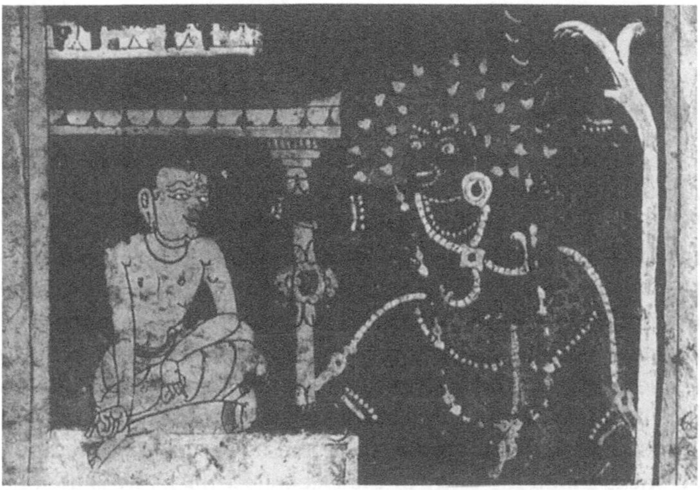

Figure 6: Revatī, 'Lady Opulence,' from Wellcome Institute MS Indic α 1936, f. 19r (courtesy of the Governors of the Wellcome Trust).

Note particularly that she appears to her victims in dreams. Kāśyapa's *Compendium* says:

> She who is both the demoness[25] and sister of the majestic Skanda first violates a child in a dream, and immediately after that she causes a disease to come upon him. Then at midday, or midnight, at dawn, or dusk, or when asleep in the nursery, one of the females mentioned before perches on him. At that, the child gives out a high-pitched shriek, and screams, trembles and shudders, is scared and feverish, becomes distressed, groans loudly,[26] becomes delirious and unstable, has stinging feelings and swelling, deteriorates, and is beset by other diseases too.

The Revatī section of Kāśyapa's *Compendium* presents a fully worked-out mythology to explain miscarriage and the early death of children.[27] The story begins with Prajāpati, Father of Creatures and creator of the world, existing before creation. After the processes of creation have been underway for a while, the gods and demons get into a fight, a theme that is ancient and widespread in traditional Indian mythology. The interesting twist given to the story in this version involves the goddess Revatī, Lady Opulence, who is brought in to fight on the gods' side. As in other versions of the tale, she kills the demons. But more than that, she notices with her divine eye that they escape to be reborn in human and animal wombs. So she transforms herself into the disease-figure Jātahāriṇī, literally 'she who takes away what has been born,' and *follows them through their rebirths, killing them again and again.*

> But Lady Opulence saw those demons in their human and animal wombs. So she turned into Jātahāriṇī, the Childsnatcher, and killed them. And so it is that Childsnatcher kills the menstrual blood, she kills the embryo (*vapus*), she kills the fetuses, she kills those that have been born, she kills those being born, she kills those who will be born, and especially anyone demonic, anyone descended from sinners, anyone tainted with sin. She is the one, Vṛddhajīvaka, Old Lifegiver. She is called Lady Opulence, Shapechanger (*bahurūpā*), Childsnatcher, Pilipicchikā. And she is called the Screamer, and she is called the Lady of the Ocean (*Vāruṇī*). She is the one who, by the power of Skanda's wish, has come into being amongst all creatures to confound sinners, for the eradication of evildoers.

This train of thinking leads inevitably to the idea, elaborated explicitly in the text, that miscarriage and child mortality happen because the soul of the infant is either a former demon, or has been tainted in some way by evil and unrighteousness. And from that it is a small step to saying that miscarriage happens to bad women. So the text presents a passage describing the kind of bad woman whom Jātahāriṇī, the Childsnatcher, catches. This passage is wonderfully vivid in its characterization.

> Now, consider a woman who has given up righteousness, pious behaviour, purity and devotion to god. She hates the gods, cows, priests, gurus, elders, and good people, she is badly behaved, egotistical, and fickle. She loves quarrels, strife, meat-eating, cruelty, sleep and sex. She is vicious, spiteful, voracious, garrulous, nonchalant, and she laughs, bawls, or laments for no apparent reason. She tells lies, is a greedy eater, is rumoured to be prepared to eat anything, does whatever she wants, and rejects conducive food and conversation. She is fiercely impious. She is cruel to other peoples' children, only cares about her own business, and is negligent about helping others. She is contrary with her husband, has no love for her children, and constantly curses them. She deeply despises her

> father-in-law, her sister-in-law, her brother-in-law, priests, and others who hold such positions. She may devastate them with her fury, or curse them. She is wicked and puts the evil eye on her co-wife, or she does black magic on her using mantras, evil herbs and rituals. And she drops the baby on his head! She doesn't know their joys and sorrows. She is malicious towards her friends, what she says is jinxed. She never makes peace offerings, she never does rituals, or meditates, or gives to charity, or makes offerings to her ancestors, or congratulates anyone, or spits, or kisses or hugs anyone, even when it is appropriate.
>
> Because of this behaviour, and because of other bad actions, past and present, such as habitually drinking, eating, sleeping and wrangling, she creates openings, caused by the unrighteousness, through which Childsnatcher fastens on to her.
>
> Then her husband starts to behave like this too!
>
> One should realize that for such a pair, Childsnatcher is incurable. If only one of the couple is unrighteous, the Childsnatcher is curable with difficulty. But if they are both righteous, upright, free from pride, and healthy, their children will thrive.

In the light of the pervasiveness of such heavily value-laden explanations, it is interesting to see in this part of Kāśyapa's *Compendium* that the author sometimes develops his thinking slightly beyond this point, and presents a form of what might be taken as spirit-contagion as a cause for miscarriage and child mortality. The idea of disease contagion is not common in pre-modern medicine from any culture, and this passage is interesting as an early occurrence of the concept in India.[28]

> Suppose a woman who is pregnant for the first time comes into contact with people whose children have died, or with other women friends who are unclean, impure, bad, who are not accepted by society, or who have been caught by Childsnatcher. Perhaps she eats with them, washes with them, exchanges clothes or ornaments. Or she treads on the places where they bathe, or pee, or leave their food offerings. Or, in particular, she treads on hair, nails, body lotion, or offcuts of old clothing which have been contaminated by menstrual blood, or she accepts leftovers of food, drink, herbs, perfume, flowers, or old sandals. If this happens, Childsnatcher will fasten on to her.

> Or suppose a woman is pregnant for the very first time, or is goodlooking, shapely, healthy, and her hips, bosoms, thighs, arms and face are chubby. Her conjugal happiness is on the increase, her hair is lovely, and her large eyes are charmingly tinted red at the corners. The line of hair on her belly is growing fast, and her hands, feet, nails, eyes, and skin have a gloss to them. She is exquisitely dainty, tender, and languid. Her womb grows steadily bigger as time goes by, her body increases in weight, and her breasts fill with milk. If wicked people, on seeing a pregnant woman like this, keep staring at her, and she fails to perform a pacification ritual, then Childsnatcher will fasten on to her.
>
> For this reason, a woman who wants a child is advised to perform voluntary rites every day, so that she can lay to rest such evil. Therefore a pregnant woman should not even eat with her own mother.

It is extraordinary that the pregnant mother can be placed in jeopardy by the presence of her own mother. But the pregnant woman's husband can be an even greater threat, even if he has taken care to be ritually pure. The text continues:

> One has to be especially careful during the first pregnancy. Through his own fault, even a wise brahmin priest who has performed many rituals and is actually engaged in a ritual can be fastened onto by Childsnatcher. Someone who is antagonistic in discussions, a hypocrite, an egotist, all such people, as well as priests, become food for Childsnatcher.
>
> When the husband goes along the road at night and gets dusty feet, then if he touches his wife during her period or when she is pregnant, Lady Opulence can take possession.
>
> If a husband makes love to a woman who has been seized by Childsnatcher, then the moment he goes to his wife, Childsnatcher fastens on to her.
>
> One should always avoid a home which has been seized by Childsnatcher. Anything received from there will make Childsnatcher seize you.

Notice the inversion: in contemporary thinking, we catch a disease, but in this text, the 'disease' catches us.

Finally, here is a description of the poor woman who has been possessed by the Lady Opulence:

> These are the forms which her deteriorating body acquires: her gaze darts about, she becomes agitated, and she does not thrive at the time she should. Her spirit is broken, she has no energy, and she suffers stabbing pains in the abdomen. She looks awful, and she is attacked by various diseases. Her sense of initiative disappears, as does her perseverance. She becomes stale, disfigured and wanton. She involves herself in everything, but succeeds in nothing. Any sense of achievement eludes her. The young of her cows, goats, sheep and buffaloes do not survive. She gets a dreadful reputation, and may become a widow.[29] Once attracted, Childsnatcher may destroy her family.

It is interesting to note that in this telling of the myth, Revatī is introduced as a champion of the gods, but ends up being a horrific demoness figure.

Conclusion

Mahatma Gandhi, speaking of the earthquake of 15 January 1934 which devastated Bihar, said, 'A man of prayer regards what are known as physical calamities as divine chastisement alike for individuals and nations . . . A man like me cannot but believe that this earthquake is a divine chastisement sent by God for our sins'.[30] The idea that disease and calamity are consequences of evil conduct has existed in many – if not most – cultures and periods. When Jenner developed smallpox vaccination in England at the end of the eighteenth century, debates raged throughout Europe about whether the disease should be suffered as a punishment from God to evildoers, or whether it was acceptable to prevent its occurrence. Throughout the Muslim Middle-East too, the ethics of avoiding, or attempting to cure, lethal diseases such as plague became a prominent subject for debate in *haḍīth* literature.[31] After all, if God had sent the disease as a punishment for evildoers, was it not it was morally wrong to seek to escape his cleansing wrath? And in Europe, it was only in the eighteenth century that Enlightenment physicians finally abandoned the Biblical idea that mental illness was caused by diabolical possession.[32] Even in contemporary times, religious fundamentalists have seen AIDS and 'mad cow' disease as divine punishments visited on an immoral society.

The rise of the fundamentalist Hindu right in India in the 1990s is perhaps the most serious political issue to have faced India since independence fifty years ago. As in other countries, fundamentalism brings with it a return to what are perceived as 'old' values and beliefs. We may conclude with the prominent right-wing Hindu fundamentalist leader, Acharya Giriraj Kishore, who heads a campaign in South India against the use of cows in the meat trade. Under the byline 'Right-wing Hindus revel in "mad-cow" scare,' CNN reported in March 1996 that the Acharya, a former professor of Indian history and Hindu activist for 50 years, saw mad cow disease as a message from God that the world should follow the Hindu way of life.[33]

> I feel that the West is being punished by God due to their brutal killing habit . . . And if the world continues to insist on eating beef, they risk inviting the wrath of the gods.

Once again, in a statement that could have been made two thousand years ago, and which has been echoed throughout the intervening period, a direct connection is made between medical suffering and the abrogation of moral law.

NOTES

1. Jeffery *et al.* (1989), citing an informant from the early 1980s.
2. For accessible introductions to the concept of *prajñāparādha*, see Dasgupta (1969: II, 415–18 *et passim*), and Weiss (1980).
3. Other important studies of this fascinating subject include Radner and Radner (1982), Gardner (1957), and Regis (1992).
4. Sagan (1996: 20 f.).
5. See, for example, the works of Kapferer (1983), Jeffery *et al.* (1989).
6. Translation: O'Flaherty (1981: 292).
7. Dasgupta (1969: 2.300) lists the names of several Atharvanic demons.
8. Bloomfield (1979: 36, 302).
9. On the formation of early Indian medical literature, see Zysk (1991).
10. The manuscripts are Wellcome MS Indic α 1936, Wellcome MS Indic α 1937, and Wellcome MS Indic β 1409. (For another image of Revatī, from a manuscript in the private collection of Murial and Jack Zimmerman, see van Alphen and Aris (1995: 32).) The first of these Wellcome manuscripts is dated to AD 1480. The second, though not dated, must be from a similar period. MS Indic β 1409 is a later manuscript, perhaps from the end of the eighteenth century. An extraordinarily similar image from an eighteenth-nineteenth century Greek manuscript is reproduced in Stewart (1991: 171). It shows a demoness called 'Beauty of the Mountains' who is inspecting a table of foods which has been put out to placate her. Each demon image is Wellcome MS Indic β 1409 is also accompanied by a picture of a placatory food offering. Like the Nepalese

demons, the bottom half of Beauty of the Mountains's body is serpentine, and the whole montage is remarkably similar to the Indian material. The textual matter contained in these manuscripts is not, in fact, Suśruta's *Compendium*, but different versions of a much later type of text in the *grahaśānti* genre (cf.Kane (1968–77: 5.719–814), describing the days and times at which these demons attack, as well as rites and prayers to avert their baleful influence.

11. See Ācārya (1992: utt.27).
12. See Ācārya (1992: utt.37).
13. Filliozat (1937: 77) notes that this passage in Suśruta's *Compendium* is almost certainly inspired by *Mahābhārata*, 'Vanaparvan', Mārk. verse 14309 ff. of the Calcutta edition.
14. Ācārya (1992: utt.37.19):
    utsannabalibhikṣeṣu bhinnakāṃsyopabhojiṣu//
    gṛheṣu teṣu ye bālās tān gṛhṇīdhvam aśaṅkitāḥ//
    tatra vo vipulā vṛttiḥ pūjā caiva bhaviṣyati//
15. See Filliozat (1937).
16. Cited from Sharma (1994: 565). This text may be compared with the following works which contain similar material: the *Uḍḍīśatantra*, the *Īśānaśivagurudevapaddhati*, the *Agnipurāṇa* and, as previously noted, the *Mahābhārata*. For these other works of this genre, see Goudriaan and Gupta (1981: 127 ff.).
17. Translation: Philostratus (1912: 317).
18. Wellcome MS Indic δ48.
19. Anonymous (1909: 570). Thite (1982) and Pingree (1997) provide further interesting materials from this work.
20. Since writing this, a translation by Tewari (1996) has been published; although dated 1996, the book appears to have become generally available from the publisher only in late 1997 or early 1998.
21. Other texts in this category include the *Bheḷasaṃhitā*, the *Aṣṭāṅgasaṃgraha* of Vāgbhaṭa, the *Navanītaka* and even the *Carakasaṃhitā* itself. None of these texts is represented by more than a few manuscripts, often fragmentary. Of Bheḷa's *Compendium* there is only a single manuscript, in the great Saraswati Mahal Library in Thanjavur, South India. The *Navanītaka* is a short text which we know only from a single manuscript found in the Taklamakan desert of Central Asia.
22. Bibliothèque National MSS 1155 et 1156 du fonds Palmyr Cordier (Filliozat 1934: 157). See also Roşu (1989: 540 f., *et passim*).
23. Hemarāja Śarman (1988).
24. See Bagchi (1942/43).
25. Read *grahaṇī*? There are problems with the manuscript readings in this passage.
26. Read *vistan-*?
27. *Kāśyapasaṃhitā* 6, the 'Revatīkalpa' (Hemarāja Śarman 1988: 187–202).
28. Cf. Conrad and Wujastyk (forthcoming).
29. Verse 29a: read *prāpnute*.
30. Tendulkar (1962: 3.304–8, 4.41–42), cited by Kane (1968–77: 5.764).
31. See Conrad (1993: 683–6).

32. Porter (1990: 66).
33. http://www.cnn.com/WORLD/9603/mad-cow/29/india/index.html (the article misprints the date).

REFERENCES

Ācārya, Jādavji Trikamji (ed.) (1992). *Suśrutasaṃhitā, śrīḍalhaṇācāryaviractayā nibandhasaṃgrahākhyavyākhyayā nidānasthānasya śrīgayadāsāryaviracitayā nyāyacandrikākhyapañjikāvyākhyayā ca samullasitā . . . Ācāryopāhvena trivikramātmajena yādavaśarmaṇā . . . saṃśodhitā.* Vārāṇasī, Delhi: Caukhambhā Oriyanṭāliyā, fifth edn.

van Alphen, Jan and Anthony Aris (eds.) (1995). *Oriental medicine: an illustrated guide to the Asian arts of healing.* London: Serindia Publications.

Anonymous (1909). *Vṛddha-Sūryāruṇakarmavipāka.* Bombay: Khemarāja Śrīkṛṣṇadāsa.

Bagchi, P. C. (1942/43). 'A fragment of the Kāśyapa-saṃhitā in Chinese.' *Indian Culture,* **9**, 53–64.

Bloomfield, Maurice (1979). *Hymns of the Atharvaveda.* No. XLII in Sacred Books of the East. Delhi: Motilal Banarsidass, repr. of 1897 edn.

Conrad, Lawrence I. and Dominik Wujastyk (eds.) (forthcoming). *Contagion: perspectives from pre-modern societies.* London, New York: Kegan Paul International.

Conrad, Lawrence I. (1993). 'Arab-Islamic medicine.' In W. F. Bynum and Roy Porter (eds.), *Companion encyclopedia of the history of medicine,* vol. 1, chap. 31, pp. 676–727. London: Routledge. 2v.

Dasgupta, Surendranath (1969). *A history of Indian philosophy.* Cambridge: Cambridge University Press, fifth edn.

Filliozat, Jean (1934). 'Liste des manuscrits de la collection Palmyr Cordier conservés à la Bibliothèque Nationale.' *Journal asiatique,* **224**, 155–73.

Filliozat, Jean (1937). *Étude de démonologie indienne: le Kumāratantra de Rāvaṇa et les textes parallèles Indiens Tibétains, Chinois, Cambodgien et Arabe.* Paris: Imprimerie Nationale.

Gardner, Martin (1957). *Fads and fallacies in the name of science.* New York: Dover.

Goudriaan, Teun and Sanjukta Gupta (1981). *Hindu tantric and śākta literature,* vol. 2.2 *of A history of Indian literature.* Wiesbaden: Harrassowitz.

Hemarāja Śarman (ed.) (1988). *Kāśyapasaṃhitā (vṛddhajīvakīyaṃ tantraṃ vā) maharṣiṇā mārīcakaśyapenopadiṣṭā . . . Hemarājaśarmaṇā . . . samullasitā* Vārāṇasī: Caukhambhā Saṃskṛta Saṃsthāna, fourth edn.

Jeffery, Patricia, Roger Jeffery, and Andrew Lyon (1989). *Labour pains and labour power : women and childbearing in India.* London: Zed.

Kane, P. V. (1968-77). *A history of Dharmaśāstra.* Poona: Bhandarkar Oriental Research Institute, second edn. 5v.

Kapferer, Bruce (1983). *A celebration of demons: exorcism and the aesthetics of healing in Sri Lanka.* Bloomington: Indiana University Press.

O'Flaherty, Wendy (1981). *The Rig Veda.* New Delhi: Penguin.

Philostratus (1912). *The Life of Apollonius of Tyana, the epistles of Apollonius and the treatise of Eusebius, with an English translation by F. C. Conybeare*, vol. 1. Cambridge, Mass.: Harvard University Press, 6th edn.

Pingree, David (1997). 'Two *Karmavipāka* texts on curing diseases and other misfortunes.' *Journal of the European Āyurvedic Society*, **5**, 46–52.

Porter, Roy (1990). *The Enlightenment*. London: Macmillan.

Radner, Daisie and Michael Radner (1982). *Science and unreason*. Belmont, CA.: Wadsworth.

Regis, Ed (1992). *Great mambo chicken and the transhuman condition: science slightly over the edge*. London: Penguin.

Roşu, Arion (1989). *Un demi-siècle de recherches āyurvédiques. Gustave Liétard et Palmyr Cordier: Travaux sur l'histoire de la médecine indienne*. Paris: Institut de Civilisation Indienne.

Sagan, Carl (1996). *The demon-haunted world: science as a candle in the dark*. London: Headline.

Sharma, Priya Vrat (ed.) (1994). *Cakradatta (Text with English Translation: A treatise on principles and practices of ayurvedic medicine)*. No. 17 in Kashi Ayurveda Series. Varanasi, Delhi: Caukhambha Orientalia.

Stewart, Charles (1991). *Demons and the devil: moral imagination in modern Greek culture*. Princeton: Princeton University Press.

Tendulkar, Dinanath Gopal (1962). *Mahatma: Life of Mohandas Karamchand Gandhi*. Delhi: Government of India, new edn. 8v.

Tewari, P. V. (1996). *Kāśyapa-saṃhitā or Vṛddhajīvakīya tantra: text with English translation and commentary*. Varanasi: Chaukhambha Visvabharati.

Thite, G. U. (1982). *Medicine: its magico-religious aspects according to the vedic and later literature*. Poona: Continental Prakashan. Publisher: A. A. Kulkarni, Continental Prakashan, Vijayanagar, Poona 30.

Weiss, Mitchell G. (1980). '*Caraka Saṃhitā* on the doctrine of karma.' In Wendy Doniger O'Flaherty (ed.), *Karma and rebirth in classical Indian traditions*, pp. 90–115. Berkeley: University of California Press.

Zysk, Kenneth G. (1991). *Asceticism and healing in ancient India: medicine in the Buddhist monastery*. New York, Bombay, etc.: OUP.

III

COMPARATIVE PERSPECTIVES ON MEDICINE AND RELIGION IN THE ANCIENT WORLD

Helen King

In ancient Greece, the main myth accounting for suffering permits a variety of answers to the question of its origin. The culture-hero, Prometheus, attempted to trick 'the mind of Zeus', the chief god of the Olympian pantheon, into taking the inferior portion of a sacrificed ox; Zeus duly took it, but planned his revenge.[1] Because Zeus is all-knowing, but not all-powerful, there is no 'theodicy problem' in the ancient pagan world. After Prometheus had stolen fire from the gods to give to the mortal men whose helper he traditionally was, Zeus caused the creation of the first woman, Pandora. Moulded by all the gods into the deceptive form of a marriageable virgin containing 'the mind of a bitch', she was sent to earth, where she opened the jar containing all the evils the world now knows: diseases, pain, grief, old age. Who is here responsible for suffering? Pandora? Zeus, who sent her? Prometheus, whose actions caused her to be made? Or all the gods, since each contributed to her creation?

The ancient Greeks are thus a particular case for the issues of this book; indeed, they form more than one case, since by the classical period of the fifth century BCE each city-state had its own constitution, preferred deities and outlook on life, although they shared a world-view or culture. This chapter raises a number of issues concerning the relationships between medical and religious approaches to health and suffering in the societies of classical antiquity, and suggests ways in which the traditional models by which we study medicine and religion in the ancient world can be challenged and refreshed by perspectives provided by materials from the social sciences.

The enterprise of cross-cultural comparison is far from straightforward. Its use in classical studies remains surprisingly controversial after years of conversation between classics and anthropology.[2] In a recent book on ancient gynaecology, for example, Lesley Dean-Jones used some brief cross-cultural references in order to emphasize the absence from classical Greece of taboos associated with menstruating women; she then proceeded to investigate ancient Greek social structures to account for this absence. In reviewing the book, Danielle Gourevitch responded to this limited and cautious use of cross-cultural comparison only by asking, 'What does it matter here what happens in this or that American Indian tribe?'[3] This debate is far from new; in his preface to *The Greeks and the Irrational* (1951), E.R. Dodds defended his own use of 'recent anthropological and psychological observations', aware that 'such borrowings from unfamiliar disciplines are, I know, generally received by the learned with apprehension and often with active distaste'. Dodds went on to criticize classical scholars of his day who were working with 'obsolete anthropological concepts'. Cross-cultural comparison which operates at the level of theory continues to attract such criticisms. There remains the real danger for classical scholars of adopting the very theories which anthropology has just discarded.[4] Traditionally, historical disciplines have turned to anthropology in a very limited way, to gain some insight into what are perceived as the more exotic areas of belief and culture, rather than when studying the political and economic framework.[5] However, there are also hazards in relying on limited comparisons based on correlating isolated features of ancient society and culture with apparently similar features in another society; what we identify as 'the same' feature may have an entirely different meaning in its own particular context.

Dodds' answer to these problems was that, 'We must work by whatever light we can get, and an uncertain light is better than none'.[6] While being aware of the dangers both of blanket application of a single social science theory to the ancient material, and of identification of features taken out of context which strike a modern observer as being similar, we can at least use cross-cultural comparison at the less ambitious level of demonstrating the range of the possible. If classicists are familiar only with ancient Greek medicine and Western biomedicine, they may have a misleading sense of what is 'normal' and what is not.

A brief example will illustrate the value of expanding classicists' sense of the range of the possible. Should the classical Greek *parthenos* be translated as 'virgin'? The belief in translation remains at the heart of any endeavour in the arts and humanities: any attempt at cross-cultural comparison questions the limits of translatability.[7] In the empiricist tradition, translation is made possible by the existence of 'nature', an external world independent of culture. The tradition takes it for granted that virgins exist, with cultures using different words for the same thing. In the relativist tradition, however, virgins do not exist; cultures put different emphasis on the existence of a hymen, the relative importance of youth, social status (unmarried/engaged/married) and sexual inexperience to the category. Virginity may be a state ended once and for all, or a renewable condition; according to the geographer Pausanias, the goddess Hera renewed hers annually by bathing in a spring near Nauplion,[8] while contemporary groups in the Sudan which practise the surgical excision of the clitoris and subsequent sealing of the vagina (infibulation) achieve something comparable in the human world by 'opening' a woman for her husband to penetrate, then 'closing' her again after the birth of a child in order to renew her virginity. Virginity is no longer physical and unique, but social and repeatable: virgins are made, not born.[9] Here, even a superficial cross-cultural comparison makes the custom recounted by Pausanias seem less exotic, suggesting that it would be fruitful to correlate renewable virginity with other social and cultural features. At the same time, it points up one difference between Nauplion and the Sudan; in the former, the renewal of virginity is open only to a goddess.

The value of cross-cultural comparison often lies more with highlighting such differences between the ancient world and other cultures than in postulating any human constants. For example, the Porters have argued that patients in the long eighteenth century were highly demanding, choosing the practitioners they wanted, discussing their treatment, and carrying out self-treatment. The dominant ethos, based on the Protestant work ethic and Locke's individualism, was 'busy, energetic, and practical'.[10] This model of the individual patient choosing within the medical marketplace is open to criticism as the product of the Thatcherite England of the late 1980s when the Porters were writing. It cannot be applied to the ancient world, far from the individualism of Thatcherite economics, but it does have the value of shifting our focus from the healers whose written theories and remedies survive, making us more aware of the alternatives – some of them 'religious' – available to patients. The points where the 'medical market-place' model fails to fit can fruitfully direct us to differences between medicine now, in the eighteenth century, and in the fifth century BCE.[11]

In the fifth and fourth centuries BCE, temple and Hippocratic medicine coexisted. 'Temple medicine' was predominantly, but not exclusively, that of the god Asklepios, but many gods and local heroes had healing, or the promotion of health,[12] among their functions; for example, Artemis was associated with women's diseases, difficult childbirth, and the transition to womanhood. The normal mode of healing in these cults was through offerings made at a local shrine; in the case of Artemis, women offered articles of clothing.[13] The category of 'Hippocratic medicine' should not be pushed too far. As it survives today, the Hippocratic corpus contains treatises from a wide time span giving a range of mutually incompatible explanations and therapies, but sharing the belief that disease is due to a disturbance in the balance of the fluids composing the body.

In the fourth century BCE, when many of the Hippocratic medical treatises were composed, around two hundred temples of Asklepios were founded in Greece. In studying the coexistence of these models of healing, I will be using cross-cultural materials from societies which are comparable in the strictly limited sense that they too demonstrate the coexistence of religious and medical healing. Even at this limited level, one valuable point of difference emerges immediately. The 'medical' model in modern anthropological studies is almost always Western biomedicine, the imported medicine of the former colonial powers. 'Western biomedicine' may appear to be a far more homogeneous system than Hippocratic medicine, but anthropologists studying it have demonstrated that it too works with a large number of different explanatory models, including 'biochemical, immunological, viral, genetic, environmental, psychodynamic, family interactionist and so on'.[14] In the classical world, it was not the 'medical' model, but the 'religious' model of Asklepios, which was imported to many parts of Greece and, in 291 BCE, to Rome. Associated by Homer with the northern Greek area of Thessaly, Asklepios does not appear to have been the object of worship at Epidauros until the early fifth century BCE, when he replaced an earlier healing deity.[15] The ancient geographer Strabo, however, claimed that Asklepios' 'oldest and most famous sanctuary' was at Trikka in Thessaly.[16] It remains far from clear whether Epidauros or Trikka was the first sanctuary, but when other cities decided to import the cult it was to Epidauros that they sent for sacred objects. Athens established a sanctuary of the god in 420 BCE, perhaps as a result of the plague's effects on Attica, or because of the enthusiasm of an Epidaurian who happened to be resident in Athens.[17] Medicine from 'outside' can be thought to have power simply because of its novelty, but Asklepios did not have the support of the colonial powers which Western biomedicine now has.

In 1983 the ancient historian Robert Parker wrote that 'A scholarly account of Greek healing gods in general seems not to exist.' That remains the case.[18] Asklepios is an exception among the healing gods of the ancient world, both because of his cult's promotion as an 'international' one[19] and because of the role of the 'divine dream' experienced by the patient at the sanctuary. Hippocratic healing took account of dreams as potentially important signs indicating the present state of the body; a dream of polluted rivers indicates bowel disturbance, and high rivers indicate an excess of blood in the body, while the patient with a swollen liver dreams of enemy warriors and believes he is fighting them.[20] However, healing in Hippocratic medicine took place in the physical world of bodily fluids and material substances. In Asklepian medicine, the patient dreamed of the god's healing acts, using surgery, drugs or touch. From the *iamata*, the inscriptions recording cures performed at the temple of Asklepios at Epidauros, we read that the god stretched out the hands of the paralysed, poured drugs into the eye to restore sight to the blind, restored the voice, tied on a headband which removed a birthmark, extracted a spearhead from the jaw, operated on an abdominal abscess, and applied drugs to the head to cure baldness.[21] Many questions about the *iamata* remain unanswered. Were they written by the priests, or at least under their supervision?[22] Dillon stresses their 'didactic nature', arguing that they should be seen not as case records, but rather as demonstrations to sceptics and doubters of the power of the god, and a warning to suppliants to pay what they have vowed – or expect divine punishment.[23] Later literary accounts of Asklepios' healing methods, in particular by the orator Aelius Aristides in the second century CE, suggest that the god sometimes gave unexpected advice, such as exercise when the patient had expected to be told to rest.[24]

Scholars in the early part of this century, operating with a model of science as progress out of superstition, thought that the temples of Asklepios pre-dated Hippocratic medicine,[25] and then envisaged a later conflict between 'the scientists of the Hippocratic period' and 'the general population . . . still close to their gods'.[26] In a recent book, revealingly entitled *Greek Rational Medicine*, James Longrigg defined 'rational medicine' as 'free from magical and religious elements and based upon natural causes'.[27] This definition should be challenged as misleadingly dependent on our own cultural concepts. We may not see the gods' anger as part of the 'natural world', but one could argue that the Greeks did. As post-Enlightenment beings, we separate medicine from both magic and religion, and call this liberation, or progress: the Greeks did not. In a highly circular argument, we study the Greeks as our cultural ancestors, looking at what impresses us, which is of course precisely what we define ourselves as being.

Indeed, rather than Hippocratic medicine breaking 'free' from temple medicine, there is evidence that temple medicine copied Hippocratic and subsequent secular medicine; for example, in the late fourth century BCE surgery was in vogue, and the Asklepios seen in dreams duly practised surgery.[28] But, being a god, he kept ahead of the real world, performing operations superior to any on offer there. When compound drugs were fashionable, Asklepios used them too, but his were invariably more effective.[29] One could argue that the successes of Hippocratic medicine actually led to an increase in the Asklepios cult, with patient expectations rising and cures for a wider range of symptoms being sought,[30] or that Asklepios' appropriation of the symbols and prestige of Hippocratic medicine was a smart career move: as Parker puts it, 'The truest explanation for the rise of Asklepios may be that he was, as it were, in partnership with Hippocrates.'[31]

There is little evidence that Greek physicians objected to temple medicine. No Hippocratic writer criticizes Asklepios – indeed, the Hippocratic oath invokes Asklepios, among other gods – and doctors were present at Asklepian temples, some serving as priests themselves.[32] Our current construction of 'priesthood' and 'medicine' sees both as 'professions', a concept utterly alien to the ancient Mediterranean, where in some states any number of priesthoods could be held by a man who was also serving on the ruling body of his state, leading its armies, and treating the medical disorders of his family or soldiers. Those whose primary identity appears to have been 'physician', at least insofar as they practised for a fee, could be exempted from civic or military service, but there was nothing to keep them from holding priesthoods. On the few occasions when a Hippocratic text tells us what religious healers do in a particular situation, what is criticized is not the invocation of the gods as such, but the search for any cause outside the human body. In *On the Sacred Disease* and *Diseases of Young Girls* the cause of the distressing symptoms is seen as the accumulation of a bodily fluid in a vital area of the body. The cause is mechanical, so the therapy must also be mechanical, removing the blockage so that the fluid can move. In many texts the Hippocratic authors recommend the use of opposites – the dry must be made moist, the hard must be softened[33] – which may be a deliberate distancing from the like-cures-like approach of magical therapy.[34]

Studies of the interaction between Hippocratic and temple medicine reveal the difficulty of bracketing out contemporary ideas about rationality and irrationality, order and chaos, sense and nonsense. The traditional images in medical history of the relationship between Asklepios and Hippocratic medicine present them as analogous either to Lourdes and the general practitioner, or to a health spa and Harley Street. The first model concentrates on the religious element of temple medicine, taking up a narrowly post-Enlightenment view to assume the 'obvious' superiority of science over religion. The second, while concentrating on temple medicine as a harmless, but socially enjoyable, experience, also accepts at face value the Hippocratic healer's assertion of his personal superiority over anything else available; whereas current work suggests that 'The boundary between the self-acknowledged doctor and the educated layman was very narrow.'[35] Seeing the sanctuaries of Asklepios as health spas accords with Vitruvius' statement of the principles on which healing sanctuaries should be sited in a healthy location, and also with the known sites of Asklepieia outside towns, although it is likely that the latter was due to a desire to separate ritual space from normal life.[36] The Roman sanctuary, on the Tiber island, may seem to us to occupy an unhealthy location, but makes sense as a way of achieving ritual separation.[37] However, the health spa model removes the religious aspect entirely; here, one could argue that the position of the Greeks as our cultural ancestors encourages us to play down their religious life. The Edelsteins provide a valuable historiographical account of modern explanations for the cures recorded for Asklepian medicine. These include seeing them as miracles (but, since they were performed by a pagan god, they must be deeds of the devil), 'natural remedies', a form of spiritual healing, or 'trickery'. A further possibility is that people were more willing to follow the treatment given because it carried the authority of the god; Galen mentions those who will obey the god, but not a doctor who gave identical advice.[38] After the tablets from the sanctuary of Asklepios at Epidauros were first published in 1883, the cures were seen as 'fraud': this was followed by a counter-reaction interpreting them as real cures, performed by the then-fashionable methods of dream interpretation or hypnosis. As the Edelsteins put it:

> The miracle, a dish so distasteful to the modern palate, had been cooked until it became acceptable and digestible; the irrational had been worked on until it finally evaporated into nothingness; the amoral had been sifted until it had cleared off a useful and orderly substance.[39]

The historiography of responses to temple medicine thus illustrates clearly how our images of the Greeks and our relative valuations of Hippocrates and Asklepios change with our own medical preferences.

Perspectives provided by materials from the social sciences may help us to look at the relationship between Hippocratic and temple medicine not by de-sacralizing temple medicine, nor by romanticizing the priests of Asklepios as 'holistic' traditional healers, nor indeed by condemning them as quacks.[40]

All formulations to date of the relationship between Hippocratic medicine and the cult of Asklepios assume that they were perceived by patients as 'alternatives', in which the patient had to follow one or the other independently, shifting between sectors only after one failed. Literary and epigraphic evidence from the ancient world only tells us of people shifting from physicians to god; since physicians did not encourage their patients to put up inscriptions, it would be unwise to claim that the reverse never occurred. Where patients moved, as in an inscription stating that a patient had consulted 36 doctors before the god, the failure of the medical sector is however stated 'in sadness rather than in anger',[41] and studies of contemporary groups who have access both to traditional healers and to Western-style clinics suggest that perception of the two sectors as clear 'alternatives' is most unlikely to have been universally the case. Tola Olu Pearce's work on Yoruba communities in south-west Nigeria suggests that, both in times of crisis and in everyday preventative care, 'people consistently combine different traditions' while also believing that particular traditions are best for particular conditions; Western medicine is used for surgery, accidents, aches and pains, while indigenous practitioners and prophets are consulted for what is perceived as mental illness.[42] These patient expectations in turn influence the services offered by practitioners, and thus the development of the various types of medical care on offer. In rural Mali, Sarah Castle concluded that the perception of traditional and Western medicine as opposed is not found: 'mothers tended to cross sectors substantially in their search for treatment'.[43] In early modern England, too, 'People used many different kinds of practitioner without being troubled about the distinctions between them.'[44] In their study of the eighteenth century, the Porters concluded that, 'Probably few sick people restricted themselves solely to regular, or to unorthodox medicine.'[45]

If Hippocrates and Asklepios were not perceived as incompatible alternatives, what differences can we identify between them which would tend to lead a patient to one rather than the other? Since both are intended to heal, it would be misleading to follow Laplantine's general suggestion that medicine aims at determining cause and cure, while religion is concerned with meaning.[46] The type of disease is a possible area of difference, as Asklepios seems to have cornered the market in five-year pregnancies, but some ancient sources clearly state that he can cure 'diseases of every kind'.[47] It is sometimes argued that access and cost are the most important variables in dealing with suffering; for the ancient world information on costs is rarely available, but doctors did charge fees.[48] However, so did temple medicine.

A further variable is the experience of the suffering patient within both sorts of healing. Kaja Finkler's work on the relationship between Spiritualist healing and Western biomedicine in Mexico today emphasizes the similarities between the systems, as perceived by the patients. In both systems, the patient presents with chronic bodily pain and is treated as passive by the healer: in both, the patient expects the healer to 'see inside' the body, either by using the technology of X-rays and blood tests, or with the aid of the spirits.[49] Looking at the situation from outside, however, Finkler argues that significant differences do exist. Spiritualist healing can start from a group consultation, whereas the biomedical encounter is one-to-one. Where Spiritualist healers blame impersonal spirits for the illness, biomedicine may implicate equally impersonal pathogens, but often suggests individual blame due to poor habits. Biomedical practitioners ask the patient questions which seem intrusive and which would be irrelevant to Spiritualist consultations: Finkler argues that, 'Whereas patients were concerned with anguish and pain often associated with culpability and unresolved contradictions, [biomedical] physicians focused on the nature of the patient's excrement and frequency of sexual intercourse.'[50] Where biomedical healers blame individual lifestyle, spiritualist healers remove blame from individuals and place it on the spirits. Finkler also argues that the interest of the biomedical practitioner in the individual, reflected in the one-to-one privacy of the contemporary medical encounter, is something which we value positively only because in our own society the individual is so highly valued at the expense of the family and the community.

How can this material apply to Asklepios and Hippocrates? Two aspects may be considered: first, the group dynamics of the medical encounter, and second the way blame and suffering are handled. When we consider group dynamics, at first sight the Asklepian medical encounter may appear to be between the individual and the god in the dream; how the priests mediated between the two is not clear. The Hippocratic encounter may look like more of a group affair; the consultation takes place within the household, not at some distant and neutral location, while we read of those in the household assisting in medical procedures.

If however we bring in a further anthropological study of a society in which temples play a role in healing, we may question the assumption that temple medicine is, by its nature, individualistic. Vieda Skultans has worked on a Mahanubhav healing temple in rural Maharashtra, where the sick stay for some time in order to gain a diagnosis and effect a cure. The diagnoses most commonly given are of spirit possession, which comes out of the blue and is relatively simple to cure, and witchcraft, which comes from other family members. In neither case is suffering the patient's fault. She has also shown the importance of gender expectations in the treatment of men and women with mental disorder. The dominant ideology – incidentally, like that of the ancient Greeks – claims that women have less will-power and self-control than men, so are more likely than men to suffer mental affliction,[51] but Skultans argues that there are more women than men in the temple not because these women are ill, but because they are staying there as caregivers to male family members, while many women patients arrive unaccompanied.[52] Some women lived at the temple as 'spiritual hostages' for the continued health of their sons, who had previously been cured there; a similar phenomenon was found in the Greek temples of Asklepios, since it was possible to travel there in order to dream on behalf of a sick family member who remained at home.[53] In Athenian healing cults in general it was possible to pray for another family member or to make a vow on another's behalf, while votive reliefs at Asklepieia often show a family group making offerings.[54] The temple is not then as 'individualistic' as one may think; anyone who travels there – particularly if going to one of the most famous shrines from a considerable distance away[55] – will presumably have had to find family support in order to leave fields, business and family in good hands. Greek temple medicine is also familiar with the idea that a family member can be the cause of illness; one of the Epidauros *iamata* involves a man for whom the god opens his chest and removes leeches, which were there because his stepmother had put them in his drink.[56] So perhaps we should reverse the provisional opposition – that temple medicine focuses on the individual, while Hippocratic medicine operates within the family – and consider instead that in religion, someone can go and dream for you, but in Hippocratic medicine, you are on your own.

As for blame, neither the priests of Asklepios nor the god himself seem to have had any interest in morality or in culpability;[57] the only time blame is mentioned is when a patient fails to give the dedication promised in the event of a cure and is then punished by the god. Otherwise, the god intervenes to heal without telling the patient why he or she is sick.[58] While the god refrains from asking questions about one's medical history, Hippocratic prognosis is based on observing the patient and asking questions in order to determine the present, the past, and the future of the condition.[59] The patient is sick because of past lifestyle, or because of the interaction between individual humoral balance and a particular combination of the location of the city, the prevailing wind and the time of year. This can be illustrated from the case histories of the Hippocratic *Epidemics*, where it has been suggested that there is a 'residual moralizing tone';[60] for example, 'She drank a purgative for the sake of conception and had twisting in the intestines'; 'The man from Baloea had become careless in his way of life'; 'Terpides' mother miscarried twins after a fall in the fifth month . . . nine years later she had terrible pains in the belly'; 'the servant of Dyseris, when she was young, whenever she had sexual intercourse suffered much pain . . . she never conceived . . . When she was sixty, she had pain from midday, like strong labour. Before midday she had eaten many leeks. When pain seized her, the strongest ever, she stood up and felt something rough at the mouth of her womb . . . another woman, inserting her hand, pressed out a stone like a spindle top, rough.'[61] The main focus in Hippocratic prognosis is on what the physician can observe in the present, and the writers sometimes doubt information given them by patients about past events;[62] but, as these cases illustrate, although recent history is the most commonly recounted, distant history can also be relevant. It is therefore possible that Asklepios may be preferred over Hippocrates because of his lack of interest in potentially embarrassing questions about the past.

In terms of providing a cure, however, Hippocrates may be more effective than Asklepios. This is not a judgement on Hippocratic pharmacology; indeed, it is often assumed that temple treatment was more pleasant than some invasive Hippocratic therapies. Medical anthropologists, most notably Arthur Kleinman, suggest that the search for meaning in suffering – whether carried out through what we would categorize as 'medicine' or as 'religion' – should be seen in terms of narrative. Explaining illness leads to reflection on one's life, in a specific cultural context.[63] Reflection leads to narrative, as previously unconnected events are perceived to have been linked in ways unseen at the time. Kleinman has shown how illness makes people today become 'archivists researching a disorganized file of past experiences'.[64] As suffering 'unmakes' the world, so the creation of a narrative reconstructs the world anew;[65] this creation can be carried out alone, but even then it may need to be given authority by a specialist, whether priest or healer. Alternatively, the patient may expect the specialist to construct the narrative, within a cultural context in which the explanation makes sense to the patient; Linda Garro noted that, where a patient in chronic pain tried many doctors, the treatment which worked best was that given by the doctor who provided a key element of the patient's explanatory model, making sense of the past, and giving options for the future.[66] The narrative itself may thus heal. However, just as there is a sort of 'placebo effect' when patient and healer agree on the diagnosis, so there can be a 'nocebo effect'; a medical diagnosis can lead a patient to behave in a 'sicker' way than before.[67]

The construction of a narrative linking past to present and providing expectations for the future is a central part of Hippocratic medicine. The theory of critical days, in which models of regular crises taken from malarial-type fevers are applied to other types of disease, gives even greater control of the future, predicting exactly when the patient will feel worse or better. But Asklepios too uses time management; votives, objects promised to the god in the event of a cure, are 'a major human strategy for coping with the future', making time manageable by creating a public, and thus social, contract of the 'if . . . then' type.[68]

When creating a narrative, how do the Hippocratics apportion blame? Wujastyk (this volume) considers the death of a child as the supreme event raising the question, 'Why does God permit this?'; in the Indian material, the mother is blamed for laying herself open to demonic powers. Sarah Castle has worked on contemporary rural Mali, an area of high childhood mortality in which over 50% of children die before reaching the age of five. Here, the death of a child may be attributed to *foondu* ('the owl') or to *heendu* ('the wind'). *Foondu* is caught if a child cries at the same moment as an owl shrieks, if dust falls from an owl on to a child, or if an owl flies over a pregnant woman. *Heendu* is caused by a sorcerer or a spirit drinking the patient's blood. The central points about both diagnoses are, first, that they are rarely given to living children and, second, that they are both seen as untreatable, although amulets and inhalation of smoke may be attempted.[69] To diagnose a living child as having *foondu* or *heendu* makes the diagnosis into a self-fulfilling prophecy. To diagnose a child post-mortem as being a victim removes any suspicion that its death was the responsibility of the mother, or the healer. An important element of these diagnoses is that they are given only by traditional healers, clerics or senior women of the patrilineage, thus reinforcing the hierarchical transmission of knowledge.[70] Here, explanations for disease are couched in such a way that they exonerate all parties, while reproducing socially-significant structures.

We do not know how Greek religion accounted for the death of a child. Wujastyk's material on Lady Opulence, represented with wings, talons and beak, and killing foetuses and young children as 'Child-Snatcher', suggests to a classicist the Greek mythical figures of the harpies (literally, 'snatchers') who, on the Xanthos tomb, are represented carrying away small human figures. But, thanks to an important article by Ann Hanson, we do know how Hippocratic medicine coped with the death of a new-born child. The Hippocratic solution to the problem refers not to gods or spirits, but to an unavoidable law of nature related to numbers. Based on beliefs about gestation, the Hippocratics insisted that the eight-months child inevitably died, while the seven-months child was at risk of death. This meant that a child born dead could be hastily redefined as an eight-months child – 'They always die – there's nothing anyone can do' – while the statement 'This is a seven-months child' became a convenient shorthand to warn everyone involved that the child may not live long. It was in the interests of doctor, mother, family, and midwives to go along with these statements and thus to avoid all blame or guilt.[71]

The advantage of using suffering as a way into the relationship between Asklepios and Hippocrates is thus that it helps us to avoid issues of rationality in looking for answers to why a patient may prefer religion or medicine. The different systems handle the issues of blame and suffering in different ways. Work on chronic pain suggests that – at least in the industrialized West – the construction of a narrative can be part of the healing process; Hippocratic medicine duly allows the creation of meaning from suffering by anchoring it to the patient's experience. In Hippocratic medicine you are on your own; you, as an individual, are the focus of enquiry. Not everyone, however, wants to feel the medical gaze; as Alcinda Onwana (this volume) has reminded us in the context of post-civil war Mozambique, not everyone wants to research their past. Both the focus on the present in prognosis and the power of numbers in Hippocratic medicine respond to this problem but, if you still fear the implications of the narrative which a Hippocratic would create for you, you may prefer what the temple offers. The patient who opts for the narrative-free neutrality of temple medicine may also have gained a much greater investment of symbolic capital from the family and friends whose support makes the journey to the temple possible, so that the network of expectations surrounding him or her makes a cure even more likely.

Acknowledgment

My thanks to Vivian Nutton for his help in improving the earlier versions of this paper; the faults which remain are entirely my own.

NOTES

1. The story is told by the mid-eighth century BCE poet Hesiod, in his *Works and Days*, 42–105 and *Theogony* 535–616. The best modern analysis of these passages is by J.-P. Vernant, 'The myth of Prometheus in Hesiod' in *Myth and society in ancient Greece* (Sussex and New York: Harvester Press, 1980; French original 1974), 168–85.
2. C. Kluckhohn, *Anthropology and the Classics* (1961); M.I. Finley, 'Anthropology and the classics' (1972), reprinted in his *The Use and Abuse of History* (2nd edition, 1986); S.C. Humphreys, *Anthropology and the Greeks* (1978); J.M. Redfield, 'Classics and anthropology', *Arion* (Spring 1991), 5–23; P. Cartledge, 'The Greeks and anthropology', *Anthropology Today* 10.3 (June 1994), 3–6; H. King 'Anthropology and the classics' in *Oxford Classical Dictionary* (1996).
3. L. Dean-Jones, *Women's Bodies in Classical Greek Science* (Oxford: Clarendon Press, 1994), 234–43; D. Gourevitch, 'Review of Lesley-Ann Dean-Jones, *Women's Bodies in Classical Greek Science* (1994)', *History and Philosophy of the Life Sciences*, 16 (1994), 499 caricatures Dean-Jones' position as 'une manie compariste qui n'apporte pas grand chose'.
4. B. S. Cohn, 'History and anthropology: the state of play', *Comparative Studies in Society and History* 12 (1980), 198–221 and 'Anthropology and history in the 1980s: towards a rapprochement', *Journal of Interdisciplinary History* 12 (1981), 227–52.
5. J.W. Adams, 'Anthropology and history in the 1980s: consensus, community and *exoticism*', *Journal of Interdisciplinary History* 12 (1981), 253–65. A sensitive study of an 'exotic' area is G. Lanata, *Medicina magica e religione popolare in Grecia, fino all'età de Ippocrate* (Rome: Eds dell'Ateneo, 1967).
6. E.R. Dodds, *The Greeks and the Irrational* (Berkeley: University of California, 1951), preface.
7. B.J. Good, *Medicine, Rationality and Experience: an anthropological perspective* (Cambridge: Cambridge University Press, 1994), 89.
8. Pausanias 2.38.2.
9. R.O. Hayes, 'Female genital mutilation, fertility control, women's roles and the patrilineage in modern Sudan: a functional analysis', *American Ethnologist* 2 (1975), 617–33; J. Boddy, 'Womb as oasis: the symbolic content of Pharaonic circumcision in rural Northern Sudan', *American Ethnologist* 9 (1982), 682–98.
10. R. Porter, *Health for Sale. Quackery in England 1660–1850* (Manchester University Press, 1989), 31; R. and D. Porter, *Patient's Progress. Doctors and doctoring in eighteenth-century England* (Stanford, CA: Stanford University Press, 1989), 8.
11. V. Nutton, 'The medical meeting place' in Ph. J. van der Eijk, H.F.J. Horstmanshoff and P.H. Schrijvers (eds), *Ancient Medicine in its Socio-Cultural Context* (Amsterdam and Atlanta, GA, 1995), 13.
12. J.D. Mikalson, *Athenian Popular Religion* (Chapel Hill and London: University of North Carolina Press, 1983), 22 and 122 n.24 distinguishes the functions of prevention and cure. On local healing cults around Athens, see Garland, *Introducing New Gods*, 132–3.

13. H. King, 'Bound to bleed: Artemis and Greek women' in A. Cameron and A. Kuhrt (eds), *Images of Women in Antiquity* (London: Croom Helm, 1983), 109–27; on dedications to Artemis Brauronia, T. Linders, *Studies in the Treasure Records of Artemis Brauronia found in Athens* (Stockholm: Svenska Inst. of Athens 4.19, 1972).
14. B.J. Good and M.-J. DelVecchio Good, 'The meaning of symptoms: a cultural hermeneutic model for clinical practice' in L. Eisenberg and A. Kleinman (eds), *The Relevance of Social Science for Medicine* (Dordrecht: D. Reidel, 1981); C. Helman, 'Disease and pseudo-disease: a case history of pseudo-angina' in R.A. Hahn and A.D. Gaines (eds), *Physicians of Western Medicine* (Dordrecht: D. Reidel, 1985), 294. Which model is used depends to some extent on the audience; see C. Helman, ' "Feed a cold, starve a fever" – folk models of infection in an English suburban community, and their relation to medical treatment', *Culture. Medicine and Psychiatry* 2 (1978), 107–37. See also A. Kleinman on 'the kaleidoscope of healers and healing practices' in North America today ('Pain and resistance: the delegitimation and relegitimation of local worlds' in M.-J. DelVecchio Good, P.E. Brodwin, B.J. Good, and A. Kleinman (eds) *Pain as Human Experience* (Berkeley: University of California Press, 1992), 205. 15. Homer, *Iliad* 2.729–32; see R. Garland, *Introducing New Gods: the politics of Athenian religion* (London: Duckworth, 1992), 116–18.
16. Strabo, *Geography* 9.5.17.
17. Evidence summarized by Garland, *Introducing New Gods*, 116–35 and R. Parker, *Athenian Religion: a History*, (Oxford: Clarendon Press, 1996), 175–85. See also S.B. Aleshire, *The Athenian Asklepieion. The people, their dedications, and the inventories* (Amsterdam: J.C. Gieben, 1989).
18. R. Parker, *Miasma: Pollution and Purification in Early Greek Religion* (Oxford: Oxford University Press, 1983), 248 n. 70. But see now F. Graf, 'Heiligtum und Ritual: das Beispiel der Griechisch-Römischen Asklepieia' in O. Reverdin and B. Grange (eds), *Le Sanctuaire grec* (Geneva: Fondation Hardt, 1992), 152–99.
19. A. Burford, *The Greek Temple Builders at Epidauros* (Liverpool: Liverpool University Press, 1969), 15.
20. E.g. *Epidemics* 1.10 (Loeb I, 180). Dreams are not always believed to be as significant as the patient fears; see *Epidemics* 4.57 (Loeb VII, 150). River dreams: *Regimen for Health* 4.89 (Loeb IV, 438). Fighting the enemy: *Regimen for Health* 4.93 (Loeb IV, 446), a passage also found in *Critical Days* 3 and *Internal Affections* 48. See H. von Staden, *Herophilus. The Art of Medicine in Early Alexandria* (Cambridge: Cambridge University Press, 1989), 306–7; a fuller discussion is S.M. Oberhelman, 'Dreams in Graeco-Roman medicine', *ANRW* II 37, 1, 121–56.
21. Literary evidence for the cult; E.J. and L. Edelstein, *Asclepius: a collection and interpretation of the testimonies* (2 vols) (Baltimore: Johns Hopkins, 1945); for these examples, see T 423.3, 423.5, 423.4 and 9, 423.6, 423.12, 423.27 and 423.19 (pp. 229–37). *Iamata* also survive from Rome, Athens and Lebena.
22. E.J. and L. Edelstein, *Asclepius*, 146–7.

23. M.P.J. Dillon, 'The didactic nature of the Epidaurian *iamata*', *ZPE* 101 (1994), 239–60.
24. T 408; E.J. and L. Edelstein, *Asclepius*, 154. On Aristides, see H. King, 'Chronic pain and the creation of narrative', forthcoming in J. Porter (ed.), *Constructions of the Classical Body* (University of Michigan Press).
25. A.J. Festugière, *Hippocrate, l'Ancienne Médecine* (Paris: Klincksieck, 1948), vii.
26. I. Veith, *Hysteria: the History of a Disease* (Chicago: University of Chicago Press, 1965), 15–16.
27. J. Longrigg, *Greek Rational Medicine: Philosophy and medicine from Alcmaeon to the Alexandrians* (London: Routledge, 1993).
28. E.J. and L. Edelstein, *Asclepius*, 166.
29. E.J. and L. Edelstein, *Asclepius*, 167.
30. Parker, *Miasma*, 250.
31. Parker, *Athenian Religion*, 184.
32. Von Staden, *Herophilus*, 8; Nutton, 'Lay attitudes', 46. See also O. Temkin, 'Greek medicine as science and craft', *Isis* 44 (1953), 216 'There is neither competition nor enmity between the god [Asklepios] and the physician'; E.J. and L. Edelstein, *Asclepius*, 139 for the god as 'a friendly ally' of the doctor; and Nutton, 'Medical meeting place', 4 on Athenian doctors' collective sacrifices to Asklepios.
33. E.g. *Nat. Hom.* 9. 1–2.
34. See A.E. Hanson, 'Talking recipes in the gynecological texts of the Hippocratic Corpus', forthcoming in *Gender and History*.
35. V. Nutton, 'Lay attitudes to medicine in classical antiquity', in R. Porter (ed.), *Patients and Practitioners* (Cambridge: Cambridge University Press, 1985), 38.
36. Vitruvius, *De architectura* 1.2.7; Graf, 'Heiligtum und Ritual', 166–7 and 198.
37. E.J. and L. Edelstein, *Asclepius*, 158 draw attention to the Roman temple being located on the Tiber island.
38. T 401; E.J. and L. Edelstein, *Asclepius*, 168–71.
39. E.J. and L. Edelstein, *Asclepius*, 144.
40. K. Finkler, 'Sacred healing and biomedicine compared', *Medical Anthropology Quarterly* 8 (1994), 179. The definition of 'quack' is of course fraught with difficulty. As Porter, *Health for Sale* shows for the period 1660–1850, a quack is always someone else. The dominant image is of someone who lacks any qualifications, knows very little, tricks patients and lies about their results. For the ancient world, there was no qualification system; in terms of Western biomedicine, very little was 'known'; frank admission that trickery of patients occurs is found in the Hippocratic corpus.
41. P. Roesch, 'Médecins publics dans les cités grecques', *Histoire des sciences médicales* 18 (1984), 290, discussed in Nutton, 'Medical meeting place', 14; Nutton, 'Lay attitudes', 47. See also T 582, a fifth-century CE account of a girl who could not be cured by the physicians and was therefore prayed for at an Asclepieion.
42. T.O. Pearce, 'Lay medical knowledge in an African context' in S. Lindenbaum and M. Lock (eds), *Knowledge, Power and Practice. The*

Anthropology of Medicine and Everyday Life (Berkeley: University of California Press, 1993), 154.

43. S.E. Castle, '(Re)negotiation of illness diagnoses and responsibility for child health in rural Mali', *Medical Anthropology Quarterly* 8 (1994), 328.
44. A. Wear, 'The popularization of medicine in early modern England' in R. Porter (ed.), *The Popularization of Medicine 1650–1850* (London: Routledge, 1992) 17.
45. Porter and Porter, *Patient's Progress*, 106–8.
46. F. Laplantine, *Anthropologie de la maladie* (Paris: Eds Payot, 1986), 350.
47. T 423.1 and 423.2 recount five- and three-year pregnancies, while T 426 from Lebena shows Asklepios curing female sterility. Strabo, in T 735, states that the god can cure all diseases.
48. In a possible reference to physicians leaving Athens in a time of crisis, a character in Aristophanes' *Ploutus* asks: 'Is there a doctor in town at the moment? There's no fee now the profession has gone' or perhaps 'With no fees, there's no skill' (407–8).
49. Finkler, 'Sacred healing', 181–2.
50. Finkler, 'Sacred healing', 185.
51. V. Skultans, 'Women and affliction in Maharashtra: a hydraulic model of health and illness', *Culture, Medicine and Psychiatry* 15 (1991), 349 and 347; for the classical material, see R. Padel, *In and Out of the Mind: Greek images of the tragic self* (Princeton: Princeton University Press, 1992).
52. Skultans, 'Women and affliction', 349. Women may enter a trance to lift illness from male relatives; sharing the affliction of a family member affirms 'the legitimacy of their connection with that family' (352).
53. The *iamata* from Epidauros include a Spartan mother sleeping at the temple for her daughter (T 423.21), and a father who dreams on behalf of a missing son (T 423.24); see also W. Burkert, *Ancient Mystery Cults* (Harvard University Press, 1987), 15–16 on Tibullus envisaging his beloved Delia sitting outside the temple of Isis in gratitude for his cure. See also Mikalson, *Athenian Popular Religion*, 22–3.
54. F. van Straten, 'Votives and votaries in Greek sanctuaries' in Reverdin and Grange (eds), *Le Sanctuaire grec*, 255–6 and 279.
55. Dillon, 'Didactic nature', 240 suggests patients would normally go to their nearest Asklepieion, but would travel to a major one if they thought it necessary. For an example see *Palatine Anthology* 6.330, discussed by Garland, *Introducing New Gods*, 133.
56. T 423.13.
57. Parker, *Miasma*, 249; Nutton, 'Lay attitudes', 47. Exceptions are inscriptions from second and third centuries CE Lydia and Phrygia, which present disease as divine punishment, cured by confession, expiation, and the transfer of the sin to animals, birds or fish; see A. Chaniotis, 'Illness and cures in the Greek propitiatory inscriptions and dedications of Lydia and Phrygia' in Van der Eijk et al., *Ancient Medicine*, 323–44.
58. Parker, *Miasma*, 249.
59. Given in this order in *Prognosis* 1.
60. L. Garcia-Ballester, 'Galen as a clinician: his methods in diagnosis' in *ANRW* II 37, 2, 1648.
61. *Epidemics* 5.42; 7.17; 7.97; 5.25 (all translations from W.D. Smith).

62. E.g. *Epidemics* 4.6.
63. Kleinman, 'Pain and resistance', 181.
64. Arthur Kleinman, *The Illness Narratives. Suffering, Healing and the Human Condition* (New York: Basic Books, 1988), 48.
65. Good, *Medicine. Rationality and Experience*.
66. Linda C. Garro, 'Chronic illness and the construction of narratives' in Good *et al.*, *Pain as Human Experience*, 130–1.
67. Cecil Helman, 'Disease and pseudo-disease: a case history of pseudo-angina' in R.A. Hahn and A.D. Gaines (eds), *Physicians of Western Medicine* (Dordrecht: D. Reidel, 1982), 323.
68. Burkert, *Ancient Mystery Cults*, 13; see also Nutton, 'Lay attitudes', 47 on the patient of Asklepios making 'a bargain for the future, not a repentance of the past'.
69. Castle, '(Re)negotiation of illness diagnoses'.
70. Castle, '(Re)negotiation of illness diagnoses', 330–1.
71. Ann Ellis Hanson, 'The eight months' child and the etiquette of birth: *Obsit omen!*', *Bulletin of the History of Medicine* 61 (1987), 589–602.

PAIN IN HIPPOCRATIC MEDICINE

Peregrine Horden

'About suffering they were never wrong,/The Old Masters,' W.H. Auden wrote in 'Musée des Beaux Arts'; 'how well they understood/Its human position . . .'[1]

It is not difficult to produce quotable 'old masters' from either classical or late antiquity on this subject of sick and suffering humanity – Aeschylus, in the *Agamemnon*, on 'wisdom through suffering', the encapsulation of a whole philosophy with pain at its focus;[2] Aristotle: 'pain perturbs and destroys the nature of the sufferer but pleasure does nothing of the sort';[3] Epicurus: 'pain does not last continuously in the flesh: when acute it is there for a short time . . . and chronic illnesses contain an excess of pleasure in the flesh over pain';[4] Seneca: 'pain is slight if not reinforced by opinion';[5] Jesus, as quoted in the *Epistle of Barnabas*: 'those who wish to see me and attain to my kingdom must lay hold of me through pain and suffering';[6] the pagan Caecilius in Minucius Felix's *Octavius*, strikingly characterizing Christians in somatic rather than doctrinal terms, as 'parched with fever, racked with pain';[7] Jerome: 'am I in good health? I thank my Creator. Am I sick? In this case, too, I praise God's will.'[8] Very particular pains, not just pain and illness in general, may be similarly 'theory-laden'. Contradicting any notion of the Virgin's Immaculate Conception, there is a tenth-century (or earlier) 'Praise of the Archangel Michael' written in Coptic: a lengthy prayer for healing in which the individual labour pains of the Virgin are not only invoked but even named.[9]

All these quotations derive from 'old masters' who give pain and suffering a 'human position' rich in ethical implication, often in the form of theodicy. In this paper, however, I am concerned with old masters of medicine, chiefly the writers of the *Corpus Hippocraticum*

(CH) but also, more briefly, Rufus of Ephesus and Galen. And these masters are different from those represented above – far more so, I suggest, than we might expect from the obvious contrast of literary genre between, for instance, high tragedy and medical treatise. The difference can be characterized under three headings.

First, *philosophy*. Hippocratic authors and physicians do not articulate any philosophically elevated theory of pain – any conception of its place in the human scheme of things. Undoubtedly they evolve physiological *explanations* of pain; but they go no further than that. Pain, for them, is no 'lived metaphysics'.[10] It is simply 'a message composed, sent, and delivered by illness'.[11] That is, the Hippocratics step aside from the religious and ethical frameworks within which pain can acquire meaning. They offer, for example, no more than occasional recognition of the possibility that an illness is of supernatural origin.[12] Nor did the passing centuries soften this outlook. At the other end of the classical period, a comparable detachment is to be found in the work of the early Byzantine medical encyclopaedists, writing in an overwhelmingly Christian environment. Perhaps in part reflecting religious change, these encyclopaedists guardedly include a few more magical remedies than their Hippocratic-Galenic authorities did; but they are otherwise difficult to distinguish from them in tone and broad intellectual outlook.[13] Their conservatism shows the narrow limits of learned medicine's accommodation to Christian theodicy in late antiquity.

Philosophies of a less elevated kind were registered no more fully. In the conclusion to his admirable account of 'Hippocratism' in antiquity, Owsei Temkin writes that Hippocratic medicine offered a counterbalance to the claims of the spirit. Especially in late antiquity, he argues, medicine sided with the majority of the people – with the rationally disciplined claims of the flesh, rather than with the extreme ideals of chastity and asceticism that, according to some modern scholarship, are such a prominent feature of the culture of the later Roman world.[14] Temkin's argument is plausible enough. But it should be noted in the present context that, at least in the major texts through which it has come down to us, ancient medicine did not explicitly discuss the high level of background pain with which most 'rationally disciplined' people were presumably resigned to living until only decades ago. Stepping aside from metaphysics, ancient medical writers were apparently no more responsive to the presumed world-view of common men and women – for whom pain was simply painful, and unwelcome, but very often unavoidable. Whatever actual doctors' practice, Hippocratic medicine does *not* see some pain as inevitable, as intrinsic to 'the human condition'.

The second of the three headings is *distinctiveness*, or rather the lack of it. The writers of CH do not, I suggest, see pain as a distinct or even an especially important subject. It blends easily into the rest of medicine. To my knowledge, no ancient doctor wrote a treatise on pain *tout court*. The eminent Muslim physician Razi preserves fragments of what he refers to as a work on pains in various parts of the body by that major first-century figure, Rufus of Ephesus. Razi is, however, likely to have been mistaken as to the literary integrity of the fragments' original.[15] Rufus, like other ancient medical authors, doubtless discussed pain *en passant* in a variety of works. For undoubtedly pain could have enormous diagnostic-prognostic significance. Indeed, *pace* Foucault, no ancient doctor of any calibre would have been so epistemically challenged as to fail to ask 'where does it hurt?'.[16] But that was only one among a number of appropriate questions, equivalent in prognostic potential: it was not necessarily the primary question. And it did not necessarily deserve a treatise to itself.

The third heading is *vocabulary*. Whatever clinically transpired between doctor and patient was (I propose) seen as too diffuse, too 'sub-theoretical', to be recorded in subtly-differentiated terminology. For the literate physicians or medical authors of the CH, pain seemed, perhaps, a subject on which there were narrow limits to what could – and therefore need – be written. There was no call for sophisticated taxonomies.

I have introduced the last of my three headings only briefly because I now want to explore it in some detail. I take it first because it is fundamental to the other two. Looking at the ways in which Hippocratic doctors wrote – or failed to write – about pain will, I believe, simultaneously show its lack of metaphysical significance for them (the initial heading) and will also begin to open up, for subsequent consideration, the second topic, distinctiveness.

The corpus of over sixty treatises associated with the name of Hippocrates was composed at sundry times over the course of a century or more, beginning *c.* 450 BC. It is the product of a diversity of authors, perhaps including Hippocrates himself, and its contents reveal a variety of genres and intellectual allegiances.[17] The Corpus does none the less exhibit a certain coherence: its authors partake of shared assumptions and beliefs. Therefore it can, for present purposes, be considered as a whole: a dossier of ancient medical thought second only to the output of Galen in size and compendiousness.[18] Given this abundance of material, we should hardly be surprised to find scholars asserting that in CH 'the semantic field of pain is extremely important' and, indeed, 'rich' – as rich as the semantic field of disease.[19]

Is that really so? With all respect to specialists in this material, I want to argue that CH's language of pain is somewhat undifferentiated, even impoverished. Far from offering its readers a rich terminology, it deals for the most part in synonyms; moreover, these synonyms are attended by only a small repertoire of adjectives and adverbs. Pain is not an especially vivid subject in CH. To support this proposition, some statistics will be helpful, though alas they will be no more exciting than the vocabulary that they represent – statistics of the kind that the splendid Concordance to CH now available makes it almost perilously easy to generate.[20]

Undoubtedly the number of references to pain in CH is considerable, larger perhaps than the number of occurrences of *nosos*, the basic word for disease or illness, and its family.[21] Four principal terms are involved. Of the immediate ('nuclear') family of *algos* and *algema* over 400 uses have been counted; members of the *ponos* family appear almost 700 times; *pathos* is favoured on some 150 occasions; there are precisely 772 uses of *odyne*.[22] We can leave aside the rare *lype* (a mere 59 entries), the single instance of the Homeric *pema*, and the obviously specialized *odis*, meaning labour pain (12 references). We should also discount the uses of *ponos* for exercise and *pathos* for emotion and so on. Still, the total number of occurrences of some kind of word signifying pain must still approach 2,000. The Hippocratic writers certainly did not keep silent on the subject. One could be forgiven for supposing that it was important to them.

Now that we have the statistics, they should be put to analytical use. Before we confront the obvious question of definition, it is worth pausing to consider whether the vocabulary shows any great historical development. For instance, *algema*-based words appear more frequently in *Epidemics V* and *VII*, sometimes dated to *c.* 350 BC, than they do in Books *I* and *III*, perhaps written some seventy years earlier.[23] But since the dating of individual Hippocratic works is fraught with controversy, it is impossible to hazard any large conclusions about when a particular term found or lost favour – and still less about why it did so.

In her ambitious *History of Pain*, the late Roselyne Rey tries a different tack. She asks which words occur how often in which treatises, and tries to infer something about the respective preferences of those two great medical schools, Cnidus and Cos, between which scholars have often attempted to divide the authorship of the Hippocratic treatises. *Odyne*, the most popular word for pain overall, appears with the greatest frequency in the supposedly Cnidian writings, *Diseases II*, *Epidemics VII* (traditionally seen as the runt of the litter), *Internal Affections*, and the gynaecological works. 'At most,' Rey writes, 'one could conclude that the so-called Cnidian treatises concentrate more on pain and that, when they do so, it is the word *odyne* that is used to convey it'.[24]

There is indeed a contrast to be drawn between the 'Cnidian' texts, with their preference for *odyne*, and the *Coan Prenotions* or Prognoses. In the latter work *algema* predominates among pain terms (being used 70 times), *ponos* is the second most-favoured (63 uses), and *odyne* is chosen on only 18 occasions. As with the chronology of the different books of *Epidemics*, however, no great hypothesis can be erected on such a basis. Rey, for instance, conjectures that *odyne* is characteristic of the supposedly more primitive Cnidians, and that they place more emphasis on pain, and on its usefulness in localizing disorders, than do their 'rationalist' Coan rivals. But it is time Hippocratic scholarship removed the dichotomy between 'primitive/archaic' and 'rational' from its conceptual armoury;[25] such thinking, one might almost say, is a vestige of a now archaic mode of thought – the mode of Victorian evolutionism. Moreover, as Lonie and others have demonstrated, none of the distinctions between the two schools that some scholars propose has ever been adequately justified; they rest more on contrasts of topic and literary form than on any differences of mentality or underlying theory.[26] I conclude, then, that the vocabulary of pain did not develop in any now obvious ways as the constituent texts of CH were slowly and spasmodically set down. Their authors' attitudes to, and vocabularies of, pain cannot be distinguished by either historical period or institutional origin.

A fashionable question to raise next would be that of whether pain is 'gendered' in CH. In modern times women are perhaps more likely to report experiencing a variety of recurrent pains than are men, although they are also more aggressive in combating pain.[27] In that, they distinguish themselves from the women patients referred to in the Hippocratic *Diseases of Women*:[28] these render themselves incurable through ignorance of the source of their condition and through being too ashamed to talk to the doctor until there is little that can be done. According to the Hippocratic writers, female pathology is determined predominantly by the reproductive system (the Hippocratic woman is essentially, as has often been noted, a tube with an orifice at either end).[29] Therefore, if women menstruate regularly, they will not suffer serious illnesses as often as men do; and that compensates to some extent for their lesser but perhaps more frequent ailments arising from innate bodily weakness.[30] Are Hippocratic female patients depicted as being more often in pain than male ones? I undertook some sample counts of the number of pain references in the case histories in *Epidemics*, and it may well be that pain is on average referred to as a symptom with greater frequency in female cases than in male. But there is no characteristic vocabulary of female pain. Nor, apart from the delusions of certain suicidal virgins (on which more below), do women's afflictions seem to be rendered particularly expressively. And that is true of both the *Epidemics* and the gynaecological works – a point which may have some indirect bearing on the continuing debate among specialists about whether women's voices are 'audible' in the *gynaikeia*.[31]

So the semantic field of pain in CH cannot be divided up by period, medical school, or gender. The major question of course remains: are there detectable differences of overtone between the various pain words? Roselyne Rey and Helen King have both argued that there are. They concede that the *algema* family need not be discussed: *algema* is indisputably an all-purpose word for pain. But they do contend that the contexts in which *ponos* and *odyne* are used allow us to distinguish the two words' respective resonances. In King's scheme, '*to an extent* [my italics], in the medical texts *ponos* is often used for long-lasting pain, dull pain; *odyne* for sharp pain, pain which pierces the body'.[32] Rey proposes in similar fashion that the verb *poneo* 'is used without any qualification to describe a general state of suffering or illness, and that when the localisation of pain is referred to, it is almost always approximate, involving the use of prepositions such as *peri* or *es*, i.e. "in the area of" or "about"'. *Odyne*, she writes, is by contrast 'almost always used in a precise sense – either by qualifying, or by giving some clue as to the whereabouts of, the pain'.[33] My own sampling of the texts, via the Concordance, provides only limited support for such conclusions. Both terms, not just *odyne*, can be used of pain in a particular part;

and the way *odyne* is localized seems hardly more precise than the manner in which *ponos* is deployed (*contra* Rey). If there is *odyne* in the hip, or throughout the belly, there may equally be *ponos* in the head or the hypochondrium. If *ponos* is for the most part chronic, dull pain (King), why do we find it qualified by *ischyros* (strong) or *sphodros* (violent) or *oxys* (sharp)? If *odyne* is sharp or piercing pain by definition (King again), it is perhaps odd that it should sometimes be qualified by an adjective such as *sperchnos* (rapid). For neither *odyne* nor *ponos*, it might be added, is the range of typical adjectives strikingly evocative: 'terrible' and 'sharp' are common; exotic analogies are hard to find. The Hippocratic authors provide little guidance as to what thinking (if any) lies behind their choice of pain words.

Rather than 'surf' the Concordance, playing with aggregates across the entire corpus, we might seek enlightenment from individual works. In absolute terms, the word *odyne* occurs more often in *Diseases II* than in any other treatise. And far from exhibiting any clear, single, meaning, it seems to be used as the all-purpose noun for pain. It is pain which can indeed be sharp, which suddenly seizes the patient's head, is violent, or presses.[34] In a rare metaphoric flight it is associated with the sensation of pricking needles or styluses.[35] It can be intense or excessive (*periodynie*). But, equally, it can also be light.[36] It can be localized with relative precision in the front of the head or, more loosely, in the side.[37] On other occasions, it clearly signifies lasting and more diffuse pain, linked to chills and fever, dizziness and heaviness. It can radiate, move gradually, or withdraw beneath the shoulder-blades.[38] This is humpty-dumpty writing: *odyne* apparently refers to whatever type of pain the author chooses. Everything depends on the context, which, as can be seen, displays some variety in this work.

More telling still, there are several passages in CH where major pain terms appear to be used synonymously. Two verbally similar *Aphorisms*, on pain in the diaphragm and the liver respectively, show *ponos* and *odyne* as equivalent;[39] while elsewhere *algema* is replaced now with *odyne* and now with *ponos* – though not in such a way as to suggest that *algema* is a general term embracing two distinct semantic sub-fields.[40] The phrase 'ponos de kai [and] odyne', which for instance occurs in *Places in Man*, does not suggest that, for the author of that particular work, there was much to choose between them.[41] Nor does the rapid shift from *algema* to *odyne* to *ponos* in a passage in the treatise on *Regimen in Acute*

Diseases betray a greater fastidiousness.[42] Indeed, in this undifferentiated lexical landscape only one manifestly specialized term can be discerned, and that is *odis* – occasionally used in CH, mainly in the gynaecological treatises, for the pain of childbirth – but never to the exclusion of *odyne* and *ponos*.[43]

What we today think of as the psychogenic pains of mental illness fail to elicit any richer descriptions. There is no mind-body problem for Hippocratic medicine; the problem arises only for its modern interpreters, handicapped by a conceptual dualism not evident in their sources. The Hippocratics' theory of mental illness was essentially physicalist, and therefore mental disorder did not seem to present any particular problem of description, aetiology or treatment.[44] As G. E. R. Lloyd has written, 'the doctors were concerned to collect cases of cold toes along with those of fear and despondency: all formed part of a total homogeneous epidemiological culture'.[45] The Hippocratics made no concessions to the Platonic view that certain kinds of madness, under divine patronage, were blessings rather than afflictions.[46] Emotions that were presumably in some way painful – the 'psychological' ingredients in somatic disorder that would later, in Galenic medical theory, be numbered among the 'non-naturals' – are therefore simply listed. Seldom do the Hippocratics give us any sustained evocation, any first-person account of 'how it felt'.

One striking exception is the often-quoted passage in a short gynaecological treatise describing the delirium of young virgins of marriageable age, virgins made ill by the retention of menstrual blood. Fears and terrors are said to be aroused in them; they become murderously inclined; delusions bid them leap into wells or hang themselves; they are more than half in love with death.[47] In Hippocratic eyes, however, such powerful emotions are still largely epiphenomenal to somatic disorders; they are not therefore generally described as in themselves painful. In one of the case histories of insanity in *Epidemics III* a woman is said to experience intense and continuous pains, but these are entirely somatic, mentioned separately from her 'psychological' symptoms.[48] In another work, it is *insensitivity* to pain in those with a physical illness that is taken as a sign that the mind also is afflicted.[49] Pain and psychological trauma are kept in separate diagnostic compartments.

The topic of insanity is a suitable point at which to relax the discussion's restriction to medical texts and bring into play the wider context of ancient Greek literature. Medical historians have often turned to literature for enlightenment as to the overtones that medical terms may possess. Helen King for example draws on the possible meanings of *ponos* in a range of texts from Hesiod to Plutarch to elicit a further medical definition: 'pain with a goal, a means to an end . . . very unlikely to be relieved in any way . . . divinely-ordained as part of the human condition'.[50] I have, by contrast, already argued that there is no evidence in CH of discriminable categories of pain of any type, let alone one so redolent of a whole philosophical anthropology. In some literary texts *ponos* undoubtedly refers to unevadable toils and pain; it is also used of the 'work' (for women) of sexual relations.[51] But not all the possible overtones of a word are necessarily present in any single use of it. And no ethical dimension to *ponos* is hinted at in the various references already surveyed. It might even have been the case that Hippocratic authors were intent on establishing their own particular, neutral, usages, purifying (in medicine at least) the dialect of the tribe.

Instead of pressing literature into the service of explaining medicine, I would prefer to emphasize the differences between the two. For beyond the medical corpus there does lie a rich semantic world of pain – a world in which more than two or three basic terms are in question, context supplies a way of gauging delicate alterations of register, physiology is inseparable from ethics, and somatic and psychological pain and distress lie on a continuum rather than either side of a conceptual chasm. There is no space here for detail. Mere allusions will have to suffice: to the representations of pain or wounding in Homer – those involving, say, Aphrodite and Agamemnon in the *Iliad* or the Cyclops in the *Odyssey*;[52] to Philoctetes' suppurating foot, its pain devouring his mind like a plague;[53] to the dementia of Io in *Prometheus Bound*; or, in a perhaps less familiar and later example, to Medea's torments of love in Apollonius's *Argonautica*:

> From her eyes flowed tears of pity, and within her the pain [*odyne*] wore her away, smouldering through her flesh, around her fine nerves and deep into the very base of the neck where the ache and hurt [*achos*] drive deepest, whenever the tireless Loves shoot their torments into the heart.[54]

How inordinately different from the Hippocratic tone of voice . . .[55] I have been suggesting that the Hippocratic vocabulary of pain is not rich or evocative – that it is replete with synonyms and predictable adjectives; also that it does not extend to psychological suffering. I now return to my second heading, distinctiveness. For the Hippocratic authors, pain is as it were all of a piece, important in the clinical encounter but perhaps in a uniformly banal and sub-theoretical way. It poses no insuperable problems, nor even ones that are very special. It is so intimately bound up with the rest of medicine as to exert no great independent leverage on the perceptions and mind of the theorist.

Granted, to feel pain in general is, for the Hippocratics, part of the human condition. We feel pain because, as *The Nature of Man* has it, we are not a unity[56]. If we were made up entirely of one element, pain would be impossible, for a unity would not exhibit change and corruption, excess and deficiency; and these, as we read in *Places in Man*, are the causes of pain.[57] But if pain arises inevitably in such disunited creatures, it does not follow that, when it does so, it must be endured. Medicine, we are told, is completely discovered; it has no frontiers left to cross.[58] Its goal is health, which is the absence of pain; and pain can be dealt with. *The Art* 3: 'I would define medicine as the complete removal of the pains (or troubles) [*tous kamatous*] of the sick.' *The Sacred Disease* 18: 'there is nothing in any disease which . . . is insusceptible to treatment'.[59] Of course, against those texts, one could cite *Prognostic* 1: 'it is impossible to cure all patients',[60] or the continuation of the passage from *The Art* just quoted: '. . . the complete removal of the pains of the sick, the alleviation of the more violent diseases [note that this still creates the impression that all minor pains can all be dealt with], and the refusal to undertake to cure cases in which the disease has already won the mastery, knowing that everything is not possible to medicine'.[61]

The resolution of the conflicting testimonies, as Heinrich von Staden proposes, is to conclude that, in Hippocratic eyes, no case is in principle hopeless, no pain *in principle* beyond removal or alleviation.[62] Hippocratic doctors did not uniformly refuse to treat those beyond help. Their underlying thought (according to von Staden's persuasive reconstruction) was that only in particular instances was a condition to be deemed untreatable. The condition – together with its attendant pains – could arise from heredity, or from some flaw in Nature; it might have been left untreated too long, or might lie beyond the skill of the individual doctor or the current resources of medicine. In that case, and if the pains were so nearly unbearable that the patient requested euthanasia, then the physician would not hesitate to assist.[63] But pains, even very severe ones, were not considered intrinsically beyond the reach of medical science.

All pain is in principle treatable because so are all diseases. Part of the reason why the Hippocratic authors are not much interested in the subtleties of pain, or very interesting when they do write about it, is that those statements about pain and disease are nearly tautologous. Having discoursed about disease, its symptoms and treatment, the Hippocratic authors have nothing of consequence to add. In *Ancient Medicine* 3, the reason medicine was founded is given as 'ridding man of the diet that caused pain, sickness and death'.[64] There, pain is a preliminary to disease or in effect a minor ailment, at the other end of the spectrum from the most serious ailment of death. In *Breaths* 1, the greatest evils are *lype*, *ponos* [two words for pain], and death. In *Places in Man* 42, 'pains are cured by opposites and there is something specific for each disease'.[65] Both texts show the approximate equivalence of pain and disease.

I must certainly avoid creating the impression that analgesia was never considered an end in itself. Precisely because of that intertwining of pain and disease, there was, I believe, no serious anxiety expressed by the Hippocratics (such as was later voiced by Caelius Aurelianus)[66] that concern with analgesia might distract from the main purpose of addressing the disease. A large repertoire of anodynes was available, for both local and general use: regimen, bathing, purgatives, fomentations, cataplasms, sneezing, and simply letting nature do the work. More remarkably, cauterizing was occasionally in order as an analgesic, for gout among other things – and it was also held by some that 'pain calms pain', can itself be an analgesic, and that if two pains occur simultaneously but in different places, the worse one cancels the other out.[67] The striking feature of this repertoire is that the treatments for pain are virtually coterminous with those for disease. Analgesics no more belong in a separate domain than do the sensations of pain against which they are directed.

Pain was thus of some concern to the Hippocratic physician, but as a subject it blended very well into the general medical context. Of course, what the patient said and showed about his or her pains might be crucial to prognosis. 'The spread of pains to the head without a sign, in the presence of fever, is fatal.' And again: 'pains which depart without obvious cause are fatal'.[68] In less extreme cases, pain might be particularly helpful in beginning to localize a disease or physical symptom, or in suggesting the direction of treatment, for instance by its position above or below the diaphragm.[69] 'When you question the patient and examine each thing carefully, do so first with regard to the state of his head, whether it is free of pain and has no heaviness in it; then the hypochondrium and the sides, whether they are free of pain . . .' and so on.[70] And yet – it is striking that in other extensive descriptions of clinical examination and diagnosis (i.e. descriptions longer than a few lines), such as that at the beginning of the treatise on *Prognosis* or in *Epidemics*, i. 3. 10, there is no mention of pain.[71] Was it taken for granted, or was it deliberately omitted? Perhaps at this learned level the Hippocratic physician was too anxious to assert his own 'professional' standing to grant the patient that limited degree of authority implicit in the description or demonstration of pain.[72] Or perhaps clinical conversation about pain was, as I have already proposed, thought too individual and subjective a matter to be added to the stock of theoretical wisdom: as remote from the rigidities of the treatise as (apparently) is a session with a psychoanalyst from a textbook on Freud.

The final question to raise – briefly – is that of how far, on this score, the Hippocratics can stand for the whole of ancient Greek medicine. The thrust of the answer depends hugely on the choice of texts to be adduced. In Aretaeus of Cappadocia's writing *On the Causes and Indications of Acute and Chronic Diseases*, we find for example some finely tuned representations of various types of headache.[73] On the other hand, in an anonymous work also dealing with acute and chronic diseases, and also of the first century AD, we encounter such bland statements as 'warmth applied by contact is fine for any pain'.[74] And we realize that we should not be seduced into associating the entire gamut of medical writing with the achievements of a few distinguished names. The legacy of Rufus of Ephesus, a greater and more famous clinician of the first century than Aretaeus, provides further warnings against expecting learned medicine under the Roman Empire to produce newly refined approaches to the problem of pain. As remarked here at the outset, Rufus may not actually have written a treatise on pain. The subject is none the less prominent in some of his case histories preserved in Arabic. For example:

> The pain did not subside but extended to the side of [a melancholic's] face . . . when I feared that it might pass to his eye and brain and that it might kill him, I asked him to have his blood

> let . . . Then, I cauterized his ribs where there was pain. The pain subsided completely . . .[75]

At first blush, pain seems important, a subject for treatment in its own right. Then, however, it becomes apparent that Rufus is virtually equating pain with disease, as the Hippocratics had often done. The relative vividness of the passage does not proclaim a novel or more sensitive theory. And in another work Rufus himself tells us why that should be so. *Questions of the Physician* runs in some detail through the ideal clinical interrogation of the patient – enquiries concerning diet, defecation, previous experience with doctors, and so forth.

> We must also ask what pains [*algemata*] the ailment is causing. It is true that one can judge in other ways when a person is in pain – by his groans and exclamations, by his uneasy movements, his embarrassment, the posture of his body . . . it is possible to recognize pains [*ponoi*] in a patient apart from his complaints.[76]

To ask where it hurt was not therefore absolutely essential, even though Rufus did not consider that the question should be lightly omitted from the clinical encounter. On the other hand, in *Questions of the Physician* he immediately went on to caution against the histrionics of the effeminate, whose representations of pain (*odyne* this time) were as bad as those of tragic actors. And, most significantly for the present argument, enquiries about pain fall well below the top of his list. Some six other topics are treated first in *Questions*.

Perhaps for similar reasons, Galen, to close with the greatest Hippocratic of them all, also had *relatively* little to say of a theoretical nature about pain. Of course, in some cases, Galen could prognosticate *solely* on the basis of questioning the patient, provided he or she were intelligent and articulate. Moreover, to underpin that virtuosity he elevated investigation of pain into a prime means of locating the affected part. On the basis of his masterly synthesis of Hippocrates and Aristotle with dashes of Platonism, and his advances in anatomy and physiology, Galen elaborated a theory of the production of pain to a degree of sophistication inevitably lacking in the Hippocratic corpus. He enriched the descriptions and extended the similes. He began classifying the different kinds of pain (including sympathetic or referred pain) according to their character and their potential for revealing not only the location of the diseased organ but also a general humoral imbalance.[77] As always, Galen is his own most best advocate:

> These organs [liver and kidneys] develop a feeling of heaviness, as if some kind of an unnatural tumor had taken hold of them. In the membrane surrounding each of the viscera mentioned above a nerve is inserted which is endowed with sensibility; when distended by the swelling of the organ it indicates to us the diagnostic classification according to the type of pain. Therefore Hippocrates was the first to write: 'pain in the kidneys feels heavy'.[78]

Hippocrates was the first to write it; Galen the first to explain it. Yet what is striking is that, despite all this, and despite the number of brief discussions of pain in his massive corpus, he seems to have devoted to the topic only one book of the one late treatise just quoted, *On the Affected Parts*. There is no reference to the significance of pain in his extended self-advertisement *On Prognosis*.[79] In comparison with the massive literary attention he paid to pulse and the almost over-refined descriptive vocabulary that he developed for that subject,[80] it is not very much. The best modern commentators on his clinical-diagnostic method find correspondingly little to say about patients' reports of pain or their involuntary signs of distress.[81]

That is surely because Galen rapidly came up against what he took to be the limits of the subject. Where his own recollected experience of pain was inadequate, he would have to rely, as he put it, either on those who did not understand their experiences or on those who understood but could not formulate their suffering in words, 'since it requires a considerable effort or cannot even be communicated verbally'.[82] Malingering, too, presented problems.[83] Hence, despite the distinctions advocated in *On the Affected Parts*, he generally seems to have used *algema*, *odyne*, and *ponos* interchangeably, just as the Hippocratics had done.[84] Pain was easier to deal with from a neurological than from a clinical point of view. The task of interpreting its verbal and behavioural representations was, on the whole, best left at the bedside and kept out of the treatises.

Did the general reluctance of ancient physicians to develop a sophisticated account of the experience of pain stem from inherent limits set to learned endeavour by the topic's irreducible subjectivity? Or was pain more deliberately marginalized? Galen would have responded to the enquiry by referring to subjectivity. He might have agreed with Virginia Woolf, had he lived to read her, on this if nothing else: that 'the merest schoolgirl when she falls in love has Shakespeare, Donne and Keats to speak her mind for her, but let a sufferer try to describe a pain in his head to a doctor and language at once runs dry'.[85] Galen would also have found congenial the twentieth-century surgeon René Leriche: 'in the suffering patient the pain is like a storm which hardly admits of assessment once it is over . . . and there you are, powerless to understand.'[86]

None the less, we must be wary of accepting either the Hippocratics' or Galen's attitude to pain as simply dictated by the inherent nature of the problem. Their attitude should, additionally, be given a cultural setting. But where? One approach, of which a great deal has lately been made, would place Galen in a context that he would not have appreciated: the emergence of Christianity. The period of the late Roman Republic and the earlier empire (the first two centuries) has been interpreted by historians of Foucauldian persuasion as witnessing a 'turn toward the body'. They have discerned an increasing literary emphasis on the representation of physical suffering – an emphasis which foreshadowed, and indeed facilitated, the cultural reception of Christianity's suffering martyrs and saints. Galen assumes a prominent role in such accounts, his fame and success suggesting a medicalization of Roman imperial society, even a medicalization of the notion of the self.[87] There is much evidence to favour such an interpretation. It is surely not coincidental – that is, not just a reflection of the greater abundance of the written evidence – that the type of quotation with which I began is easier to find in the age of Galen than in that of Hippocrates. Yet the history of pain in medicine suggests at least as much continuity as development in the centuries separating the two presiding genii of the subject. Pain does *not* come to dominate Roman medical 'discourse' in the manner predicted by the Foucauldians.

A rather different backdrop may be more appropriate. It has sometimes seemed tempting to divide the history of pain, if only implicitly, into three phases.[88] The third and most recent one began as recently as the 1960s and 1970s. It has witnessed the establishment of pain clinics for chronic sufferers, the founding of the journal *Pain*, a celebrated pain questionnaire, the burgeoning of an anthropological literature which attends to the culturally determined ways in which the afflicted fashion significant narratives around their pains,[89] and a steady increase in the number of doctors who do *not* separate mental suffering from somatic pain or confine treatment to the latter. Before all this, in Phase Two, came the advances in neuro-anatomy of the nineteenth and earlier twentieth centuries and the 'laboratory revolution' in medicine. It is this period, we have in effect been told, which first banished pain to the margins of medical interest and encouraged the view that non-somatic pain was unreal.[90] Phase One, which stretches back to antiquity, is therefore, on this account, pre-lapsarian: a phase in which power lay with the patient, and in which the holistic approach of humoral medicine ensured a much greater degree of attention to patients' suffering and its relief. Phase Three can thus be presented as to some extent a return to Eden – not (admittedly) to a paradise in which there is no pain, but at least to one in which pain is again accorded due status.

Galen and the Hippocratic authors, as I have been construing them, refute the ideas underlying all such nostalgic historical schemata. In their seeming indifference to the pains of mental illness, in their reluctance to give pain too prominent a place in diagnostic enquiry, in their unwillingness to elaborate a vocabulary of pain, above all in their refusal to philosophize about it, they can (in retrospect) be seen as performing two salutary tasks. First, they hinder our general attribution to Phase One of too great an interest in the causation or relief of pain.[91] But second, paradoxically, they also in a sense align themselves with the age of the laboratory, more readily seen as their cultural and intellectual antithesis. And this alignment seems appropriate: in each of the two ages, that of the Hippocratics and that of the laboratory, learned medical aspirations were, though expressed very differently, perhaps quite similar – aspirations towards scientific rationality and the prestige that went with it, aspirations towards authority over the patient, and thus over everything that he or she said as well as did. About suffering they were never wrong, the Old Masters?[92]

NOTES

1. Edward Mendelson (ed.), *The English Auden* (London: Faber and Faber, 1977), 237.
2. *Agamemnon*, line 177, with Eduard Fraenkel, *Aeschylus: Agamemnon*, 2 vols (Oxford: Clarendon Press), ii. 106.
3. *Nicomachean Ethics*, iii. 12.

4. Epicurus, *Key Doctrines*, 4, trans. A.A. Long and D.N. Sedley, *The Hellenistic Philosophers*, 2 vols (Cambridge: Cambridge University Press, 1987), i. 115.
5. *Moral Letters*, lxxviii. 13, with P.H. Schrijvers, 'Pijn, waar is je overwinning? Over de 78e Brief van Seneca', in H.F.J. Horstmanshoff (ed.), *Pijn en Balsem, Troost en Smart: Pijnbeleving, en Pijnbestrijding in de Oudheid* (Rotterdam: Erasmus Publishing, 1994), 185–95.
6. Vii. 11. Cf. *Acts*, xiv. 22.
7. *Octavius*, 12, trans. Judith Perkins, *The Suffering Self: Pain and Narrative Representation in the Early Christian Era* (London/New York: Routledge, 1995), 38–9.
8. *Letters*, xxxix. 2. Cf. Darrel W. Amundsen, *Medicine, Society, and Faith in the Ancient and Medieval Worlds* (Baltimore/London: Johns Hopkins University Press, 1996), ch. 5.
9. Marvin Meyer and Richard Smith (eds), *Ancient Christian Magic: Coptic Texts of Ritual Power* (New York: HarperCollins, 1994), no. 135, p. 335.
10. Cf. David Melling, this volume; John Bowker, *Problems of Suffering in Religions of the World* (Cambridge: Cambridge University Press, 1970).
11. David B. Morris, *The Culture of Pain* (Berkeley/Los Angeles: University of California Press, 1991), 74.
12. James Longrigg, *Greek Rational Medicine: Philosophy and Medicine from Alcmaeon to the Alexandrians* (London/New York: Routledge, 1993), 26 n.1 with refs.; G.E.R. Lloyd, *Magic, Reason and Experience: Studies in the Origins and Development of Greek Science* (Cambridge: Cambridge University Press, 1979), ch. 1.
13. Vivian Nutton, 'From Galen to Alexander: Aspects of Medicine and Medical Practice in Late Antiquity', *Dumbarton Oaks Papers*, xxxviii (1984), 8–9.
14. Owsei Temkin, *Hippocrates in a World of Pagans and Christians* (Baltimore/London: Johns Hopkins University Press, 1991), 256; Peter Brown, *The Body and Society: Men, Women and Sexual Renunciation in Early Christianity* (New York: Columbia University Press, 1988); Simon Goldhill, *Foucault's Virginity: Ancient Erotic Fiction and the History of Sexuality* (Cambridge: Cambridge University Press, 1995); Perkins, *The Suffering Self*.
15. Charles Daremberg and Charles Emile Ruelle (eds), *Oeuvres de Rufus d'Ephèse* (Paris: Imprimerie Nationale, 1879), nos 256–324; J. Ilberg, 'Rufus von Ephesos: ein griechischer Arzt in trajanischer Zeit', *Abhandlungen der philologisch-historischen Klasse der Sächischen Akademie der Wissenschaften*, xli. 1 (1931), 38–42. I am grateful to Vivian Nutton for advice.
16. Michel Foucault, *The Birth of the Clinic* (Tavistock: London, 1973), xviii.
17. No aspect of the *Corpus Hippocraticum* is free from continuing debate. I do no more than attempt to summarize the conventional scholarly wisdom. The most accessible means of entry into CH is through Paul Potter, *Short Handbook of Hippocratic Medicine* (Quebec: Editions du Sphinx, 1988), and G.E.R. Lloyd (ed.), *Hippocratic Writings* (Harmondsworth: Penguin, 1978).
18. The standard edition, Carl Gottlob Kühn, *Claudii Galeni: Opera Omnia*, 22 vols (Leipzig: Cnobloch, 1821–33), is only the upper part of an

iceberg. In what follows all references to CH will be by volume and page number in the standard edition of E. Littré (hereafter L), *Oeuvres complètes d'Hippocrate*, 10 vols (Paris: J.-B. Baillière, 1839–61).

19. Simon Byl, 'Le traitement de la douleur dans le *Corpus* hippocratique', in J.A. López Férez (ed.), *Tratados Hipocráticos* (Madrid: Universidad Nacional de Educacion a Distancia, 1992), 203, a study to which I am greatly indebted.
20. Gilles Maloney and Winnie Fromm (eds), *Concordantia in Corpus Hippocraticum*, 5 vols (Hildesheim/Zurich/New York: Olms-Weidmann, 1986).
21. Byl, 'Traitement', 203, has larger aggregates.
22. Cf. Roselyne Rey, *The History of Pain* (Cambridge, MA/London: Harvard University Press, 1995), 18.
23. On the dating, L. Conrad *et al.*, *The Western Medical Tradition* (Cambridge: Cambridge University Press, 1995), 22.
24. Rey, *History*, 19.
25. Contrast Lloyd, *Magic*, subtly distinguishing tradition and naturalism in Hippocratic ideology, with Longrigg, *Greek Rational Medicine*.
26. I.M. Lonie, 'Cos versus Cnidus and the Historians', *History of Science*, xvi (1978), 42–75, 77–92.
27. A.M. Unruh, 'Gender Variations in Clinical Pain Experience', *Pain*, lxv. 2–3 (1996), 123–67.
28. I. 62, L viii.126.
29. Useful conspectuses: Lesley Dean-Jones, *Women's Bodies in Classical Greek Science* (Oxford: Clarendon Press, 1994); Ann Ellis Hanson, 'The Medical Writer's Woman', in David M. Halperin *et al.* (eds), *Before Sexuality: The Construction of Erotic Experience in the Ancient Greek World* (Princeton, NJ: Princeton University Press, 1990), 309–38.
30. Dean-Jones, *Women's Bodies*, ch. 2, esp. 119, 125.
31. Helen King, 'Self-help, Self-knowledge: in Search of the Patient in Hippocratic Gynaecology', in Richard Hawley and Barbara Levick (eds), *Women in Antiquity: New Assessments* (London/New York: Routledge, 1995), 135–48.
32. Helen King, 'The Early Anodynes: Pain in the Ancient World', in Ronald D. Mann (ed.), *The History of the Management of Pain* (Carnforth, Lancashire/Park Ridge, NJ: Parthenon Publishing Group, 1988), 58.
33. Rey, *History*, 19.
34. 60 (L vii. 93), 6 (14) with 21 (36); 14 (27); 60 (93).
35. 66 (L vii. 101), 73 (111).
36. 14 (L vii. 25), 15 (167).
37. 8 (L vii. 16), 27 (44), 55 (87).
38. 4 (L vii. 12), 16 (30); 20 (33), 23 (38).
39. Vi. 40, vii. 52 (L iv. 572, 592); Byl, 'Traitement', 203.
40. Byl, 'Traitement', 203–4.
41. 7 (L vi. 290).
42. 7 (L ii. 268–72), *pace* King, 'Early Anodynes', 60, which seems to me overingenious. I am very grateful to Helen King for allowing me to read, in advance of its publication, a paper that elaborates some of the

material there: 'Chronic Pain and the Creation of Narrative', forthcoming in Jim Porter (ed.), *Constructions of the Classical Body*.

43. Cf. again King, 'Early Anodynes', 60. In the early second century AD, Soranus still used both *odyne* and *ponos;* cf. his *Gynaecoloy*, ii. 6–8.
44. P.N. Singer, 'Some Hippocratic Mind-Body Problems', in López Férez (ed.), *Tratados Hipocráticos*, 131–43.
45. G.E.R. Lloyd, *The Revolutions of Wisdom: Studies in the Claims and Practices of Ancient Greek Science* (Berkeley/Los Angeles/London: University of California Press, 1987), 23.
46. E.R. Dodds, *The Greeks and the Irrational* (Berkeley/Los Angeles/London: University of California Press, 1951), ch. 3.
47. L viii. 468. Helen King, 'Bound to Bleed', in Averil Cameron and Amélie Kuhrt (eds), *Images of Women in Antiquity*, rev. ed. (London: Routledge, 1993), 109–27.
48. Xvii. 11 (L iii. 134).
49. *Aphorisms*, ii. 6 (L iv. 470).
50. King, 'Early Anodynes', 59–60, seeming to me to confuse (a) pain which cannot on a particular occasion be relieved, (b) pain which can *never* be relieved, (c) pain which *should* not be relieved.
51. Anne Carson, 'Putting Her in Her Place: Woman, Dirt, and Desire', in Halperin *et al.* (eds), *Before Sexuality*, 149.
52. *Iliad*, v. 336f., xi. 251f.; *Odyssey*, ix. 387f. F. Mawet, *Recherches sur les oppositions fonctionelles dans le vocabulaire homérique de la douleur* (Gembloux: Académie Royale de Belgique, 1979).
53. Sophocles, *Philoctetes*, lines 705–6. Philip van der Eijk, 'Pijn en Doodsstrijd in de Griekse Tragedie: Sophocles' *Philoctetes*', in Horstmanshoff (ed.), *Pijn en Balsem*, 71–83. For wider context and many further references: Bennett Simon, *Mind and Madness in Ancient Greece* (Ithaca/London: Cornell University Press, 1978); Ruth Padel, *In and Out of the Mind: Greek Images of the Tragic Self* (Princeton, NJ: Princeton University Press, 1992); Padel, *Whom Gods Destroy: Elements of Greek and Tragic Madness* (Princeton NJ: Princeton University Press, 1995).
54. Iii. 761–5, trans. Richard Hunter, *Jason and the Golden Fleece*, World's Classics (Oxford/New York: Oxford University Press), 84 (modified slightly). Mawet, 'Evolution d'une structure sémantique: le vocabulaire de la douleur – Apollonios de Rhodes et Homère', *L'Antiquité Classique*, 1 (1981), 499–516; Richard Hunter, *The 'Argonautica' of Apollonius* (Cambridge: Cambridge University Press, 1993), ch. 3, § 3.
55. *Pace* Padel, *In and Out of the Mind*, 50: 'doctors are as fascinated by pain and its causes as are epic and tragedy'.
56. 2 (Lvi. 34).
57. 42 (L vi. 334–6).
58. *Places in Man*, 46 (L vi. 342).
59. L vi. 394, trans. Lloyd, *Hippocratic Writings*, 251.
60. L ii. 110, trans. Lloyd, *Hippocratic Writings*, 170.
61. Adapted from Lloyd, *Hippocratic Writings*, 140.
62. Heinrich von Staden, 'Incurability and Hopelessness: the *Hippocratic Corpus*', in Paul Potter *et al.* (eds), *La maladie et les maladies dans la Collection hippocratique* (Quebec: Editions du Sphinx, 1990), 75–112.

63. Amundsen, *Medicine, Society, and Faith*, chs 2, 4; Ludwig Edelstein, *Ancient Medicine* (Baltimore/London: Johns Hopkins University Press, 1967), 11 f.
64. L i. 578.
65. L vi. 90, vi. 334.
66. Caelius Aurelianus, *On Acute and Chronic Diseases*, I.E. Drabkin (ed.) (Chicago: University of Chicago Press, 1950), Chronic Diseases, ii. 79 (p. 616).
67. *Aphorisms*, ii. 46 (L iv. 482). Byl, 'Traitement'; King 'Early Anodynes'.
68. *Coan Prenotions*, 366, 364 (L v. 660–2).
69. *Aphorisms*, iv. 31, 32 (L iv. 512).
70. *Regimen in Acute Diseases, Appendix*, 9 (L ii. 436f.), trans. Paul Potter, *Hippocrates*, vi, Loeb Classical Library (Cambridge MA/London: Harvard University Press and Heinemann, 1988), 285.
71. L ii. 110f., 668f.
72. The competitively rhetorical aspect of Hippocratic writing is well brought out by Lloyd, *Magic*.
73. *Chronic Diseases*, i. 2, Carolus Hyde (ed.), *Corpus Medicorum Graecorum* [hereafter CMG] (Berlin: Academy of Sciences, 1958), 36–7. Cf. Caelius Aurelianus, *Chronic Diseases*, i. 4 (pp. 610f., Drabkin).
74. Ivan Garofallo (ed.), Brian Fuchs (trans.), *Anonymi Medici de Morbis Acutis et Chronicis* (Leiden/New York/Cologne: Brill, 1997), vi. 10 (p. 44).
75. The standard edition of Rufus's *Krankenjournale* is by Manfred Ullmann (Wiesbaden: Harrasowitz, 1978). I quote a translation by Michael W. Dols from an Oxford Arabic MS: Dols, *Majnun: The Madman in Medieval Islamic Society* (Oxford: Clarendon Press, 1992), 479.
76. Hans Gärtner (ed.), *Rufus von Ephesos: Die Fragen des Arztes an den Kranken*, CMG Supplement 4 (Berlin: Academy of Sciences, 1962), 8 (p. 38).
77. Rosa Maria Moreño Rodriguez and Luis García Ballester, 'El dolor en la teoría y práctica médicas de Galeno', *Dynamis*, ii (1982), 3–24.
78. *On the Affected Parts*, ii. 4, trans. Rudolf E. Siegel (Basel: S. Karger, 1976), 47 (ed. Kühn, viii. 78–9), with *Epidemics VI*, i. 5 (L v. 268).
79. Vivian Nutton (ed.), *Galen: On Prognosis*, CMG, v. 8. 1 (Berlin: Academy of Sciences, 1979).
80. C.R.S. Harris, *The Heart and the Vascular System in Ancient Greek Medicine* (Oxford: Clarendon Press, 1973), ch. 7.
81. Vivian Nutton, 'Galen at the Bedside: the Methods of a Medical Detective', in W.F. Bynum and Roy Porter (eds), *Medicine and the Five Senses* (Cambridge: Cambridge University Press, 1993), 7–16; Luis García Ballester, 'Galen as a Medical Practitioner: Problems in Diagnosis', in Vivian Nutton (ed.), *Galen: Problems and Prospects* (London: Wellcome Institute for the History of Medicine, 1981), 13–46, esp. 26–30.
82. *On the Affected Parts*, ii. 7 (p. 51, Siegel; viii. 89, Kühn).
83. Galen's brief discussion of it is edited by Karl Deichgräber and Fridolf Kudlien in CMG, v. 10. 2. 4 (Berlin: Academy of Sciences, 1960), 113f.
84. Richard J. Durling, *A Dictionary of Medical Terms in Galen* (Leiden/New York/Cologne: E.J. Brill, 1993).

85. Woolf, 'On being Ill', *Essays*, Andrew McNeillie (ed.), iv (London: Hogarth Press, 1994), 318.
86. Quoted by Morris, *Culture of Pain*, 28.
87. Cf. Perkins, *The Suffering Self*, ch. 6.
88. The implication of Morris, *Culture of Pain*, which provides abundant supporting references.
89. Cf. Byron J. Good, *Medicine, Rationality, and Experience* (Cambridge: Cambridge University Press, 1994), chs 5–6.
90. Cf. Eric J. Cassell, *The Nature of Suffering and the Goals of Medicine* (Oxford/New York: Oxford University Press, 1991); Andrew Cunningham and Perry Williams (eds), *The Laboratory Revolution in Medicine* (Cambridge: Cambridge University Press, 1992).
91. Rey, *History of Pain*, chs 1–3, esp. pp. 26–7; Barbara Duden, *The Woman beneath the Skin: A Doctor's Patients in Eighteenth-Century Germany* (Cambridge, MA/London: Harvard University Press, 1991), 87–91; Porter, this volume.
92. I am grateful for references and advice to several 'modern masters' of the subjects touched on here: Edward Hussey, Jane Lightfoot, Vivian Nutton, and particularly Helen King, who has kindly tolerated my incursion into her field and my friendly disagreement with some of the conclusions of her stimulating work.

MEDICINE FOR THE SOUL: THE MEDIEVAL ENGLISH HOSPITAL AND THE QUEST FOR SPIRITUAL HEALTH

Carole Rawcliffe

It has long been recognized that the medieval English hospital was chiefly, sometimes almost exclusively, concerned with the promotion of spiritual health.[1] In marked contrast to the larger institutions of continental Europe, medicalization came late, and during the Middle Ages little in the way of professional treatment was available to the sick, impotent and aged poor who constituted the great majority of patients.[2] Standards of physical care were extremely variable: mismanagement, financial problems and corruption took their toll, as did the social, economic and demographic crises of the fourteenth century.[3] Yet despite these difficulties some of the richer hospitals, such as St Leonard's, York, were able to provide their patients with plain but nourishing food, medication based on home-grown herbal preparations, high-quality nursing and a relatively clean environment with adequate bedding and heating.[4] Such a regime was entirely in keeping with recommendations for the management of the body made by medieval physicians: peaceful surroundings, a moderate diet and the avoidance of stress figured prominently in the advice manuals produced for those who could afford the services of a physician. The holistic approach to healing adopted in the larger, quasi-monastic hospitals of medieval England was thus remarkably similar to that of the *regimen sanitatis*, with its emphasis on mental as well as physical equilibrium.[5] The cure of souls – including those of founders and benefactors – was, however, accorded absolute priority, and may without exaggeration be described as the *raison d'être* of the institutions examined in this essay.

Here the patients measured time by the hours of the Christian liturgy, their days and nights punctuated by the regular rhythm of the *opus Dei*. A sequence of chants, prayers and readings unfolded eight times every twenty-four hours: that is for matins at two or three in the morning, lauds at first light, at prime when the sun rose, at terce, at sext and at nones, at the evening office of vespers, and, finally, at compline or sunset. This soothing and often melodious routine, which may itself have proved extremely therapeutic, was interspersed by masses celebrated as often as three or four times a day, and, on occasion, the solemn office of the dead which might extend over two days or even a whole week.[6] Time not thus occupied would be spent in prayer for the salvation of benefactors and patrons, an obligation shouldered in particular by the almsmen and women of fifteenth and early-sixteenth century England. The transition from comparatively large open ward infirmaries, in which patients often slept two to a bed, to far smaller and more selective almshouses for the frail, elderly and respectable poor allowed greater privacy and with it an opportunity for the cultivation of a more personal, intimate kind of spirituality.[7] Residents of the London almshouse founded by the famous mercer, Richard Whittington (d. 1424), for example, were encouraged to pray or read devotional literature in the quiet of their rooms, albeit after those who were still mobile had attended a daily service for the soul of their patron. A measure of the importance placed upon the religious life of the house may be found in regulations excluding anyone who suffered from madness or other 'intolerable infirmities', including leprosy[8]. The refusal by some English hospitals and almshouses to admit infectious or potentially disruptive individuals (such as pregnant women) was in part a practical measure intended to husband limited resources and provide appropriate surroundings for the performance of the Christian liturgy.[9] But there were other, more profound reasons for branding certain categories of people as undesirable. Might they contaminate a sacred place with the miasma of sin?

Before considering in greater detail the nature and variety of 'ghostly medicine' on offer in English hospitals, it is important to appreciate the way in which inhabitants of a pre-Cartesian world reacted to sickness and pain. Since body and soul were held to be inextricably linked, spiritual health assumed overwhelming importance. And this factor is crucial to our understanding of institutional relief for the poor, as well as medical practice for the rich, before the seventeenth century.[10] In a society which often regarded physical suffering as a punishment for sin, the condition of the soul came, of necessity, to influence every aspect of diagnosis and medical treatment. So much so, that a ruling of the fourth Lateran Council of 1215 threatened medical practitioners with excommunication if they attended anyone who had not first made a full confession, or had at least sworn to do so. Under the heading 'that the sick should provide for the soul before the body', it reads:

> As sickness of the body may sometimes be the result of sin . . . so we by this present decree order and strictly command physicians of the body, when they are called to the sick, to warn and persuade them first of all to call in physicians of the soul so that after their spiritual health has been seen to they may respond better to medicine for their bodies; *for when the cause ceases so does the effect*.[11]

This injunction was taken very seriously. There is ample evidence to suggest that surgeons, as well as patients, confessed before an operation, which, in view of the high risks involved, is entirely understandable.[12] Had earthly medicine been cheaper, less painful and more reliable, the Church would have exercised far less control over the minutiae of practice. As it was, English hospital patients, who were generally spared the uncertain benefits of phlebotomy, purgation and the rigours of humoral therapy,[13] or even (as the fourteenth century French physician, Bernard Gordon, proposed) medical experimentation, had little choice but to offer up their souls for treatment.[14]

Because they were sometimes very small, temporary structures, which functioned as little more than soup kitchens or night shelters, it is now impossible to tell how many hospitals and almshouses were actually set up in medieval England. The names of some 1,100 institutions are known, ranging in size from a handful capable of accommodating 100 or more patients, to the great majority with facilities for a dozen or fewer (although some of these offered outdoor relief as well). Generally speaking, the older, larger houses founded before 1300 either followed or took their inspiration from monastic rules, especially those of the Augustinians, which placed particular stress upon the integration of charitable work with divine worship. Of the rest, all but the meanest and most isolated could call upon the regular services of at least one priest or chaplain, who might serve in an attached chapel or visit from a neighbouring church.[15] A glance at the architecture of surviving hospitals, such as St Giles's, Norwich (1249), which

Plate 1: The south front of St Giles's hospital, Norwich. The sick poor lay in the infirmary at the west end, local parishioners worshipped in the nave in the centre of the building, and the priests celebrated in the chancel, added in *c.* 1383. *Photograph by courtesy of the Royal Commission on Historical Monuments.*

had a staff of between eight and thirteen priests in the 1320s, reveals their fundamentally religious nature **[Plate 1].**

Each and every priest, aptly described as a physician of the soul, had at his disposal a pharmacopoeia of spiritual cures, the best and most powerful of which was the medicine of Christ's body and blood as revealed in the sacrament of the mass. The mere sight of the Host at the moment of elevation was deemed to ease the torment endured by all sinners in purgatory, and also to relieve the more immediate symptoms of earthly disease:

My deadly wounds are dire and deep,
I have no place to soothe the pain.
And smarting will not suffer me to sleep
Until the physician applies his balm.
He must be a curate, a tonsured priest,
Able to say his mass with ease;
Or else the medicine has no power
To grant us leave to live at peace.[16]

In the East Anglian *Play of the Sacrament,* composed around 1460, a drunken and incompetent quack serves as a comic foil to Christ, the Divine Physician, who appears dramatically at the climax with a promise of health and redemption for penitent unbelievers. Desecration of the Host is here punished with physical torment which only Christ can alleviate through the miracle of the Mass. In a telling juxtaposition of profane and sacred medicine, which must

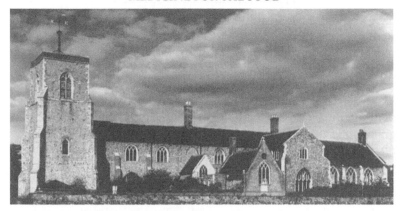

have amused the local audience, the spiritually bankrupt charlatan, with his 'threadbare gown and tattered hose', is said to live just outside St Saviour's hospital at Bury St Edmunds.[17]

Yet the two medicines were not always at odds. Jacques de Vitry may have complained in the early-thirteenth century of 'the blindness of the sick who call to their bedsides the physicians of the body rather than the physicians of souls, preferring mud to treasure, straw to grain, dregs to wine and the body to the soul', but on other occasions he spoke a language more closely attuned to the physical needs of the sick.[18] Late medieval religious literature abounds in a rich variety of medical and surgical metaphors, reflecting the symbiotic relationship which had developed between the Church and the late medieval medical profession. At a basic level the physician who diagnosed too much choler in the urine sample and urged his patient to follow a more moderate regimen, and the priest who warned against the sin of wrath were in complete accord: self-indulgence was bad for the health and lethal for the soul. Not for nothing did Whittington's almshouse threaten gluttons, inebriates and backbiters with expulsion.[19] The idea of treating the body as a discrete entity was totally alien to the medical practitioner, while the priest (who might himself have read medicine) considered it entirely fitting to pronounce upon matters of health. But the body was no more than a shell, albeit one made in the divine image, while the soul was immortal. Here, in the realm of spiritual medicine, the hospital came into its own **[Plate 2]**.

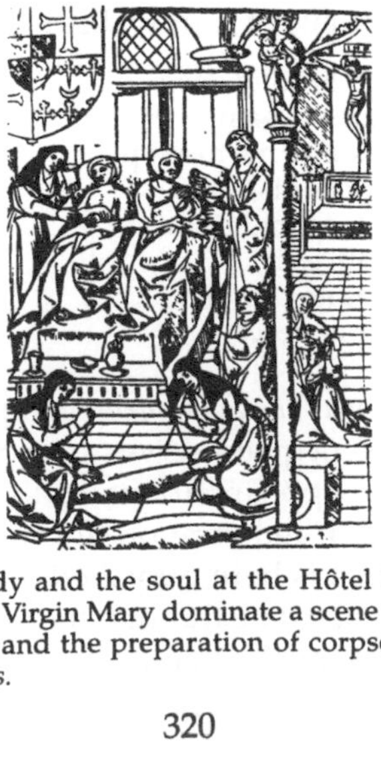

Plate 2: Food for the body and the soul at the Hôtel Dieu, Paris, *c.* 1500. The Crucifix and statue of the Virgin Mary dominate a scene which depicts the administration of the last rites and the preparation of corpses for burial. *Bibliothèque Nationale, Paris, Ms. Ea Rés.*

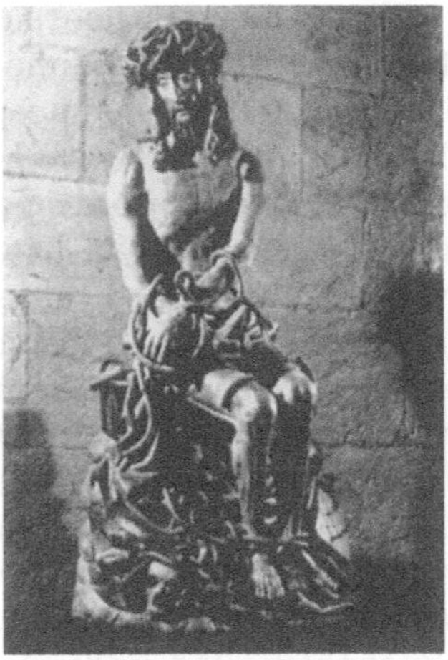

Plate 3: Christ the Physician tasting the 'bitter cup' of the Passion at the Hôtel Dieu, Beaune, Burgundy. The twisted ropes reinforce the idea of temporal suffering, but Death and its begetter, Original Sin, have been overcome.

The theme of *Christus Medicus*, Christ the Physician, first elaborated at length by St Augustine of Hippo (d. 430), is a recurrent one in the art of the medieval European hospital.[20] The painfully realistic late-fifteenth century lime-wood carving of the tortured Christ, crowned with thorns, which still stands at the west end of the *salle des pauvres* in the Hôtel Dieu, Beaune, recalls Augustine's description of the Passion as a 'bitter cup' of medicine tasted by the physician to reassure his patient **[Plate 3]**.

> He taught us . . . to drink now the cup of bitterness, and to receive afterwards health everlasting. Drink, O sick one, of the bitter cup in order to become well, you whose internal organs are diseased without exception. Do not fear to drink. For to dispel your fear the physician drank first, that is, the Lord drank first the bitterness of the Passion . . . fearlessly let us put ourselves in the hands of such a great physician, convinced beyond doubt that he will never apply a remedy that does not benefit us.[21]

And the skull at his feet served to remind the dying that they, too, would be delivered from the consequences of Original Sin by this panacea. More modest but no less therapeutic images of the crucifixion were placed in all but the meanest of English hospitals, in clear view of the patients. Because so little material evidence now survives, it is easy to forget the importance of Christian iconography in these institutions, where wall paintings and stained glass would have intensified the devotional atmosphere. Even with its slender resources, the small *leprosarium* of St Margaret and St John at Wimborne in Dorset was able to afford a painted chapel, while other, richer hospitals were decorated with hangings as well.[22]

Late medieval devotion to the popular cult of the five wounds of Christ is particularly significant in a context of healing, not least because it provides some remarkable examples of the use of medical symbolism by the authors of homiletic literature. At the crucifixion, *Christus Medicus* had placed himself in the hands of the surgeon, so that his blood might be used to cure the sinful. The early-thirteenth century *Ancrene Riwle*, written in English for the guidance of female recluses, refers to the practice of *antipasis*, which presupposes a fairly sophisticated understanding of the phlebotomist's craft:

> When a man is ill, he is not let blood in the diseased part, but in a part that is healthy, in order to heal the part which is diseased. But in all the fevered world there was not found any healthy part, among all mankind, which might be let blood, except only the body of God, which was let blood on the Cross, and not merely on the arm, but in five places, in order to heal mankind of the disease to which the five senses had given rise. Thus the living, healthy part drew out the bad blood from that which was diseased, and so healed that which was sick.[23]

Understandably, given the grim nature of the iconography (at least to modern eyes), the cult of the five wounds has been described as a manifestation of the introspective piety and obsession with death so characteristic of a society reeling under the onslaught of bubonic plague; and it played an increasingly important part in the liturgy for the dead and the dying.[24] This was certainly the case at St Giles's hospital, Norwich, where liturgical practices can be reconstructed in unusual detail thanks to the survival of a unique combination of manuscripts and material remains.[25] Masses of the five wounds in multiples of five were regularly celebrated in the chancel; and on some of the bosses of its ceiling are depicted the instruments of the Passion[26]. A routine part of the healing process in this period comprised the use of charms and prayers invoking appropriate incidents in the life of Christ or the saints; and those used in the treatment of wounds catalogue at great length each of the five sustained by Christ on the Cross.[27] Some hospitals refused to admit *vulnerati* [the wounded], who were tainted with blood, difficult to nurse and potentially troublesome,[28] but those which did almost certainly relied heavily on healing rituals of this kind. The recitation of specific prayers for the relief of less morally questionable conditions, such as deafness, blindness, toothache, ringworm and aching bones would almost certainly have been performed by nurses rather than priests, this being an activity traditionally associated with female healers. The fourteenth-century surgeon, Guy de Chauliac, who was himself a papal chaplain, contemptuously dismissed the 'women . . . and many idiots or fools, who refer patients with all manner of diseases to saints alone, on the basis that God inflicts pain as it pleases him, and he will remove it as he wills'.[29] Such attempted cures had at least the merit of being painless, and were especially suited to the religious milieu of the medieval hospital.

In the wake of Christ the Physician came his nurse, the Virgin Mary, a ubiquitous presence in the wall paintings, statuary and altar-pieces of hospital chapels and infirmaries throughout Christendom. A large fourteenth-century wall painting of the Annunciation may, for example, still be seen in the chapel of St Nicholas's hospital, Harbledown; the Virgin and child stand protectively above the gatehouse of the hospital of St Cross, Winchester; and a circle of bosses depicting scenes from the life of the Virgin embellish the side chapel of St Giles's hospital, Norwich.[30] Her image may likewise be found, among many others, on the seals of William Elsing's hospital for the blind in Cripplegate, London, the hospital of St Thomas the Martyr at Beck (Norfolk), the *leprosarium* of the Holy Trinity in Knightsbridge (Middlesex) and the hospital of St John the Baptist, Bridgwater (Somerset), as well as the scores of institutions specifically dedicated to her.[31] As a mediatrice between sinful humanity and God, she occupied a special place in the liturgy for the dead, and was consequently deemed to bring hope and comfort to the sick. She served, moreover, as a role model for the hospital sister, as Henry, duke of Lancaster (d. 1360), explained in a mystical tract on the subject of sacred medicine. This was written shortly before he reformed the statutes of the hospital of the Annunciation of St Mary in the Newarke, Leicester, which had been founded by his father. Having contemplated the variety of painful remedies available to cure his seven 'putrefying and dangerous wounds' (the seven deadly sins), he drew consolation from the prospect of convalescence:

> Since I have been given such a good nurse, who cares for me so tenderly in my sickness and binds up my wounds so carefully and so well, it would be quite outrageous if I were not patient; nor could it be beyond her skill to cure me however ill I might be. This kind nurse is the gentle Virgin Mary, our Blessed Lady and your gentle mother, dear Lord . . . and I am greatly bound to thank you with all my heart, since it pleased you to entrust me to such capable hands.[32]

The duke spoke on behalf of all medieval sinners, irrespective of wealth, but his words assume particular significance in the context of the contemporary English hospital. Since the services of physicians and surgeons were only occasionally available to the sick paupers who found refuge there, the quotidian round of prayer and liturgy came to dominate their lives. At the duke's own hospital of St Mary in the Newarke, for example, the original foundation statutes of 1330 stipulated that every newcomer was to confess his sins before gaining entry. Once admitted, he was to lie in the body of the hospital church so that he could hear 'all the divine offices' and witness the elevation of the Host at a special mass to be celebrated each day in full view of all the bedridden inmates.[33] Nor, it may be noted, were the latter able to escape the priest's watchful eye.

Duke Henry was also anxious to assuage the physical sufferings of the sick poor, and to this end he may well have donated relics to the hospital. A conviction that the earthly remains or personal effects of holy men and women possessed curative properties guaranteed the lasting popularity of celebrated healing shrines, such as those at Canterbury, Walsingham and York, while also encouraging smaller institutions to acquire relics as and when they became available. Hospitals were naturally anxious to form their own collections, the most famous English example being that of St Bartholomew's in London, which included a reputed fragment of the True Cross and body parts of the patron saint (who had been skinned alive). A twelfth-century history of its foundation lists a number of miraculous cures attributed to these sacred objects, which attracted enormous crowds and correspondingly large donations.[34] One of the most interesting accounts of the use of relics in an English hospital comes from a list of the miracles performed by Gilbert of Sempringham (d. 1189), a piece of whose wooden staff was presented by John de Lacy (d. 1190) to his new foundation at Castle Donington. At least two individuals are said to have been cured by it soon afterwards: the master, himself a victim of paralysis, and, significantly, a local physician who had a fever and was given water in which the staff had been immersed to drink. The physician's presence is explained not because he had been visiting the infirmary, but because he had gone 'to search among the powerful herbs and roots that were kept there for a means of restoring his health'. On this occasion, at least, it appears that earthly as well as spiritual medicine was being widely administered.[35]

Were such relics used, along with the constant repetition of *Aves* (the Hail Mary) and *Pater Nosters* (the Lord's Prayer), in healing rituals for the patients? In some cases they appear to have been regarded as a means of generating a supplementary income from visitors rather than treating the sick poor, although it was no doubt assumed that close proximity to them would in itself be therapeutic. St Giles's hospital, Norwich, possessed the heart of the founder, Bishop Walter Suffield, who had left it as a legacy in his will. The gift reflects his great attachment to the place, but he may also have nursed a secret hope of being canonized and thus regarded it as a potentially valuable asset. Sad to say, the hospital's relics were together raising no more than about twenty shillings a year during the fifteenth century, by which time local interest had waned.[36] Yet despite changing fashions in popular piety, the ownership of relics continued to arouse fierce, sometimes unscrupulous competition among the clergy. In 1391, an investigation into abuses at a rather less famous hospital dedicated to St Bartholomew, this time near Oxford, found that the fellows of Oriel College had removed a comb owned by St Edmund, a piece of the skin of the patron saint, the bones of St Stephen and a rib of St Andrew the Apostle 'which had remained from old times as relics for the adornment and honour of the chapel'. Three decades later similar losses of 'many relics, ecclesiastical ornaments, books and jewels' were being investigated at the hospital of St Mary, Ospringe.[37]

Elaborate liturgy, statues, stained glass, images and relics might bring comfort and hope of a better life in the next world, but in the last resort the patient had to come to terms with his or her own conscience. The idea of hospital patients as 'unseen congregations whose white rows lie set apart above', lingers on in Philip Larkin's powerful poem, 'The Building', in which he speaks of men and women 'all here to confess that something has gone wrong', and admit their 'error of a serious sort'.[38] Confession and absolution of sins, the first stage in the healing process, were deemed essential before any member of the laity could actually receive communion, and, most important of all, make the 'good death' so necessary for salvation. To die without 'shrift and housel' was to be condemned to a long spell in purgatory, or even eternity in hell, a fate which hospitals such as St John's, Ely, which insisted upon confession and communion upon admission, promised to avert.[39] Fear of purgatory, where atonement was made for any sins for which penance had not been done on earth, was real and earnest, since its pains differed only in duration from the unending torments of the damned. No sixteenth-century congregation could listen unmoved as Bishop John Fisher catalogued the agonizing disorders, such as untreated toothache, the stone and gout, which were, he claimed, as nothing compared to the fate awaiting sinners in the next life.[40] A widespread belief that St Giles had intervened to secure divine forgiveness for the Emperor Charlemagne, whose sins were so great that he dared not confess them, added greatly to the popularity of his cult in the Middle Ages, and (along with his reputation as a friend of the sick poor) made him a common dedicatee of hospitals. As 'theriac [a powerful drug] and medicine' to men and women with diseased souls, he held out a promise of spiritual healing.[41]

Henry, duke of Lancaster, was one of many hospital patrons who insisted upon confession before admission, for reasons made clear in his *Book of Sacred Medicines:*

> Just as it is in Nature that, when a man is wounded or hurt in the mouth, the tongue assists him quickly and well to heal his wound, and thus keeps it clean, Gentle Lord, have mercy on me and give me grace so I can, with my own tongue, ease the foul wound in my mouth and thereby cleanse it of its encrusted filth: that is to say, by reciting the foul sins committed by my own mouth, along with all the others, in the true confessional, with a desolate heart. And so I may cure my diseased mouth with my own mouth . . . [42]

Given the stress placed in the medieval *regimen sanitatis* upon the psychological state of the patient, it is not surprising that medical practitioners sometimes claimed to detect a marked improvement in physical health after confession.[43] Hospital chaplains were no doubt also well aware of the physiological benefits which it imparted, although their first priority was clearly spiritual. They were lancing the boils and apostumes of sin: as John Fisher observed, 'the more the filth and matter is hidden, the more the corruption and venomous infection grows, piercing and infecting the very bones'.[44] At St Leonard's hospital, York, one or two chaplains were supposed to make a tour of the wards every night, comforting the sick and encouraging them to repent and confess.[45] Since they were modelled upon the ordinances of the Florentine hospital of Santa Maria Nuova, which made elaborate provision for the administration of the sacraments, regulations drawn up by Henry VII's executors for his new foundation at the Savoy in London were unusually specific on this score. In 1512, the executors secured a papal indult allowing the master and no fewer than six priests 'to hear confessions within the hospital of all who are ill there, and to absolve them from sins however grave, even if forgotten, both at the point of death and when death is expected'.[46] The clerical staff also secured permission to hear the confession of pilgrims, who were attracted to the Savoy by the promise of an unusually generous indulgence, remitting years of penance already enjoined upon them for past sins in return for charitable donations. The sale of indulgences, which was to incite the wrath of Martin Luther a few years later, provided many English hospitals with a supplementary income from men and women seeking to buy a speedy passage through purgatory.[47]

That chronically sick, long-stay patients should confess regularly was a matter of concern to patrons, since the intercessionary prayers they were supposed to say for the Christian departed would thus be rendered more efficacious. Rules devised for the *leprosarium* of St James, Westminster, in 1267, ordered the infirm sisters and healthy lay brothers alike to confess together every week and take the Sacrament four times a year, while also performing a quotidian round of devotions for the souls of past benefactors. This requirement was later modified, in accordance with customary lay practice, to allow for communion just once a year. But the master alone was henceforth to act as confessor, any unlicensed resort to other priests being punishable by a month's fast on reduced rations.[48] St James's was a leper hospital; and the ambivalence felt towards victims of this disease provides some fascinating insights into medieval reactions to extremes of physical suffering. Although it is possible to cite many examples of brutality and prejudice (fostered in part by the vituperative language used by many twelfth- and thirteenth-century clergymen in describing Jews, heretics and other social outcasts as moral lepers, polluting the body politic), responses were more complex and liable to change than has sometimes been allowed.[49] Christ had loved the leper, and much spiritual merit was to be gained from helping the most deformed and rejected members of society. As holy men and women, such as Francis of Assisi (d. 1226) and Elizabeth of Hungary (d. 1231), showed by their example, the leper served as an earthly symbol of Christ's suffering – *Christus quasi leprosus* – and was to be revered accordingly. Elizabeth's charity was, however, tempered by concern for the immortal souls of her charges: patients in her hospital at Marburg who refused to make a full confession ran the risk of being whipped.[50]

Terrible as the leper might appear, the physical decomposition apparent in the later stages of *lepromatous* leprosy promised a release from the pains of purgatory: in a transitory state between life and death, he or she suffered on earth and ascended directly to heaven, without having to endure the torments of the refiner's fire.[51] St Hugh of Lincoln (d. 1200) described the leper as 'a lucent pearl in the crown of the Everlasting King',[52] while the French theologian, Eudes de Châteauroux (*c.* 1270), expressed himself more trenchantly. When preaching a sermon in *domo leprosorum* [in the house of the lepers] he explained that God had separated his congregation from the society of healthy men 'out of love, as a man shuts up his wife and jealously removes her from the company of other women who might corrupt her through the their bawdy talk and lewd suggestions'. Indeed, just as the possessive spouse might cut off his wife's hair or slice off her nose, in order to keep her to himself, so the leper had been forced, by disfigurement, to forgo his love of earthly pleasures.[53] So to some people, at least, leprosy was a calling, an inducement to leave the world and follow a life of contemplation, in preparation for celestial rewards to come. Far from forcibly confining their inmates, many of the earlier quasi-monastic English *leprosaria* threatened those who were disruptive or disobedient with expulsion. Life within their walls revolved around the service of God and the purification of the soul through prayer and the *opus Dei*. We get a glimpse of life in such an institution from the *Vita* of

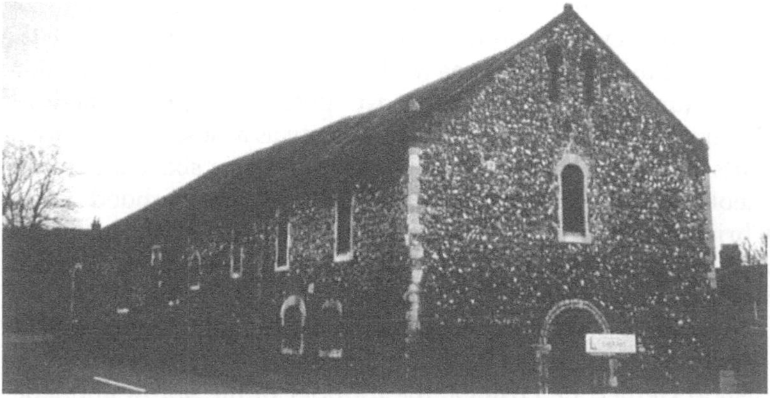

Plate 4: The leper hospital of St Mary Magdalen on the outskirts of Norwich from the west, infirmary end (*c.* 1119, but heavily restored). The patients lay on two floors, with an uninterrupted view of the altar in the chapel to the east.

William of Norwich, which describes how the body of the saint was discovered in 1144. A shooting star appeared near the leper house at Sprowston **[Plate 4]**, and was sighted by the wife of a high ranking Norman official:

> she who for the love of God has her dwelling hard by St Mary Magdalen's attending upon the sick; and, engaged in such services, lives as a beggar for the salvation of her soul. But the sick people of that place in the same night as they were getting up for the midnight office in the silence of the night, when Legarda showed it them, saw the brightness of that same light.[54]

The poor inmates of such places were not, however, the only hopeful beneficiaries of what, in practice, constituted the spiritual equivalent of intensive care. Founders, patrons and staff, too, sought to derive lasting merit from their almsdeeds. The medieval hospital was, in fact, the concrete expression, in bricks and mortar, of the Seven Comfortable Works, through the performance of which medieval men and women hoped to obtain 'health in body, grace in soul and everlasting joy'.[55] The works in question, as listed by Christ in St Matthew's gospel (XXV, vv. 32–6), were a constant theme of medieval preachers: feeding, clothing and giving drink to the poor, visiting prisoners, caring for the sick and sheltering the homeless were all charitable activities undertaken by hospitals, as, of course, was providing a proper burial for the dead, which took its inspiration from the Old Testament Book of Tobit.[56] If, in Bishop John Fisher's words, sin was a 'grievous sickness' infecting all the organs of the body, strong as well as weak, with a lethal infection, then almsdeeds were the most potent of prophylactics.[57] Reiterating the medieval view of the body as a close community of parts bound together in mutual support, another sixteenth century theologian observed that in the 'blessed brotherhood under Christ . . . the benefits of the head are shared by all the members; and any good work performed by one such member wonderfully redounds to all the rest'.[58]

Whereas the sick poor were clearly dependent upon the rich for charity on earth, in the next life, the roles would be reversed. As Bishop Herbert de Losinga, the founder of the Sprowston leper house, reminded the wealthy citizens of Norwich: 'The holy poor are lean with hunger, and shiver with cold, but hereafter in heaven they shall be kings, and in the presence of God shall sit in judgement upon your crimes and those of all the wicked.'[59] Almost as much as eternity in hell, the prospect of a lengthy sojourn in purgatory served to concentrate the mind and free the purse strings. Leaving little to chance, the founders of hospitals were pedantic and exacting in the matter of intercessionary prayers and masses. The statutes of the hospital of St Margaret, outside Gloucester, which date from about 1200, demanded that each of the brothers and sisters should say one hundred *Aves* and another hundred *Pater Nosters* both before and after the main meal 'for all their benefactors, living and dead'.[60] Many of the almshouses founded in fifteenth-century England imposed far heavier burdens upon inmates carefully selected from the ranks of the respectable and acceptable poor. William Pykenham (d. 1497), archdeacon of Suffolk, required the almsmen and women of his foundation at Hadleigh, where he was rector, to say two full psalters of the Blessed Virgin (a grand total of 300 *Aves* and fifteen *Pater Nosters*) each day without fail, along with a variety of other devotions. Although the sick and feeble were temporarily excused attendance in chapel, it is clear that such an arduous round of devotion would necessarily have precluded the moribund or severely disabled.[61] It also placed a serious question mark over the fate of those who did not conform to a strict moral and social code. Because of the growing emphasis upon the *quality* as well as the quantity of prayers said on their behalf, founders became increasingly preoccupied with the moral character of patients and almsmen, on the assumption that God would incline his ear more readily to the prayers of the righteous.

If, as theologians reminded them, the lame beggar, leaning on his crutch of alms, led the rich man, blinded by wealth, to the banquet of heaven, the latter still clearly expected to take a seat above the salt.[62] For in the last resort, his spiritual health came first. In an age notable for its pervasive culture of 'good lordship', clientage and protection, hospitals performed a vital role as spiritual intermediaries, whose function was to 'labour' or intercede with the almighty on behalf of miserable sinners, just as a courtier might agree to solicit a royal pardon for one of his retainers. John Somerset, physician to Henry VI, who knew at first hand how to cultivate a royal patron, earned a great reputation as a philanthropist during his lifetime, endowing an almshouse for nine poor men at Brentford in Middlesex, in 1446, with the profits of his lucrative practice. Yet when he himself came to list his many charitable activities, four years later, he placed first the 'dedys of devotion' involved in setting up a chantry chapel and fraternity nearby, dedicated to the nine orders of angels and the immortal souls of his royal and baronial patients.[63] The masters and brethren of St Giles's hospital, Norwich, naturally endorsed this scale of values. Royal letters patent of 1451 allowing them to acquire additional estates to the value of £20 a year describe the first and overwhelming claim on their time and resources as 'the divine service which has to be celebrated in the hospital church every day . . . for the praise of God and honour of St Giles, *and the soul's health of the founder*'.[64]

As part of a survival strategy, designed to adapt itself to difficult financial circumstances, and, above all, to appeal to the spiritual aspirations of the wealthy citizens of Norwich, St Giles's refashioned itself as a grand collegiate foundation. Its spectacular new chancel boasted two organs (with a third in the lady chapel), a costly and elaborate decor and a choir skilled in polyphony: here was an appropriate setting for the lengthy requiem masses and other offices of commemoration which its patrons now demanded **[Plate 5]**. A few bedesmen may have joined the increasingly elaborate festivals and ceremonies, which are described in the hospital's own, unique processional **[Plate 6]**, but there is reason to believe that the sick poor may have been obliged to vacate the former infirmary, at the west end of the church, for premises in a less conspicuous part of the precinct.[65] Throughout England,

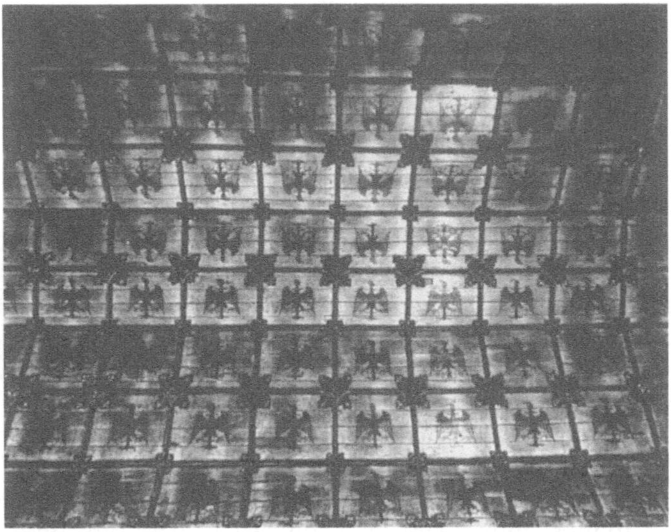

Plate 5: The ceiling of the chancel of St Giles's hospital, *c.* 1383. With 252 wooden panels and some 232 gilded bosses, it reveals the level of artistic patronage enjoyed by the larger urban hospitals of medieval England. *Photograph by courtesy of the Royal Commission on Historical Monuments.*

hospitals of this type were the recipients of a new kind of patronage, which took the form of architectural embellishments, plate, vestments and service books, designed to enhance the performance of rituals dedicated to the salvation of the men and women who hoped thus to buy their way out of purgatory.[66] Prayers and masses had always been said for the Christian departed, but now this aspect of life in the English hospital became an end in itself. Even during the late 1530s, after the first wave of Protestant reform had led to the dissolution of several of the larger monastic hospitals, the master of St Giles's stubbornly upheld the terms of Henry VI's grant. When suing Robert Wace in Chancery for 'unlawful and crafty practice to let and hinder the celebration of . . . divine service and deeds of [spiritual] charity', he emphasized that religious observance had been the chief and most serious casualty. It was in this way, he reminded the court, that all English hospitals not only praised God, but also brought 'relief and comfort, and health of soul to a great number of the King's highness's faithful subjects, both poor *and rich*'.[67] The wealthy had, indeed, more often than not become the intended beneficiaries of the medicine dispensed in these institutions: with eternal salvation as the prize at

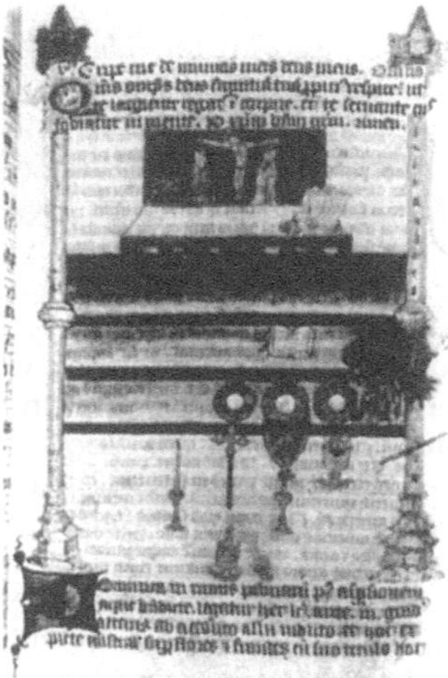

Plate 6: The Processional of St Giles's hospital contains the only known surviving set of medieval diagrams instructing the clergy (represented by tonsured heads and items of ecclesiastical furniture) how to conduct processions. This illustration shows the blessing of palms on Palm Sunday; note the painting of the Crucifixion on the high altar. *British Library, Department of Manuscripts, Add. Ms. 57,534, fo 32r.*

stake, a modest investment in good works among deferential paupers must have seemed well worth the cost.

NOTES

1. This is the theme of Rotha M. Clay's pioneering study, *The Mediaeval Hospitals of England* (London: Cass, 1909, reprinted 1966), which has recently been updated and enlarged by Nicholas Orme and Margaret Webster, *The English Hospital, 1070–1570* (New Haven/London: Yale University Press, 1995). An important continental dimension is supplied in Peregrine Horden's comprehensive review article, 'A discipline of relevance: the historiography of the medieval hospital', *Social History of Medicine*, i (1988), 359–74.
2. See, for some comparative examples, Danielle Jacquart, *Le Milieu Médical en France du XIIe au XIVe Siècle* (Geneva: Hautes Etudes Médiévales et Modernes, series 5, xlvi, 1981), 120–1; Annie Saunier, *'Le Pauvre Malade' dans le Cadre Hospitalier Médiéval: France du Nord 1300–1500* (Paris: Editions Arguments, 1993); John Henderson, 'The hospitals of late-medieval and Renaissance Florence: a preliminary survey', in Lindsay Granshaw and Roy Porter (eds), *The Hospital in History* (London/New York: Routledge, 1989), 63–92; and Katherine Park, 'Medical assistance in renaissance Florence', in Jonathan Barry and Colin Jones (eds), *Medicine and Charity before the Welfare State* (London/New York: Routledge, 1991), 26–45.

3. Miri Rubin, 'Development and change in English hospitals, 1100–1500', in Granshaw and Porter, *The Hospital in History*, 41–59; *eadem*, 'Imagining medieval hospitals', in Barry and Jones, *Medicine and Charity*, 14–25.
4. Patricia Cullum, *Cremetts and Corrodies: Care of the Poor and Sick at St Leonard's Hospital York in the Middle Ages* (York: University of York, Borthwick Paper, 79, 1991), 15–18; Rubin, 'Development and change', 50–1; Roberta Gilchrist, *Contemplation and Action: The Other Monasticism* (London/New York: Leicester University Press, 1995), 32–8.
5. Succinctly described by Luis Garcia-Ballester, 'Changes in the *Regimina Sanitatis:* the role of the Jewish physician', in Sheila Campbell, Bert Hall and David Klausner (eds), *Health Disease and Healing in Medieval Culture* (New York: St Martin's Press, 1992), 118–31; and Peter Murray Jones, *Medieval Medical Miniatures* (London: British Library, 1984), chapter vi, *passim*.
6. Carole Rawcliffe, 'Gret criynge and joly chauntynge': life, death and liturgy at St Giles's hospital, Norwich, in the thirteenth and fourteenth centuries', in *eadem*, Richard Wilson and Roger Virgoe (eds), *Counties and Communities: Essays on East Anglian History* (Norwich: Centre of East Anglian Studies, 1996), 37–55.
7. Marjorie K. McIntosh, 'Local responses to the poor in late medieval and Tudor England', *Continuity and Change*, iii (1988), 220–3; Orme and Webster, *The English Hospital*, 136–46.
8. William Dugdale, *Monasticon Anglicanum*, 6 vols (Caley ed., London: Longman, 1817–30), vi(2), 744–7.
9. Martha Carlin, 'Medieval English hospitals', in Granshaw and Porter, *The Hospital in History*, 25; Rubin, 'Development and change', 49. Whittington was, however, unusually sympathetic towards the plight of unmarried mothers, and endowed an eight-bedded ward for their private use at St Thomas's hospital, Southwark: James Gairdner (ed), *The Historical Collections of a Citizen of London* (London: Camden Society, new series, xvii, 1876), ix.
10. Considered at length in Darel W. Amundsen, 'The Catholic tradition', in *idem* and R.L. Numbers (eds), *Caring and Curing: Health and Medicine in the Western Religious Tradition* (New York/London: Macmillan, 1986), 65–107; and also by Katherine Park, 'Medicine and society in medieval Europe, 500–1500', in Andrew Wear (ed.), *Medicine in Society* (Cambridge/New York: Cambridge University Press, 1992), 59–90.
11. Norman Tanner (ed.), *Decrees of the Ecumenical Councils*, 2 vols (Washington DC: Georgetown University Press, 1990), i, 245–6. This ruling was reiterated in a papal bull of 1566: Richard Palmer, 'The Church, leprosy and plague in medieval and early modern Europe', in W.J. Shiels (ed.), *The Church and Healing* (Oxford: Studies in Church History, 19, 1982), 85.
12. Carole Rawcliffe, *Medicine and Society in Later Medieval England* (Stroud: Alan Sutton, 1995), 95.
13. Classical medical theory, followed closely in the Middle Ages, drew heavily upon the belief that health depended upon a careful balance of

four bodily fluids or humours (blood, phlegm, black bile and yellow bile). Excess or deficiency would cause illness, and the physician's task was to prevent this: Nancy G. Siraisi, *Medieval and Renaissance Medicine: An Introduction to Knowledge and Practice* (Chicago/London: University of Chicago Press, 1990), 101–6.

14. Gordon suggested that, after animals, hospital patients might be used to test new forms of treatment, which, if successful, could then be tried on 'lesser brethren', a telling indication of the position of the sick poor in the great chain of being: Luke E. Demaitre, *Doctor Bernard de Gordon: Professor and Practitioner* (Toronto: Pontifical Institute of Medieval Studies, 51, 1980), 128.
15. Orme and Webster, *The English Hospital*, 35–41; Rawcliffe, 'Life, death and liturgy', 41–2. See also, for comparative purposes, Saunier, '*Le Pauvre Malade*', pp. 91–117.
16. Carleton Brown (ed.), *Religious Lyrics of the Fifteenth Century* (Oxford: Clarendon Press, 1962), 273.
17. Rawcliffe, 'Life, death and liturgy', 37.
18. Nicole Bériou, 'Les lépreux sous le regard des prédicateurs d'aprés les collections de sermons *ad status* du XIIe siècle' in *eadem* and Francois-Olivier Touati, *Voluntate Dei Leprosus: Les Lépreux entre Conversion et Exclusion aux XIIème et XIIIème Siecles* (Spoleto: Testi, Studi, Strumenti, 4, 1991), 67. De Vitry expressed a keen interest in hospital reform: see Jean Imbert, *Histoire des Hopitaux en France* (Toulouse: Privat, 1982), 48–50.
19. Dugdale, *Monasticon*, vi(2), 744–7.
20. See, for example, Andree Hayum, *The Isenheim Altarpiece: God's Medicine and the Painter's Vision* (Princeton: Princeton University Press, 1989).
21. Rudolph Arbesmann, 'The concept of *Christus Medicus* in St Augustine', *Traditio*, x (1954), 15.
22. Elizabeth Prescott, *The English Medieval Hospital 1050–1640* (London: Seaby, 1992), 16, 21; Rubin, 'Development and change', 54; Miriam Gill and Helen Howard, 'Glimpses of glory: paintings from St Mark's Hospital, Bristol', in Laurence Keen (ed.), *'Almost the Richest City': Bristol in the Middle Ages* (Leeds: British Archaeological Association Conference Transactions, xix, 1997), pp. 97–106.
23. M.B. Salu (ed.), *The Ancrene Riwle* (Exeter: Exeter Medieval English Texts and Studies, 1990), 50.
24. See, for example, Paul Binski, *Medieval Death: Ritual and Representation* (London: British Museum Press, 1996), 126–34 and plate vii.
25. Carole Rawcliffe, *The Hospitals of Medieval Norwich* (Norwich: Studies in East Anglian History, ii, 1995), 91–134.
26. Norfolk Record Office, press G, case 24, shelf A, Great Hospital (previously St Giles's hospital) general accounts, 1465–1501, account of the steward for 1500–1; Norwich Consistory Court, reg. Alpe, fos 49v–50r.
27. As, for instance, British Library, Department of Manuscripts, Sloane Ms. 468, fos 56v–59r.
28. Miri Rubin, *Charity and Community in Medieval Cambridge* (Cambridge/New York: Cambridge University Press, 1987), 300–1.

29. Rawcliffe, *Medicine and Society*, 95.
30. Prescott, *The English Medieval Hospital*, 21 and plate 31; Orme and Webster, *The English Hospital*, 120; Rawcliffe, *Medicine and Society*, plate 3. See also, Grace Goldin, *Works of Mercy: A Picture History of Hospitals* (Erin, Ontario: Boston Mills Press, 1994), 31–2.
31. British Library, Department of Manuscripts, Seals, lxiii.54, lxix.6, lxviii.17, lxxi.56; *Catalogue of Seals in the Department of Manuscripts of the British Museum. I* (London: British Museum, 1887), 422–826, *passim*.
32. Henry of Lancaster, *Le Livre de Seyntz Medicines* (Arnould ed., Oxford: Basil Blackwell, 1940), 233.
33. A.H. Thompson, *The History of the Hospital and the New College of the Annunciation of St Mary in the Newarke, Leicester* (Leicester: Leicestershire Archaeological Society, 1937), 18.
34. Norman Moore (ed.), *The Book of the Foundation of St Bartholomew's Church in London* (Oxford: Early English Text Society, clxiii, 1923) is an early-fifteenth century English translation of the twelfth century original.
35. Raymonde Foreville and Gillian Keir (eds), *The Book of St Gilbert* (Oxford: Clarendon Press, 1987), 304–9. The incompetence or venality of the medical profession was a standard *topos* in such accounts, often exaggerated to enhance the reputation of the healing saint: Ronald C. Finucane, *Miracles and Pilgrims: Popular Beliefs in Medieval England* (New York: St Martin's Press, 1995), 63–8.
36. Rawcliffe, *Hospitals of Medieval Norwich*, 97.
37. *Calendar of Inquisitions Miscellaneous, V, 1387–1393* (London: HMSO, 1963), no. 313; *Calendar of Patent Rolls, 1416–1422* (London: HMSO, 1911), 208. The jewels at Ospringe may have been set in reliquaries or have been used to embellish the relics themselves (as, for example, the alleged remains of St Elizabeth of Hungary in the hospital of that name, Vienna, depicted in Goldin, *Works of Mercy*, 30), but they may also have been held to possess healing properties in their own right: Richard Kieckhefer, *Magic in the Middle Ages* (Cambridge/New York: Cambridge University Press, 1989), 102–5.
38. Philip Larkin, *High Windows* (London: Faber and Faber, 1974), 24–6.
39. Eamon Duffy, *The Stripping of the Altars: Traditional Religion in England, c.1400–c.1590* (New Haven/London: Yale University Press, 1992), 310–15; Rubin, 'Development and change', 50.
40. Alan Kreider, *English Chantries: The Road to Dissolution* (Cambridge, Massachusetts/London: Harvard University Press, 1979), 41.
41. Rawcliffe, *Hospitals of Medieval Norwich*, 95–6.
42. *Livre de Seyntz Medicines*, 180–1. Since confession was seen as a cleansing of the soul, it is not surprising that ritual washing and perhaps even total immersion played their part in the life of the hospital: see, for instance, Bériou, 'Les lépreux', 58; Gilchrist, *Contemplation and Action*, 37–8. Recommended in the *regimen sanitatis*, bathing was also held to be physically therapeutic: Imbert, *Histoire des Hopitaux*, 29, 120, 127.
43. Palmer, 'The Church, leprosy and plague', 86.
44. J.E.B. Mayor (ed.), *The English Works of John Fisher* (Oxford: Early English Text Society, extra series, xxvii, 1876), 27.

45. Cullum, *Cremetts and Corrodies*, 8.
46. Katherine Park and John Henderson '"The first hospital among Christians": the ospedale di Santa Maria Nuova in early sixteenth century Florence', *Medical History*, xxxv (1991), 179–80; M.J. Haren (ed.), *Calendar of Entries in Papal Letters Relating to Great Britain and Ireland, XVIII, 1503–13* (Dublin: Irish Manuscripts Commission, 1989), no. 102.
47. Orme and Webster, *The English Hospital*, 60–1, 97–8, 206.
48. British Library, Department of Manuscripts, Cotton Ms. Faustina A III, fos 319v, 321r; Gervase Rosser, *Medieval Westminster 1200–1540* (Oxford: Clarendon Press, 1989), 300–10.
49. Both Robert I. Moore, *The Formation of a Persecuting Society* (Oxford: Basil Blackwell, 1987), 47–80, and Francoise Bériac, *Histoire des Lépreux au Moyen Age: Une Société d'Exclus* (Paris: Imago, 1988), *passim*, see the leper as an early victim of the Church's repressive policies. A less sweeping view, which dates a hardening of attitudes to the mid-thirteenth century may be found in Francois-Olivier Touati, 'Les léproseries aux XIIème et XIIIème siècles: lieux de conversion?', in *idem* and Bériou, *Voluntate Dei Leprosus*, 3–32.
50. Granger Ryan and Helmut Ripperger (eds), *The Golden Legend of Jacobus de Voragine* (New York: Arno Press, 1969), 685. The ambiguous, often conflicting responses to leprosy in the Middle Ages are examined in S.N. Brody, *The Disease of the Soul: Leprosy in Medieval Literature* (Ithaca/London: Cornell University Press, 1974).
51. A liminal situation reflected in the actual location of *leprosaria*: see Gilchrist, *Contemplation and Action*, 38–48.
52. Decima L. Douie and Hugh Farmer (eds), *The Life of St Hugh of Lincoln*, 2 vols (London: Nelson, 1961–2), ii, 12–14.
53. Johannes Baptist Schneyer (ed.), *Repertorium der Lateinischen Sermones des Mittelalters, IV, 1150–1350* (Münster: Aschendorff, 1972), no. 615, discussed by Beriou, 'Les lépreux', 74–8, 95–100.
54. Thomas of Monmouth, *The Life and Miracles of William of Norwich* (Jessopp and James eds, Cambridge: Cambridge University Press, 1896), 31. The layout of this hospital is described by Gilchrist, *Contemplation and Action*, 45, 47, 48.
55. From the preamble to the foundation statutes drawn up in the 1440s by the duke and duchess of Suffolk for their almshouse at Ewelme: *Historical Manuscripts Commission. Ninth Report. Part I* (London: HMSO, 1883), 217.
56. Rawcliffe, *Hospitals of Medieval Norwich*, 13–18.
57. *The English Works*, 12.
58. William Allen, *A Defense and Declaration of the Catholike Churchies Doctrine touching Purgatory* (Antwerp: John Latius, 1565), fos 132r–32v. For the idea of 'anatomical cohesion', see Marie-Christine Pouchelle, *The Body and Surgery in the Middle Ages* (Oxford: Polity Press, 1990), 114–16.
59. Edward M. Goulburn and Henry Symonds (eds), *The Life, Letters and Sermons of Bishop Herbert de Losinga*, 2 vols (Oxford: Parker, 1878), ii, 242–7.
60. *Historical Manuscripts Commission, Twelfth Report, Appendix IX* (London: HMSO, 1891), 426–7.

61. Dean Spooner, 'The Almshouse Chapel, Hadleigh', *Proceedings of the Suffolk Institute of Archaeology*, vii (1891), 379–80. For an even more exacting regime, see the regulations drawn up by the duke and duchess of Suffolk in the 1440s for their almshouse at Ewelme: *Historical Manuscripts Commission, Ninth Report, Part I*, 217–22.
62. Siegfried Wenzel (ed.), *Fasciculus Morum: A Fourteenth-Century Preacher's Handbook* (Pennsylvania/London: Pennsylvania State University Press, 1989), 541.
63. Thomas Hearne (ed.), *Thomae de Elmham Vita et Gesta Henrici Ouinti* (Oxford: *e Theatro Sheldoniano*, 1727), 338–50; *Calendar of Patent Rolls, 1446–52* (London: HMSO, 1910), 29; Public Record Office, London, C1/19/65.
64. *Calendar of Patent Rolls, 1446–52*, 475.
65. Rawcliffe, 'Life, death and liturgy', 37–51.
66. See, for instance, inventories of the hospital of St Giles, Kepier, County Durham (Public Record Office, CP40/1009, rots 581Av–581Br); of St Nicholas's hospital, Harbledown (Charles Cotton (ed.), *The Canterbury Chantries and Hospitals* (Canterbury: Kent Records, 12, supplement, 1934), 41–2); and of the two Winchester hospitals of St Mary Magdalen and St Cross (respectively, British Library, Department of Manuscripts, Harleian Ms. 328, fos 28r–30r, and Prescott, *The English Medieval Hospital*, 31–2).
67. Public Record Office, C1/965/58.

FEAR, ANXIETY AND THE PLAGUE IN EARLY MODERN ENGLAND

Andrew Wear

Introduction

Fear of plague was widespread. It led to social disruption: the destruction of trade, of local government, and violence between city and country people as the former, when they took the age-old advice to flee far, to stay away a long time, to come back slowly, fled into the countryside. Fear of contagion also led to the breakdown of religious and social norms such as the family and neighbourly duties of looking after the sick. Given the impact that fear of the plague had upon society, it would not be surprising if religious and medical writers, who were often aware of the social and political dimensions of plague (such as the controversial policy of 'shutting up', or the question of whether flight was allowable) might try to restrain fear and anxiety.

In this paper I shall discuss how medical and religious writers condemned fear of plague as socially disruptive. But I also want to argue that they gave recognition to the fear felt by many, and provided them with some means of easing it. Religious writers led their readers to the safety of Christianity and a Christian life; medical writers, who were especially aware that fear left one susceptible to plague, suggested counters to fear. More generally, there was a recognition that many sought ways to gain some sense of control and safety over their lives at a time of plague, and that they were anxious about the everyday minutiae of their lives. Such concern was tacitly accepted and advice was given on how to make daily life both spiritually and physically safe and less fearful. Fear of plague was cautioned against, but also recognised and accepted.

Meanings of Fear

My initial reaction when thinking about this paper was that to have been afraid of plague was a perfectly natural and normal reaction, so natural as to be largely unremarkable. But fear was not a neutral emotion; as Robert Burton pointed out, in ancient times it was worshipped as a God by the Lacedaemonians, and its effects brought misery and terror upon people.[1] It had social and personal effects: 'It hinders most honourable attempts, and makes their hearts ache, sad and heavy. They that live in fear are never free, resolute, secure, never merry, but in continual pain . . . ever suspicious, anxious, solicitous, they are childishly drooping without reason, without judgement, especially if some terrible object be offered'.[2] Burton made it clear that some were naturally fearful or more fearful than others, reacting with fear at some terror. Fear in European culture has also often been seen to merge with cowardice.

In the Christian tradition based on the Bible there have been a variety of meanings attached to fear, ranging from the positive to the negative and from the personal to the social. Fear has been seen positively as an expression of a sense of obedience to higher authority: 'The fear of the Lord is the beginning of wisdom', Psalm 111,10, and the next Psalm also has, 'Praise ye the Lord. Blessed is the man that feareth the Lord, that delighteth greatly in his commandments.'[3] The fear of the righteous bound them to God's law and expressed their obedience to it. But the Christian's fear, as well as being an aspect of the one-to-one relationship between the individual and God, extended to society and its powers. Rulers being ordained of God were also to be feared with the same type of fear. As the Epistle to the Romans put it, 'Let every soul be subject unto the higher powers. For there is no power but of God: the powers that be are ordained of God. Whosoever therefore resisteth the power, resisteth the ordinance of God: and they that resist shall receive to themselves damnation . . . Render therefore to all their dues; tribute to whom tribute is due; custom to whom custom; fear to whom fear; honour to whom honour.'[4] Fear, in other words, is not something that is limited to the individual who feels it, it can also have social consequences. The compiler of the concordance of the Geneva Bible noted other senses of fear. It could be a punishment of God. Amongst the curses for disobedience in the 28th chapter of Deuteronomy, which was a central text for any discussion of Christianity and plague as it referred to all the variety of plagues,[5] was the curse of fear: 'And thy life shall hang in doubt before thee; and thou shalt fear day and night, and shalt have none assurance of life.'[6] There was also 'carnall and worldly', almost cowardly, fear as when Pilate heard the Jews calling for Christ to be crucified.[7] Or, even more negatively, fear was a sin as in Revelations 21,8: 'But the fearful, and unbelieving, and the abominable and murderers and whoremongers, and sorcerers, and idolaters, and all liars, shall have their part in the lake which burneth with fire and brimstone: which is the second death.' And, there was also 'natural' fear which was allowable and to be expected, as when the disciples saw Jesus 'walking on the sea, they were troubled, saying, It is a spirit; and they cried out for fear'.[8]

Fear was not, therefore, likely to have been a simple concept for Christians in early modern England. It related to the individual psyche and to its relations with God and society, it had positive and negative connotations and also neutral ones. The cultural meaning of plague was likewise multifaceted, it was a disease suffered by the individual but also by society at large being defined as 'a popular' disease,[9] and it had both religious and medical causes and cures. It was the disease above all others which showed God's power and his punishment of sin. 'What payne or punishment', wrote Thomas Phayer in the *Treatyse of the Pestylence* (1546), 'can ther be ymagined to put us in remembraunce of oure owne wyckednesse, cause us to detest our abhominable livynges, and to call for mercye wyth lamentable hertes, more then this only plage and scurge of god commonlye called ye Pestilence. Is there any sycknesse that is halfe so violent, so furious and so horryble, as this sycknesse is?'[10]

Prayer and repentance might affect a cure, but plague was also believed to be a contagious disease in which a plague poison spread throughout the air and produced in Phayer's words 'a corrupte and venymous fever of pestilence very contagious to all that are aboute them, for the venymous ayer it selfe is not halfe so vehement to enfect as is the conversation or breath of them that are enfected alreadye'.[11] Medicine provided preventive strategies and cures, and it did so without conflicting with religion, for God could, it was argued, bring on plague by secondary, natural means, and he had provided of his mercy medicines on earth to cure diseases, moreover all had a Christian duty to look after their health.[12]

Social and Moral Consequences of Fear of Plague

Fear of plague led to actions which were perceived as unchristian and immoral. On 9 July 1665 Ralph Josselin, the minister at Earl's

Colne in Essex noted in his diary 'the plague feares [makes afraid] the London [people] they flie before it and the country feares all trade with London'.[13] The response of country people was notorious for its hostility to Londoners fleeing plague, whilst the latter were condemned as runaways, leaving obligations and responsibilities to the rest of the community, especially the poor who would have nowhere to run to. Thomas Dekker, the great literary chronicler of English plagues, wrote in *A Rod for Runawayes, Gods Tokens of his feareful Iudgments* (1625):

> to you the great Masters of Riches, who have forsaken your Habitations, left your disconsolate Mother [the City] in the midst of her sorrowes, in the height of her distresse, in the heavinesse of her lamentations. To you that are merry in your Country houses, and sit safe (as you thinke) from the Gun-shot of this Contagion, in your Orchards and pleasant Gardens; into your hands doe I deliver this sad Discourse, to put you in minde of our miseries, whom you have left behind you. [14]

Dekker wrote that flight from plague was permitted but only as long as it did not harm others:[15]

> We are warranted by Holy Scriptures to flie from Persecution, from the Plague, and from the Sword that pursues us: but you flye to save your selves, and in that flight undoe others.[16]

The poor who depended on the rich for food would starve:

> How shall the lame, and blinde, and half-starved be fed? They had wont to come to your Gates: Alas! they are barred against them . . . These must perish . . . You are fled that are to feed them, and if they famish, their complaints will flye up to heaven, and be exhibited in the open Court of God and Angels, against you . . . This is not good, it is not charitable, it is not Christian-like.[17]

Dekker's solution to the dilemma was that charity should be forced from the rich by the city authorities who would keep them in their houses, 'untill they leave such a charitable piece of Money behinde them, towards the maintenance of the poore, which else must perish in their absence'.[18] The fear of the plague and its consequences was thus opposed but it also was recognised and to some degree accepted by Dekker and by religious and medical writers who compromised between two Christian principles, the one of self-preservation and the other of charity.

Country people also came in for Dekker's condemnation. Throughout his plague writings he told stories of how the 'run-nawaies' fared at the 'unmerciful hands of the Country-hard-hearted *Hobinolls* who are ordained to be their tormentors'.[19] An inn stopped up every window and hole when a Londoner called for help as he fell ill, villagers feared to bury a Londoner despite a forty shilling reward, the sight of a Londoner led country people to stop their 'noses before he comes neare them the length of a furlong' and to turn him back with staves refusing him hospitality and offering the open fields instead.[20] Dekker wrote that 'A Spaniard is not so hateful to a Dutch-man as a Londoner to a Country-man'.[21] Londoners, it was believed, brought infection with them into countryside: 'They [country people] are verily perswaded, no Plagues, no Botches, Blaynes, nor Carbuncles can sticke upon any of their innocent bodies, unlesse a Londoner (be he never so fine, never so perfumed, never so sound) brings it to them.'[22] The result was suspicion, violence, lack of charity, and a denial of the most fundamental obligation of the living to the dead, burial.

From the time of Boccaccio onwards writers had chronicled how basic social and religious norms were broken and ignored at a time of plague. Any discussion of fear and anxiety at such a time has to recognise the very simple point that they caused such responses. Certainly Dekker was aware of this:

> You see therefore how dreadfull a fellow Death is, making fooles even of wisemen, and cowards of the most valiant; yea in such a base slavery hath it bound mens sences, that they have no power to looke higher than their owne roofes, but seeme by their turkish and barbarous actions to believe that there is no felicitie after this life, and that (like beasts) their soules shall perish with their bodies.[23]

The sense of brute unreason could be found, in Dekker's view, in the lessening of humanity fear brings, such as when objects of social exchange were rejected out of an irrational fear of contagion. Dekker poked fun at how some, 'receiving mony here, have tyed it in a bag at the end of their barge, and so trailed it through the Thames, lest plague sores sticking upon shillings, they should be naild up for counterfets when they were brought home'.[24]

The apothecary William Boghurst wrote in his *Loimographia. An Account of the Great Plague of London in the Year 1665* (written in 1666 but not published until 1894) that the 'vain fear' of the people 'is soe great and sinful that it stops and shuts up all Counsel, Reason, Charity, Truth etc. and makes people fall upon such vain and ridiculous courses'.

> First, what care was taken about letters. Some would sift them in a sieve, some wash them first in water and then dry them at the fire, some air them at the top of a house, or an hedge, or a pole, two or three days before they opened them. Some would lay them between two cold stones 2 or 3 days, some set them before the fire like toast, some would not receive them but on a long pole. Concerning money, some would take none . . . Some would needs take it in water and wash it. But for clothes, they were so gravelled that they would not once come near them if they came from London, especially linnen and woollen . . . Some have stopped the key-holes of their doors, and avoided the occassions, of action and communication with all people and creatures . . .[25]

Such fears were widespread, John Allin, who had been ejected as minister of Rye in 1662, wrote in 1665 to Phillip Fryth 'I am afrayd to write to Mr Miller [of the death of Miller's brother-in-law], least hee should bee afrayd of my letter',[26] and in a letter to another former parishioner in Rye, Samuel Jeake: 'It is some refreshing to mee to thinke you are yet willing to receive a line from mee. It was an affliction to mee that I knew not to whom I might send a letter with acceptance (except Mr Fryth onely). I am afrayd that some of my friends there are this day too much afrayd where no feare need to bee, for were my penn infectious my hand would soon let it drop.'[27]

What Dekker and others did when recounting such 'unreasonable' fears was to link them to uncharitable actions, so that the unreasoning fears of contagion (in the medical sense) and uncharitable actions (in the religious sense) seem to be all one aspect of a barbarous unreason in the face of plague. Religious writers employed the same technique as Dekker. Andreas Osiander's sermon on *How and Whither a Christen Man Ought to Flye the Horrible Plage of the Pestilence* (1537) addressed a central problem for Christians. Fear and flight brought on moral and social disorder, caused by the universal denial of the duty of charity to others:

'howe unwysely and unchristenly they do, that out of inordinate feare, of thys plage leave theyr callynge and office, maliciously wythdrawyng the love, helpe and faythfulnesse, which they (out of gods commaundement) are bounde to shewe unto theyr neghbours, and so do synne grevously agaynste the commaundement of God'.[28] Osiander discussed the fear of plague, calling it childish and making it appear ridiculous by describing how people were afraid of ordinary household goods and stating that this was the same type of fear that made them avoid other people. He wrote that:

> men maye heare on every syde, that some do shone and flye not onely the syck, but also the whole: Yet (that yet more foolyshe is) even the platters and candlestyckes which come out of straunge houses, as though death dyd surely styck therein. And (out of such fonde chyldyshe feare) it commeth, that not onely some syck folkes be suffred to dye away wyth out all kepynge, helpe and comforte, but the wemen also greate wyth chylde be forsaken in theyr nede . . . Yet a man maye heare also, that the chyldren forsake theyr fathers and mothers. . . .[29]

Religious writers not only decried 'irrational' fears and unchristian actions. They often created an 'us and them' division, for plague was sent to punish the ungodly, and the godly might be preserved or, because of the mysterious working of God's will, die alongside the sinners.[30] For instance, the puritan writer Henry Holland in his *Spiritual Preservatives Against the Pestilence* (1593) wrote that there were those who had an animal-like fear of the plague or had no fear at all, whilst others, 'such as feare the Lord', had a proper fear.[31] The former were the sinful majority whilst the latter were his readers who might share the sense of being God's chosen. Christians were supposed to fear God at all times, and such fear showed at a time of plague when God sent plague as a punishment, and as a means to repentance. But it was necessary to be especially careful to distinguish Christian fear both from unchristian fear and from the impious lack of fear. Holland wrote:

> Manie have a brutish feare as it seemeth, because of the losse of our long peace and prosperitie; but some again on the other side, are so foole-hardie, that they feare nothing, and thinke these loving warnings of the Lord [the initial few deaths] to be but ordinarie, and therefore not to be feared.[32]

The consequences of an improper fear or of no fear at all were both spiritual and secular, a refusal to repent and disobedience of plague orders: 'and neither regard as Christians anie amendment of life, nor as good Citizens good and wise orders appointed for the preservation of this honorable Citie, and for the health of the Lordes people'.[33] Not all religious writers accepted the secular regulations for plague: the policy of 'shutting up', for instance, produced amongst some strong disagreement. However, at a time when there was a belief that the laws of God and of nations should be equivalent it was easy to portray those who did not have the proper fear of the Lord as breaking both religious and secular norms. Those who had unreasonable fear or brutish lack of fear, lay outside the bounds of religion and of lawfully regulated society.

In his treatise Holland offered to his 'christian Reader some comfortable spiritual helpes'.[34] What were such 'helpes' that might allay unreasonable fears? Religious writers were all agreed that as the first cause of plague was God, He could also take plague away or protect the individual. The medicine of repentance could cure the disease of the body, or at least the disease of the soul, together with the associated fear. A Christian life in the face of plague also provided protection from illness. In any case, the protection of God was offered to all Christians, especially in the words of Psalm 91 whose verses Holland used as the framework for his treatise:

2. I will say of the Lord, He is my refuge and my fortress: my God; in him will I trust.
3. Surely he shall deliver thee from the snare of the fowler and from the noisome pestilence . . .
5. Thou shalt not be afraid for the terror by night; nor for the arrow that flieth by day.
6. Nor for the pestilence that walketh in darkness; nor for the destruction that wasteth at noonday.

A complete acceptance of God stilled fears of the plague. I.D. 'the preacher of Gods word' and author of *Salomon's Pest-House Or Towre Royall* (1630) assured his readers that 'this place [God] is better than the earthly, where the fearefull sonnes of men dwell which feare the apparel, houshold-stuffe, yea and thy letters'.[35]

Nothing is clear-cut in theology, however. William Gouge, the noted London puritan minister, asked 'how is then that the righteous as well as the unrighteous die of the Plague?' Part of his answer was that the 91st Psalm could not be used to argue that God especially protected the faithful from plague. His protection was no greater than what he offered against the dangers of war or of wild beasts. 'Experience,' he wrote, 'giveth evidence that many that have manifested true outward fruits of a sound faith, upright conscience, honest heart, and entire repentance, have died of the Plague.' Rather than call them 'no true believers', Gouge concluded instead that the godly died from plague, but unlike the ungodly, they went to heaven.[36] Not all agreed, therefore, that God was a complete 'refuge' and 'fortress' to the faithful in time of plague. They had to help themselves by the medicines of prayer and repentance as well as by putting their faith in God.

What is striking about the religious response to plague, whether from lay people like Dekker or from clergymen, is that 'irrational' fear, the fear that leads to unchristian and antisocial acts, is condemned but that Christian fear is recognised, and that religious writers tried to provide means of reassurance. Did the same type of discourse appear also in medical writings? Condemnation and recognition of fear were certainly present, as were some means of coping with it. What is also striking is that fear was seen as pathological, it could bring on plague.

Medicine and fear of the plague

When Osiander tried to convince his readers not to yield to 'naked feares' he repeated a commonly held view that 'experience shewe also that they which be so sore afrayed, do communly miscarry [catch plague]'.[37] Over a century later Pepys also seems to have held a similar view when he recounted how Sir Anthony Browne's brother had been put 'into a fright had almost cost him his life' when he came across a maid servant with the plague who looked 'very ill, and in a sick dress and stunk mightily as she was being conveyed in a coach to a pest-house'.[38] Pepys also reported his own 'extraordinary fear' when he learnt that his servant Will was 'ill of the head-ake'.[39] Medical opinion held that fear and melancholy could allow a person to catch plague. Controlling one's fear was, therefore, a means of avoiding plague (though as fear was not generally held to be the only way of getting plague, a lack of fear did not provide immunity).

Pepys worried about becoming melancholic. On the 14th of September 1665 he noted that he had 'matter for as much content on one hand and melancholy on another as any day in all my life'.

His money and plate were 'all safe in London' and the plague deaths had decreased by over 500,[40] on the other hand within the City walls plague had increased, 'and likely to continue so' and he added, 'is close to our house there'. He recorded a long list of happenings that brought plague close and which he feared could induce melancholy. Among them were:

> my meeting dead corps's of the plague, carried to be buried close to me at noonday through the City in Fenchurch-Street – to see a person sick of the [plague] sores carried close by me by Grace-church in a hackney-coach – to hear that poor Payne my water [man] hath buried a child and is dying himself . . . doth put me in great apprehensions of melancholy, and with good reason. But I put off the thoughts of sadness as much as I can; and the rather to keep my wife in good heart, and family also.[41]

Melancholy was a mental condition, which although almost natural to half the world in Robert Burton's view, was in Pepys' and many other's opinion best avoided. It affected the imagination, and Burton summarised medical opinion when he recounted cases where the 'force of the imagination'[42] made people ill and, 'Sometimes,' he added, 'death by itself is caused by force of phantasy. I have heard of one that, coming by chance in company of him that was thought to be sick of the plague (which was not so), fell down suddenly dead.'[43] Fear, Burton believed, was closely associated with the power of the imagination for it 'makes our imagination conceive what it list . . . and tyrannizeth over our phantasy more than all other affections'.[44] The 'fantasy' of illness could actually produce in the body the physical disease itself, this reflected the very close connection between the body and the mind in early modern medicine. Burton wrote that the power of the imagination 'works not in sick and melancholy men only, but even most forcibly sometimes in such as are sound: it makes them suddenly sick, and alters their temperature [the humoral constitution of the body, its physical reality in medical eyes], in an instant . . . it will produce real effects'.[45] As we will see, Van Helmont developed this view so that fear became a major cause of plague. Most medical writers on plague, however, did not write that fear created plague but that it allowed it to enter the body. In their advice on how to prevent plague based on the 'six non naturals' of regimen which included mental states (the 'passions', 'affections' or 'accidents' of the mind),[46] they recommended that anything that produced sadness, depression or anger was to be avoided. Thomas Phayer wrote:

> Ye must beware of al thynges that shulde make you to be pensive, heavye, thoughtfull, angrye or melancholycke, for all such thynges are ynough to enfecte a man alone.
> Passe the tyme ioyfullye in good thinges honest and decent . . .[47]

Fear and anxiety were especially dangerous in medical eyes, although one would think it was a natural reaction of a population faced with an event, as the physician William Bullein put it, 'whereof thousands have and shall die. A pitifull case how it commeth among people sodainly'.[48] But physicians warned of its physiological effects upon the body which could let the plague venom enter. Bullein, in his *Dialogue against the Fever Pestilence* (1578, 1st ed. 1564), through 'Medicus' advised 'no anger or perturbations of the mynd, especially the passion called feare, for that doth drawe the spirites and blood inwards to the hart, and is a very meane to receive this plague'.[49] Other aspects of the six non-naturals had similar effects. Bullein, after warning against fear, also ordered: 'neither use actes venerous, nor bathyng, either with Fume, stove or warme water (for this cause) – they all doe open the pores of the bodie' [and allow the plague poison to enter].[50] The injunction not to be fearful was usually part of the long list of positive and negative commands about regimen and lifestyle aimed at the individual in a time of plague. However, the plague was not simply a physical disease. It had strong religious and moral connotations. God and sin were implicated in its causation, creating a complex set of associations which coloured advice on ways of living. The avoidance of fear and the injunction to be of a merry heart were not only part of a healthy life they were also an aspect of the pure uncontaminated life.

Stephen Bradwell in his *Physick for the Sicknesse, Commonly Called the Plague* (1636) gave an extended account of fear during plague which set out a number of its dimensions. At a general level fear, wrote Bradwell, produced dire effects upon the body and especially upon the heart and brain, two of the principal organs of the body. As with other mental states, the medicine of the time described fear in organic, physical, terms and this, no doubt, made it easy to accept that fear could be a reason why a person might catch plague. Bradwell wrote, using the military metaphors often employed to describe the invasion of plague:

> Of all Passions, Feare is the most pestilently pernicious . . . Feare enforces the vitall Spirits to retire inward to the heart: By which retyring they leave the outward parts infirme, as appeares plainly by the palenesse and trembling of one in great feare. So that the walls being forsaken (which are continually besieged by the outward ayre) in comes the enemy boldly; the best spirits that should expelled them having cowardly sounded retreat: In which with-drawing, they draw in with them such evill vapours as hang about the outward pores; even as the Sunne drawes toward it the vapours of the Earth. And hence it [is] that Feare brings Infection sooner than any other occassion.[51]

The patient's fear led to the 'cowardice' of his or her body's defenders. The metaphorical language comes close to condemning the patient for being afraid; the vital spirits, which classical and early modern medicine stated were produced in the heart and conveyed life and motion to the body through the arteries, were seen as simultaneously part of the *persona* and separate from it. Such ambiguity reflects the intimate, yet separable, relationship between the physical parts of the body and its moral character at this time, which made it easy to attribute moral characteristics to the former.

Bradwell offered medical advice on what to do about fear. Partly it was up to the individual. As with other aspects of regimen such as diet, exercise, sobriety, etc., the individual had to look after him or herself. Bradwell wrote, 'This therefore, and all other *Passions* must (by a wise watching over our selves) be beaten off whensoever they but offer to set upon us.'[52] In this case, perhaps because of the close association of plague with sin and God's vengeance, Bradwell pointed his readers in the direction of the medicine of religion by using the traditional distinction between the soul and the body.

> But these are diseases of the Soule, whose Physicians are Divines. They must Purge out the Love of this World, and the distrust of GODS Providence, minister the Cordials of Faith, Hope, Patience, and Contentednesse; and Ordaine the strict Dyet of Holy Exercises.[53]

At the mundane, bodily level Bradwell wrote that the physicians of the body could apply superficial remedies to the soul:

> Wee that are Physicians to the Body are but Chyrurgians to the Soule; we can but talke of Topicall remedies; as to apply Mirth, Musicke, delightfull businesse, good Company, and lawfull Recreations; such as may take up all time from carefull thoughts and passionate affections.[54]

The tradition of extended medical metaphors used in a religious context – expressions like 'Purge out the Love of this World' – allowed Bradwell to express the religious and medical dimensions involved in the prevention of fear, and indeed the ready availability of this language and the powerful ideology that lay behind it may have led him to the view that ultimately fear was a matter that related to the soul and to its remedy, religion. Moreover, the general context into which Bradwell's discussion of fear of plague was placed was that of regimen. And advice on regimen often had a moral element. Bradwell's warning about fear was preceded by a strong condemnation of overeating and overdrinking in times of plague, which combined medical, religious and moral elements.[55]

The belief that fear could bring on plague lasted through from before the sixteenth century to Pepys' time.[56] Its longevity strengthens the case that it was part of the nexus of beliefs that were deployed to preserve the social and moral order, which was continually perceived to be under threat at a time of plague. However, unlike the discussions of the consequences of fear upon family and neighbourly duties, the case for this is largely based on inference. Many of the medical admonitions against fear were explicitly aimed at the individual and his or her welfare rather than at the good of society. Nevertheless, anything that helped prevent plague and put the individual into good order, as the prohibition of fear did, would appear to preserve social order. The longevity of the belief might also have something to do with the fact that radical as well as conservative medical writers supported it. Paracelsus thought that plague could be brought on by the imagination,[57] and Van Helmont gave great prominence to the belief that fear caused plague, when in his *Tumulus Pestis*, translated as *The Plague-Grave* in 1662, he argued that 'the plague is bred in us by an Image of terrour'.[58] He wrote that there were two types of plague, one from infected air, and the deadlier, truer, from fear: 'For Plagues which are bred onely through terrour, are more swift and more terrible than those which proceed from an infected air: for this perhaps strikes many to the heart.'[59] The imagination could produce 'in us a new generation, or transmutation of one thing into another'. The process reads somewhat like our modern ideas on mass hysteria, but Helmont was arguing that *all* cases of the worst type of plague were caused by fear, whereas the modern concepts of conversion hysteria or hypochondria are that a third party should be able to differentiate between the real case of the disease and the imagined one. Helmont, on the other hand, argued that the *archaeus*, the controller of the body's processes, turned the image of the disease into reality:

> the poyson of the Pest is made not only from an apprehension, and conceit of terrible effects, but because there concurreth together with those, a certain unseperable belief whereby any one being affrighted, and sore afraid in fearing doth imagine and slenderly believe that he hath now contracted something of the pestilential poyson: From whence (but not before) the Image of the Plague being conceived by this kind of terrour, becomes operative and fruitful. For that terrour with a credulous suspition applyeth the Soul thus affrighted, unto the Archaeus, that it may cloath this Archaeus with the Image of the conceived Terrour.[60]

The poison of the plague was both a physical and a spiritual poison. It was the 'poyson of terrour', but it also came from the physical objects that were commonly suspected of carrying plague: 'Yet any subject whatsoever, whether it shall be air, a garment, or any other more solid body (although ignorant of dread) which may be seasoned with an odour, may in like manner be the subject on which the products of a dreadful imagination may be imprinted.'[61] Helmont thus made fear *the* causal agent of plague, but he also integrated this idea with popular and 'learned' (that is orthodox, university-based Galenic) conceptions of the aetiology of plague. He kept to the general belief in contagion from the environment and from people, and he shared, for instance, in the common suspicion of southern air.[62] It was easy, therefore, for Helmontian ideas to be taken up to a greater or lesser extent by a range of medical writers of widely differing persuasions.

In England George Thomson, the radical Helmontian physician who wanted to set up a Society of Chemical Physicians in opposition to the Galenic London College of Physicians, had stayed on in

London during the 1665 plague. When he wrote up his experiences he full-heartedly took up Helmont's ideas. He suggested fear as the main cause of plague, and when, famously, he carried out a dissection on a plague body following Helmont's example, he described graphically how the poison atoms of plague entered his own body from that of the corpse, and once inside frightened the *archeus* which then created 'the perfect Idea and Image of this sickness'.[63] However, except for committed Helmontians like Thomson, fear remained one out of the many possible causes of why a particular individual might catch plague once a plague epidemic had begun.

William Boghurst, who like Thomson, stayed at his post during the plague of 1665, had read Helmont as well as Galenic authors, but he supported the new 'Epicurean or Corpuscular Philosophy',[64] and referred approvingly to 'that illustrious Virtuoso Mr Boyle'.[65] Despite his belief in the 'new science', like many other medical writers who were constructing a new 'medicine' in the light of novel chemical, mechanical and corpuscular theories, he kept to much that had been included in traditional medicine. One minor aspect was the belief that fear could bring on plague. Although sceptical, in an enlightened manner, of many previous popular and medical beliefs that had been thought to be precipitating causes of plague,[66] Boghurst did not doubt that fear in a plague outbreak was a potent cause of plague. It is as if this particular belief transcended, or bridged, the huge philosophical divide noted by historians between the sixteenth century and the later seventeenth century. This is understandable as the avoidance of fear was part of regimen, and traditional beliefs about regimen remained an essential aspect of medicine well into the eighteenth century. Moreover, plague was still perceived to be transmitted by a plague poison, albeit now composed of corpuscles, which entered through the pores and attacked the heart, a process which fear could bring about and hasten. The belief about fear was too well integrated in long-lasting medical structures and in theories about plague (and in social interests?) for it to be subjected to sceptical criticism as a 'superstitious' popular belief. It may also be that Helmont's imprimatur gave it a new currency, and when medical writers wrote that they had observed the effects of fear, they brought a traditional belief into the world of experience, showing it to be an observed fact, and hence, according to Baconian epistemology, true.

Boghurst mentioned the fear of plague in a number of different contexts and his treatise allows us to pick out different aspects of the issue. A question to ask about the medicalisation of fear is whether the patient's fear was used by medical practitioners as a way of blaming the patient and excusing their own failure. To some extent this was the case. Boghurst wrote that a 'naughty heart' together with fear could undo all medicine's efforts:

> Those that tooke never so good Antidotes and preservations and followed wholesome rules, if they had a naughty heart, it betrayed and frustrated all that which was done. Many falling into the disease and dying of it, especially those that were much dejected and afrayd to dye, dyed the sooner.[67]

Although blaming the patient for medicine's failure was a common trope at the time, especially in discussions of regimen, this is an extreme version of it. The patient has taken all the right medicines and obeyed all the rules of regimen, yet his or her character has let them down. Normally, it was the disobedience of the patient in taking prescribed medicines or in keeping to a recommended diet that explained medical failure.[68]

Did Boghurst consider fear treatable? He observed during the epidemic that 'Cheerfulness and courage of heart and spirit did chiefly uphold some in this disease, verifying Solomon's saying viz., a merry heart doth good like a medicine, whereas melancholy and dejection of spirits was the overthrow of many.'[69] However, some aspects of fear seemed incurable. Boghurst listed 'Melancholy, Frightfull Dreames'[70] as 'evil signes in the plague'[71] along with many other obdurate subjective and physical signs such as 'great thirst', 'sleeping with the eyes half open, half shutt', and 'greenish black' urine.[72] He wrote that:

> some would dream they were among Graves and Tombs in Churchyards, others that they tumbled down from some high place and fell amongst coffins, others cryed out in their dreams that they were all on fire, and these were harbingers of destruction, for they commonly proved more true than they did at other tymes in health.[73]

The inner life of the sleeping mind seemed impervious to interference, especially when it was a by-product of plague. But in early modern medicine symptoms were often synonymous with the causes of disease. So, though Boghurst noted that sighing was an involuntary effect of plague, he treated it by altering the subjective state of the patient, and so cured her not only of the sighing but also of the plague:

> But I had one patient at Westminster, a maid, that promised very ill at the beginning with a very bad countenance and frequent sighing, but I bid her instead of sighing, humm it up, and ordered her friends that they should talk to her and make her as chearefull and merry as they could, and alwaies chid her for sighing, so with two vesicatoryes and 2 or 3 cordialls she got over all and lived, which scarce one in ten did being so afflicted.[74]

More generally, Boghurst advised his readers not to listen to 'every idle tale they hear, which fills their heads with vain fears disturbing their apprehension and doeing mischief'.[75] He warned against a sense of collective fear fuelled by 'lying stories'. Boghurst also gave general advice on how to avoid melancholy. He did so because, like modern demographers, he had noted that whole families died from plague, and he believed that 'one great cause why this disease sweeps away whole families is because they grow Melancholy and discontented, one friend for another, especially being shut up brings a sad cloud upon their spirits'. The 'common and effectual' means that he advised 'when any one perceives himself very fearfull and Melancholy' were 'Company, Wine and Musick and any other lawfull diversions' and a 'Stoickal life'.[76] The classical medical doctrine of opposites cure opposites could not be applied exactly, for there was something about plague that required sober behaviour, so if the fear was great, the merrymaking could not be equally great. Boghurst wrote:

> As for musick, some may think it very unreasonable at such a tyme, which requires a contrary temper of spirit, and consequently unlawful, but I think noe man need bee soe nice and narrow spirited, as to question the lawfulness of private solace and Chamber Musick, especially when it is used for such a good purpose, and sure noe man thinks that I mean your wild wanton hackney fiddlers, whose employment is altogether to be condemned at such a tyme.[77]

Boghurst acknowledged that there were times when the fact of fear had to be accepted. His perception that fear was really dangerous in a plague time was a major consideration when he gave advice on whether to flee from plague and who it was who should flee,

Boghurst wrote 'But to speak a little more of flight, I think those who are very fearfull ought especially to fly, and that quickly.'[78] However, the needs of the fearful could not be allowed to destroy the family unit, or the bonds of obligation between masters and servants. As with much advice on how to act during plague there was a dialectic between medical and moral imperatives, and Boghurst took care to add: 'but for parts of families to fly is altogether to bee condemned; – for a man to fly, and leave his wife, children, and servants, or the wife to doe the like, or the Master and Mistress and children to fly and leave the servants or any part. Either let all stay or all go, or else but only children.'[79] Fear of plague was viewed in medical or moral terms and often in both.

Boghurst also gave precise advice on how to go into an infected area, if a person should make the attempt depended in Boghurst's opinion on whether they were fearful. He wrote that those that were not afraid could stay in an infected town two hours and half an hour in an infected house at the most. Visiting the dying required preventive medicines, such as drinking half a pint of sack, holding a clove of garlic or nutmeg in the mouth. But, he added, 'if you bee very fearfull 'tis best to stay away and save your life though you lose a legacy'.[80]

The very precise description of how to take precautions before visiting the sick was part of the larger enterprise undertaken by medical writers of providing detailed instructions on how to lead one's life and how to avoid the contagion of the plague. What windows to leave open, how to walk in the streets, when the bed linen of a plague victim became safe or could be made safe were part of the vast catalogue of advice and precautionary admonitions offered by medical writers to those fearful of the plague. Like religious writers, they offered advice, preservatives and medicines that promised protection from plague and assuaged the general sense of fear, but like religious writers they also singled out fear and condemned it as well as recognising its existence. Such rejection and acceptance may make us read controlling impulses into the religious and medical accounts, prohibitions, and exhortations concerning the fear of plague. Control of fear when the order of society was threatened would be expected. Plague was the one disease that produced government regulation in matters of public health at a time when there was little if any regulation in health matters. But not all writers expressed the ideological needs of established society, the materials about fear could be used for critical and subversive purposes as by Nicholas Culpeper in his brief *A Treatise of the Pestilence* (1655). Culpeper believed that fear could cause plague: 'in the first place let such as would avoid this Disease, avoid the fear of it, for fear changeth the blood into the nature of the thing feared, the imagination ruling the spirits natural as is manifest in Womens conception'.[81] His theory was not the standard Galenic one, but one drawn from Arabic, alchemical and Helmontian traditions, and, as befitted a radical in medicine and religion, he condemned the consequences of fear: lack of charity on the part of individuals, but also on the part of the authorities:

> A word or two now to satisfie men concerning the common fear of Infection, which makes many rich men, which might and ought to maintain poor visited people; yea many Physicians, whose duty it is to administer Physick to them, flee away, so that in a time of great Infection, you may hear more cry out for lack of Bread and means necessary, then for Anguish of the Disease.
> Hence also came that unnatural and inhumane custom of shutting up of Houses that once Visited, thereby sadding and dejecting their Spirits and thereby making way for the disease.[82]

'J.V.' whose *Golgotha* (1665) argued 'against the Cruel Advice and Practice of Shutting-Up'[83] presented a picture of the healthy shut up in a hermetically sealed house,[84] filled with 'horror of heart' and bowed 'under soul sinkings', while they were in 'this dismal likeness of Hell', they 'receive the impression of a thousand fearful thoughts of the long night they have to reckon before release'. 'Hence,' he concluded, 'are a thousand thoughts created to such, swoondings, faintings, fears (fitting for infection naturally) as have occassioned some already to lose their precious lives'.[85] The same point was made from the establishment side by Nathaniel Hodges who organised the College of Physicians' and the City of London's provision of medical help during the plague of 1665. He believed in general that fear rendered people's 'Constitutions less able to resist the Contagion', and that they could die by the force of their imagination.[86] On the specific question of the advisability of replacing the practice of shutting up by building pesthouses outside of the city, he wrote, 'the Consternation of those who were thus separated from all Society, unless with the infected, was inexpressible; and the dismal Apprehensions it laid them under, made them an easier

Prey to the devouring Enemy'.[87] Opinion of all sorts was moving against the policy of shutting up, and in 1666 it was officially changed by the Privy Council.

Shutting up was the specific issue where the belief or knowledge that fear could cause plague was employed as part of a socio-political argument. The more general social dimension to fear was where, as we have seen, fear, taken in a looser and less medical sense, was associated with uncharitable and unchristian actions. But to focus only on the social aspects of fear is to take too one-dimensional a view.

Fear, as I pointed out at the beginning, is a personal emotion, though it can have social and religious meanings. What is striking about the early modern discussion of fear is that there was an acceptance that some were constitutionally more liable to it and that there was space for natural fear. In the long night of terror inside a shut up house it was natural to be afraid. Burton added that 'especially in the dark', did fear tyrannize 'over our phantasy'.[88] Plague itself as Psalm 91 stated was 'the pestilence that walketh in darkness', 'the terror by night'. As Samson Price put it, in a sermon preached on 29 January, 1626, plague 'is the terrour by night, breeding many terrours and feares in the night; the night being a solitary time, solitarines increaseth feares . . . a time of feare in regard to the weakness of the imagination or of terrible dreames, or sudden affrights: a time terrible to travelers, where the least noise amazeth them'.[89] The plague was like the night, a time when it was natural to be afraid.

There was also an acceptance that some people were more fearful than others. George Thomson wrote that the brave escaped from plague, 'If the phantasie of man and the *Archeus* be magnanimous, stout, free from any Idea, vain conceit of fear and terrour, having a strong and valiant perswasion that neither can suffer injury in this kind: then the contagious effluviums cannot take place in such a body to offend it.'[90] But a man could have an imagination 'strongly fortified against the Infection' and yet be let down by a weak Archeus.[91] In any case, he wrote, most people were afraid, for 'few' were 'exempted from some pusillamity and distrustful thoughts either of the mind or the *Archeus*'.[92]

Fear was to be expected, and the majority in a plague time were fearful. It was a natural reaction, and also more natural for some than for others. Yet there were also warnings about the moral consequences and medical dangers of fear. The idea of balance, of moderation so prevalent in European culture in medicine and morality, is probably the key to understanding what seem to be conflicting messages about the meaning of fear of the plague. To stress one aspect (from the personal, natural, moral, social, medical) is to distort the early modern sense of the fear of plague and to hide the resolution of the problem by medical, religious and moral commentators, which lay in moderation, a rejection of extreme fear and of its opposite, a lack of fear, and a recognition and acceptance of moderated, restrained, fear. The verses of George Wither on *The History of Pestilence*, which I hesitate to subject anyone to, can bring this paper to a close by illustrating the multifaceted aspects of fear of the plague and their resolution in moderation. Wither asserted that fear could cause plague:

> So some there bee soe fearefull that their Feare
> Corrupts the blood where noe Infections were
> Begettes that Plague within them, which they shunn,
> And makes it followe, when they from it runn[93]

But he recognised the value of the 'Christian . . . feare of them':

> That are with holy Dread, imploy'd about
> Such means, as worketh true Salvation out;[94]

Nor did he condemn moderate, prudent and natural fears which distinguish us from creatures with brutish unreason:

> ffor while our Feare preserves a moderation,
> It is a very necessarie Passion.
> And stands for Sentinell, to bid us arme.
> When any Foe doth seeme to menace harme.
> Nor doe I checke that naturall Feare . . .
> . . . ffor want of that is mere Stupiditie,
> And, such cann neither feele a miserie,
> Nor tast Gods Mercyes, with more profit than
> The brutishe Creatures (wanting Reason) cann[95]

Wither accepted that some by nature appeared more fearful than others, but as long as their resolution held, despite their appearance, he would not, he declared, call them cowards. Wither wanted a middle way. Fear was recognised and accepted so long as it did not prevent 'lawfull action'. The admirable person was the one who knowing danger and fear persevered in the right actions. There was a recognition of the personal dimension of fear but not at the expense of moral and social expectations. Although, Wither wrote, he has 'a quaking *Arme*' yet he 'Walkes with a stedfast minde':[96]

Wither went on to emphasise the need for balance by repeating the point that a lack of fear was foolhardy or a 'brutishe fearlesnes'[97] that was essentially unchristian and blind to God's judgements. He may not have been much of a poet, but in relation to the fear of the plague Wither did a good job as a cultural reporter.

In the end, whether one interprets the religious and medical construction of fear at a time of plague as an example of morality and medical theory being put into the service of social interests and even being created by them is a matter of personal judgement. The evidence, however, is not strong enough to prove the case. What is apparent is that the advice that was offered was humane in accepting the reality of fear, that society as represented by religious and medical writers shied away from uncontrolled raw fear, and they sought to bring it within 'rational' discourses.

I would like to thank Dr Natsu Hattori for her helpful comments.

NOTES

1. Robert Burton, *The Anatomy of Melancholy*, ed. Floyd Dell and Paul Jordan-Smith (New York: Tudor Publishing Co., 1948), 227–8. On the historical aspects of fear see Jean Delumeau, *La Peur en Occident (xive–xviiie Siècles)* (Paris: Fayard, 1978) especially 98–142 on the typologies of fear during plague; and *La Péché et la Peur* (Paris: Fayard, 1983).
2. Burton, *Anatomy of Melancholy*, 227.
3. Psalm 112.1.
4. Romans 13 .1,2,7.
5. Deuteronomy 28.59.
6. Deuteronomy 28.66.
7. St John 19.6 'When Pilate therefore heard that saying, he was the more afraid.'
8. Matthew, 14.26.
9. See for instance Stephen Bradwell, *Physick for the Sicknesse, Commonly Called the Plague* (London: B. Fisher, 1636), 1; Nathaniel Hodges, *Loimologia, Or an Historical Account of the Plague in London in 1665*, translated by John Quincy (London: E. Bell and J. Osborn, 1720), 29.
10. Thomas Phayer, *Treatyse of the Pestylence* in the *Regiment of Lyfe* (London: W. Tilletson, 1546), sig. L3^r.
11. Ibid, sig. M3^r.
12. See Ibid., L4^r; Bradwell, *Physick for the Sicknesse*, 1–3; James Manning, *A New Booke. Intituled I am for You All, Complexions Castle* (Cambridge: J. Legat, 1604), 4–6; the crucial Biblical text was Ecclesiasticus 38.4: 'The Lord hath created medicines out of the earth.'

13. A. Macfarlane (ed.), *The Diary of Ralph Josselin 1616–1683* (Oxford: Oxford University Press for the British Academy, 1976), 519.
14. Thomas Dekker, *A Rod for Run-awayes* in F.P. Wilson (ed.), *The Plague Pamphlets of Thomas Dekker* Oxford: Clarendon Press, 1925), 145. Page references to other plague works of Dekker will be to Wilson's edition.
15. On the question of whether it was Christian to flee plague, and the differences between Lutheran and Calvinist writers see O. Grell, 'Conflicting Duties: Plague and the Obligations of Early Modern Physicians Towards Patients and Commonwealth in England and the Netherlands' in A. Wear *et al.* (eds), *Doctors and Ethics: the Earlier Historical Setting of Professional Ethics* (Amsterdam: Rodopi, 1993), 131–52.
16. Dekker, *Rod for Run-awayes*, 148.
17. Ibid., 148–9.
18. Ibid., 149.
19. T. Dekker *The Wonderfull Yeare* (1603), 32.
20. Ibid., 41–2, 56–7, *Rod for Run-awayes*, 154.
21. Dekker, *Rod for Run-awayes*, 152.
22. Ibid., 154.
23. Dekker, *Wonderfull Yeare*, 59.
24. Ibid., 59.
25. William Boghurst, *Loimographia An Account of the Great Plague of London in the Year 1665*, ed. J. F. Payne (London: Shaw and Sons, 1894), 53–4.
26. William Durant Cooper, 'Notices of the Last Great Plague, 1665–6, from the Letters of John Allin to Philip Fryth and Samuel Jeake', *Archaelogia*, xxxviii (1857), 1–22, p. 8.
27. Ibid., 15.
28. Andreas Osiander, *How and Whither a Christen Man Ought to Flye the Horrible Plage of the Pestilence* (London: I. Gough, 1537), sig. A5^{v}.
29. Ibid., sig. A5^{v}.
30. Ibid., sig. C4^{r}.
31. Henry Holland, *Spiritual Preservatives Against the Pestilence* (London: R. Thomas, 1593), Epistle to the Reader, sig. A8^{r}.
32. Ibid., Epistle Dedicatory, sig. A5^{r}.
33. Ibid., sig. A5^{r}.
34. Ibid., Epistle to the Reader, sig. A8^{r}.
35. I.D., *Salomon's Pest-House or Towre-Royall* (London: T. Harper, 1630), 23, see p. 3 on the meaning of 'place'.
36. William Gouge, *God's Three Arrowes: Plague. Famine, Sword* (London: E. Brewster, 1631), 21–2.
37. Osiander, *How and Whither*, sig. A6^{v}.
38. Samuel Pepys, *The Diary of Samuel Pepys*, Robert Latham, William Matthews (eds), 11 vols (London: Bell and Hyman, 1970–83), vol. vi, 181.
39. Ibid., 6, 174.
40. Ibid., 6, 224.
41. Ibid., 6, 225.
42. Burton, *Anatomy of Melancholy*, 220.
43. Ibid., 222.

44. Ibid., 228.
45. Ibid., 222.
46. The non-naturals were air, diet, exercise and rest, sleep and waking, the evacuations, the passions of the mind. They had been used to organise advice on regimen from the time of Galen.
47. Phayer, *Treatyse of the Pestilence*, sig. N3[v].
48. William Bullein, *A Dialogue Against the Fever Pestilence From the Edition of 1578*, Mark W. Bullen and A.H. Bullen (eds) (London: N. Trübner for the Early English Text Society, 1888), 39.
49. Ibid., 39.
50. Ibid., 39.
51. Bradwell, *Physick for the Sicknesse*, 37.
52. Ibid., 37.
53. Ibid., 38.
54. Ibid., 38.
55. Ibid., 10,22,23.
56. See Rosemary Horrox, *The Black Death*, (Manchester: Manchester University Press, 1994), 107, 55; the earliest English printed book on the plague, *A Litil Boke for the Pestilence*, [London, [1485?] by 'Canutius', Bengt Knutsson bishop of Västerias, Sweden closely based on that of Jean Jacmé [Horrox, 173] written in *c.* 1364 warned against 'drede' and recommended the reader 'to be mery in the herte', fol. 7[r]. See also Dorothea Singer, 'Some Plague Tractates', *Proceedings of the Royal Society of Medicine*, ix (1916), 21–24.
57. W. Boraston, 'A Necessary and Briefe Relation of the Contagious Disease of the Pestilence' in Thomas Vicary, *The Englishmans Treasure* (London: B. Alsop and T. Fawcet, 1633), 246, citing Paracelsus, *De Occulta Philosophia*.
58. J.B. van Helmont, 'Tumulus Pestis or the Plague-Grave' in *Oriatrike Or. Physick Refined* (London: L Lloyd, 1662), 1119.
59. Ibid., 1132.
60. Ibid., 1119–1120.
61. Ibid., 1129.
62. Ibid., 1129, 1126.
63. George Thomson, *Λoimotomia; or the Pest Anatomised* (London: N. Crouch, 1666), 32–8, 78–9.
64. Ibid., 5.
65. Ibid., 11.
66. Ibid., 17–18.
67. Boghurst, *Loimographia*, 29.
68. On the whole, medical writers did not use the patient's fear to excuse therapeutic failure. Much more typical of the reasons given are those listed by the Frenchman Theophilus Garencieres who also practised in London in 1665 and who believed that fear allowed 'the Pestilential spirit' to print his character upon the humours: 'The cause why so few escape are these. The scarcity of able Physitians willing to attend that disease, the inefficacy of common remedies, the want of accommodation, as Cloaths, Fire, Room, Dyet, Attendants, the wilfulness of the Patient, his Poverty, his neglecting the first Invasion, and trifling away

the time till it be too late; A vapouring Chymist with his drops, an ignorant Apothecary with his Blistering Plaisters, a wilful Surgeon with his untimely Lancing, an impudent Mountebancke, an intruding Gossip, and a carelesse Nurse'. Theophilus Garencieres, *A Mite Cast into the Treasury of the Famous City of London*, 3rd ed. (London: T. Ratcliffe, 1666), 6,3.

69. Boghurst, *Loimographia*, 29.
70. Ibid., 39.
71. Ibid., 31.
72. Ibid., 34,35,39.
73. Ibid., 39.
74. Ibid., 40.
75. Ibid., 65.
76. Ibid., 65.
77. Ibid., 66.
78. Ibid., 60.
79. Ibid., 60.
80. Ibid., 73.
81. Nicholas Culpeper, 'A Treatise of the Pestilence' in *Culpeper's Last Legacy* (London: N. Brooke, 1655), 118.
82. Ibid., 114.
83. J.V. *Golgotha* (London: J. Clark, 1665), title page.
84. Ibid., 12.
85. Ibid., 9–10.
86. Hodges, *Loimologia*, 3, 137.
87. Ibid., 7; see also Paul Slack, *The Impact of Plague in Tudor and Stuart England* (London: Routledge and Kegan Paul, 1985) 250–1.
88. Burton, *Anatomy of Melancholy*, 228.
89. Samson Price, *Londons Remembrancer* (London: T. Harper, 1626), 32.
90. Thomson, *Aoimotomia*, 138.
91. Ibid., 137.
92. Ibid., 138.
93. George Wither, *The History of the Pestilence (1625)*, ed. with introduction by J. Milton French (Cambridge Mass: Harvard University Press, 1932), 70.
94. Ibid., 71.
95. Ibid., 71.
96. Ibid., 72.
97. Ibid., 72.

IV

WESTERN MEDICINE AND PAIN: HISTORICAL PERSPECTIVES*

Roy Porter

Introduction

As part of their 'back to basics' campaign in the early '90s, Conservative Party politicians attempted to retrieve what might be called the positive view of pain that Mrs Thatcher had associated with Victorian values. 'No pain, no gain', 'if it's not hurting, it isn't working': those were the slogans of the day.[1] Such starkly punitive outlooks run counter not just to liberal cultural and moral values but also to certain trends in modern medicine, which, albeit rather belatedly, is now engaging with the problem of pain as never before. Powerful new physiological explanations have emerged, notably the 'gate' theory, developed from the 1960s by Ronald Melzack and Patrick Wall. Discarding as simplistic the old mechanical 'fire-alarm' theories, they emphasized how, when messages from the nerve ends reach the spinal cord, a fine tuning takes place regulating the degree of pain suffered; this is, pain can be enhanced or inhibited by brain signals. Emphasizing the symbiosis of physiological and psychological factors, 'gate theorists' have shown how pain's intensity depends on circumstances – depression may make us supersensitive. With the aid of new interactive approaches like this which stress how pain is not a mere sensation but a perceptual product, modern medicine can at last begin to shoulder its responsibilities for pain control. This is manifest in the widespread setting

* It had been our hope that Roselyne Rey would contribute a lecture to the conference and essay to this book. The brilliant young French medical historian, already distinguished for her researches on the history of the nervous system, had recently published her *Histoire de la douleur*, translated as *The History of Pain*, easily the best treatment to date. Alas it was not to be, as she died in 1995, at a tragically early age, of cancer. She is much missed. This article is dedicated to her memory.

up of pain clinics, in pain counselling, and in the foundation of the International Association for the Study of Pain and its journal *Pain*.[2]

This is surely the right way forward, but the tardiness of these developments means there is much ground to make up. Indeed, pain always was a poor relation in Western medicine. Suffering, so Christian teachings had ruled, was the just deserts of sinners – like the poor, pain would always be among us. Hence it was easy for doctors to decide that pain management was best left to sufferers themselves, or to priests or nurses, while the heroic surgeon did *his* job and sawed or slashed on. Half a century ago, John Alfred Ryle, the founder of social medicine, declared that one of the great mistakes of scientific medicine was that through embracing a mechanical model of the body it had discarded consciousness and shelved the pain problem.[3] With both clinical and humane ends in mind, Ryle called for fresh study; and things have indeed improved. Yet saving lives has always been sexier than managing pain; from arthritis to cancer, pain relief remains far from perfect; and cock-eyed protocols get in the way – heroin, for instance, is medically unavailable in the USA in cases of terminal cancer, etc., lest, it seems, the dying get addicted.[4] An ingrained medical puritanism lives on in this country too. Reflecting on his inveterate loathing of doctors, the columnist Jeffrey Barnard, smitten with pancreatitis, recently observed that 'most of all I hate them for their meanness and narrow-mindedness about dispensing pain relief'.[5]

Much of the trouble derives from the fact that we have inherited a puzzling legacy. When pain has (rather rarely) been addressed by medical scientists – rather than simply being accepted as an unfortunate side-effect – their mental programming has not always been conducive to understanding. In *The Basis of Sensation* (1928), Edgar Adrian rightly stated that:

> Whatever our views about the relation of mind and body, we cannot escape the fact that there is an unsatisfactory gap between such events as the sticking of a pin into my finger and the appearance of a sensation of pain in my consciousness. Part of the gap is obviously made up of events in my sensory nerves and brain.[6]

No doubt; but by then insisting that 'the psychological method by itself can tell us nothing at all', the Nobel prize-winning neurophysiologist was led to conclude that it was the laboratory that would provide the answers. In other words, for Lord Adrian and others of his training and programming, all true pain was physical pain, and it would finally be explained by scientific investigation; psychological pain was at bottom flimflam.[7]

Clinicians too have often sought to distinguish authentic pain from other sorts of distress judged to be (merely) of an emotional or psychological basis – those, as they say, 'all in the mind'. 'Real pain, especially severe pain', insisted the prominent mid-century American physician, Walter Alvarez:

> Points to the presence of organic rather than functional disease. On the other hand, a burning, or a quivering, or a picking, pricking, pulling, pumping, crawling, boiling, gurgling, thumping, throbbing, gassy or itching sensation, or a constant ache, or soreness, strongly suggests a neurosis.[8]

Through such reductionist strategies, scientific medicine, aided by a smattering of Freud, has sought to rescue 'real pain' or 'healthy pain' from (mere) 'suffering' – the former legitimated by falling within the domain of medical science. Cold comfort, this, for sufferers, even if it helped the doctors to cope.

Pain, Roselyne Rey justly observed, has been and remains poorly understood because it 'has no clearly defined status', all such divisions between 'real' and 'subjective' pain, founded upon archaic Cartesian body/mind dualisms, being quite problematic.[9] For isn't all pain irreducibly subjective? No physician can pop a thermometer into the brain or X-ray the heart, and thereby measure pain as if it were a fever or a fracture. Whatever its nature or function, pain is felt – indeed, as is stressed in David Morris's recent study *The Culture of Pain*, it is best envisioned not as a raw physical sensation but as an experience – that is, feeling filtered through culture. Not least, the dubious desire amongst no-nonsense medics to distinguish 'physical' from 'mental' pain invariably discounts 'psychosomatic disorders' and sows seeds of suspicion about malingering. We will get an insight into the paradoxes of modern attitudes, which frequently sound offhand or dismissive, only if we understand their history.[10]

Pain in the Past

Figuring earlier experiences of pain is itself highly problematic, both personally and philosophically, subjectively and scientifically.

For pain never comes pure; it is always mediated through particular models of mind-body relations and disease theories, and through the individual sufferer's consciousness. Moreover, it is hard to put words and names to most emotions and experiences. When in 1810 the novelist Fanny Burney underwent mastectomy without anaesthetic and wrote of 'the most torturing pain . . . when the dreadful steel was plunged into the breast – cutting through veins – arteries – flesh – nerves', we can vicariously and feebly share her agonies.[11] But what of that dauntless early Victorian essayist and economist, Harriet Martineau? She took to her bed for five years, complaining of unbearable abdominal torments whose roots were then, and remain today, quite obscure. Can we even begin to guess what she was going through?[12]

'Language,' reflected the late-Enlightenment physician, Thomas Beddoes, 'has not yet been adjusted with any degree of exactness to our inward feelings.'[13] Miss Martineau's aching womb entered the public domain, and she was assuredly no slouch at what post-modernists now call 'writing the body';[14] for all that, however, the historian is left a bewildered bystander. And sometimes words have completely failed those racked by pain. Here's William Tildesley, a seventeenth-century diarist: 'June 15, In great payne; June 16, In paines alover; June 17, In great payne'. By default Tildesley perhaps achieved a lapidary eloquence. Such enforced muteness may even help to explain why many codes of conduct, most notably Stoicism, have prescribed dignified silence as the victory of brain over pain.[15] Indeed since the Holocaust conventional wisdom has often deemed that the most hideous pain (rape, torture, genocide) is necessarily unspeakable, and any verbalization profanation. The best is silence.[16]

As well as these humanistic dilemmas, theoretical difficulties abound when the historian addresses pain in the past. The assumption often made by doctors that pain as physiological tracer and pain as inner agony should be looked upon as distinct entities may be quite anachronistic. After all, medical teachings dominant from Hippocrates to the Renaissance regarded maladies holistically, viewing the 'physical' and the 'spiritual', outer and inner, as a continuum mediated through such concepts as the humours and temperaments.[17] Cartesianism, and subsequently the new pathological anatomy that dominated French hospital medicine from around 1800, were assuredly meant to put paid to such 'confusions': every disease was to be anchored in its lesion.[18]

Yet the reverse seems to have been the result: for all their trumpeted path-lab proficiency, physicians found themselves encountering pain clusters frustratingly impossible to match up with bedside or post-mortem lesions. Those averse to taking the easy way out and dismissing such symptoms as (merely) psychosomatic or as the tell-tale marks of fakes, frauds and (female) hysterics, pioneered the concept of the 'syndrome' and formulated intermediate explanatory categories like neuralgia, functional disorder or chronic 'pain without lesion' – though, as already noted, hard-liners deplored such perhaps face-saving formulae.

Medical theory and laboratory science have often tried to put pain out of mind, but that has never been so easy at the bedside. Down the centuries, pain has been the normal *entrée* into and crux of medical encounters. Every culture, group and individual has distinctive pain thresholds, beneath which it is normal to grin and bear it.[19] But unexpected pain, strange, erratic, searing, intense or protracted modes of discomfort have led sufferers to seek primary care, desperate for relief and fearing that pain reveals some deeper malady. Within old-style medicine, the physician used to 'take the history' and encourage patients to speak their pain: its nature, location, onset, duration, intensity, periodicity and quality. Whilst clinicians had always felt the pulse and gauged eye- and skin-colour, hands-on physical examination and instrumental testing became standard practice only fairly recently; even in mid-Victorian times it was noted by Dr Peter Latham that 'not only degrees of pain, but its existence, in any degree, must be taken upon the testimony of the patient'.[20]

Scientific Medicine

Things were changing, however, thanks to the emergence of what Michel Foucault dubbed the new 'clinical gaze'. The traditional bedside question – 'What is the matter?' – gave way to the modern: 'Show me where it hurts'; in other words, there was a diagnostic switch from subjective symptoms to objective signs, involving a shift in power from patient to physician.[21] And with the help of new diagnostic aids – stethoscopes, ophthalmoscopes and, from a century ago, X-rays – it became feasible to pin down pain to specific bodily sites and pathological events (joint degeneration, toxins, and so forth).[22]

Such views – amounting to what Max von Frey called the 'doctrine of specificity' – have various conceptual underpinnings.[23] The birth of neuro-anatomy in the Scientific Revolution was important, developed by key figures like Thomas Willis, who coined the term 'neurologie'. In the eighteenth century the great Göttingen physiologist, Albrecht von Haller, clarified the distinction between muscles (endowed with irritability, the property of contracting under stimulus) and nerves (which alone possessed sensitivity, the power to communicate feeling). William Cullen and his Edinburgh contemporaries, John Hunter in London, and the Montpellier 'vitalists' further explored the relations between sensation and the nervous system. Early in the nineteenth century, François Magendie in France and Charles Bell in Britain established the sensory/motor division of the spinal roots as fundamental to nervous organization. Neurology thereby mapped pain onto the body.[24]

Neurology and Philosophy

Experimenters sliced and snipped, but they also looked to philosophy, their theory of the 'reflex arc' being underpinned by a Cartesian model of the body machine. Espousing the mechanical philosophy, Descartes had pointed to the automatic withdrawal of a limb from a flame. Heat impacted upon the skin, causing signals to speed to the brain like a tug on a bell-rope. Pain was the ringing, a literal fire-alarm for self-preservation. This physiological representation of pain as a beneficial reflex mechanism, a warning system, appealed to anatomists, reinforcing their adaptationist, natural theological 'all is for the best' vision of the perfect design of the organism. Neurology provided confirmation that human responses were not random but governed by well-designed natural laws of 'motion' and 'motivation'. By way of spin-offs in applied psychology, the Enlightenment educationalist, Helvétius, and the utilitarian Jeremy Bentham deemed that mankind was programmed to react to the stimulus of pleasure and the sanction of pain – the latter being, according to Bentham, 'the only evil'. A science of motives was therefore feasible, to be fine-tuned by the felicific calculus. Resourceful distribution of pleasure and pain in a prison, school or other controlled milieu – a 'just measure of pain' – would train subjects to behave in desired, regular, and predictable ways. Through such psychologies of applied pain,

Enlightenment sensationalists paved the way for the audacious meliorist cruelties of modern behaviourist and conditioning psychologies.[25]

The triumph of such sensory-motor models of nervous organization rendered it conceptually easy, albeit experimentally fiendishly tricky, for nineteenth-century physiologists to study the pathways linking pain to the central nervous system. Inspired in part by phrenology, understanding grew of pain-tracks and the localization of functions in the brain. Through exquisite vivisection experiments (sometimes performed upon themselves) involving severing nerve fibres, a string of ingenious investigators from Pierre Flourens to Henry Head and Charles Sherrington laid bare the central nervous system's intricate mechanisms. By 1900, the sensory-motor alterations which, it had become known, could be effected by severing spinal nerve roots, were being produced by slicing segments off the brain. Like a canary at a coal face, pain was the surest demonstration of the body's nervous circuitry: no pain, no physiological research.[26]

One problem that long puzzled observers was the differential sensitivity to pain of various bodily parts: why were fingertips or lips so much more responsive than the skin on the back? Why was pain not directly felt in diseased internal organs like the liver? Neurologists like Frey were able to show that these effects were products of the differential distribution of nerve endings. Pain was also discovered to possess a labile quality, defying crude bell-pull reflex models. Bodily surfaces could become unresponsive or hyperaesthesic, as in tickling – a reminder of the fact that one standard test for possession during the great early-modern witch-craze had been insensitivity to pain, discovered by applying a candle flame or sticking pins into the suspect. The new neurophysiology proved that such bizarre occurrences had been quite authentic – not as the Devil's doings, of course, but as products of neurophysiological abnormalities. From the 1860s the notable Parisian neuro-anatomist Jean-Martin Charcot experimented on hysterics' reactions to pain-stimuli, using hypnosis to induce anaesthesias and hyperaesthesias. Others explored the 'phantom organ' and conversely sensation loss in an intact part – occurrences recently given a wry autobiographical twist in Oliver Sacks's *A Leg to Stand On*.[27]

At the crossing-point between physiology and philosophy, new insights into the protective role of pain have always posed fresh conceptual problems. If pain was integral to the reflex response, could it (asked a succession of thinkers from Enlightenment materialists like La Mettrie to Victorian physicians like Thomas Laycock) strictly be said to be the *cause* of activity? Or was it only 'noises off', a scream in the machine? Pain, some argued, was not the *motivation* for retracting one's foot from the fire, but simply the psychological voice-over to stimulus-and-response reflexes, implicitly echoing the old Cartesian denial of animal conciousness: kick a dog and it would yelp but feel no pain at all.[28]

Philosophical questions have likewise been raised by modern investigations which show how pain's substrate lies in the biochemistry of the brain. A research tradition sparked by Henry Dale's investigations into the brain-modifying properties of ergot revealed the role of chemical neurotransmitters in pain inhibition. Eventually it was discovered that endorphins are released that override the normal protective pain mechanisms, notably at times of great excitement or danger, explaining why soldiers are often oblivious to appalling wounds in the heat of battle. Such discoveries have proved suggestive for the molecular modelling of drugs like antihistamines and, more recently, Prozac. But as a result of such work, is consciousness finally being shown to be just a trick of brain chemistry?[29]

Pain and Consciousness

By no means all styles of healers, however, have embraced these biochemical or neurophysiological models of pain. For some, pain is still viewed, *pace* Lord Adrian, as immediate proof of the sovereignty of the psychological. The nineteenth century brought studies of pain-inducing or -inhibiting conditions like hypnosis, trance, hysteria and voodoo, which parapsychologists still claim defy reductionist explanation, while psychoanalysis touted solutions of its own. Freud explained both 'hysterical' anaesthetizations and diseaseless symptoms (like persistent coughs) as somatic conversions, consequent upon repression of primary psychological disturbance. The cunning of the unconscious, it is suggested, displaces emotional conflict or insupportable anguish by translating them into more manageable, or more personally and socially acceptable organic modes. This view was taken to its logical conclusion by Freud's sometime follower, Georg Groddeck, who held that all physical pain was, at bottom, psychogenic, to be glossed as nonverbal language: thus neck pain pointed to a 'pain in the neck'.[30] In his early *Pain and Pleasure: A Study of Bodily Feelings* (1957), Thomas Szasz comparably suggested that pain functioned as a communication system particularly well-adapted for attracting attention in a highly medicalized society such as ours. Biomedical critics may counter that such psychological explanations are trivializing and false – many scholars have argued that psycho-analysis's famous hysterical patients like Bertha Pappenheim ('Anna O') were actually suffering from physical illnesses – but the enduring value of psychological theories is that they reach out to the richer domains of philosophy, language and subjectivity which personalize the barbs of pain.[31]

The Meaning of Pain

Regardless of such disputes, it has been axiomatic within biomedicine that 'real' pain has a purpose: if in some pie-in-the-sky Utopia snake-bites and frost-bite, toxins and infections provoked no such pangs, our survival would be jeopardized. For modern Darwinian doctors like the American Randolph Nesse, pain is a healthily adaptive evolutionary response to danger.[32]

Why, then, is it so often chronic or insupportable? Are not such pains disproportionate to their functions, a monstrous form of overkill? A spanner was thrown into medical consensus on this subject by the leading (but in the English-speaking world neglected) interwar French bio-philosopher, René Leriche. In his dissenting view – he may sound like the Devil's advocate – neither diagnostically nor prognostically has pain ever served much purpose, while 'in certain chronic cases it seems to be the entire disorder which, without it, would not exist'. Leriche was wont to mock conventional medical pieties about 'good pain':

> Defence mechanism? Welcome warning? . . . When the pain does arrive, it is already too late . . . The pain has only made the whole battle, lost early on in the game, sadder and more unbearable.[33]

In challenging orthodox views of 'healthy pain' – it was as foolish an idea as the medieval notion of laudable pus – Leriche did for medicine what the Enlightenment did for Christian theodicies at large, and Voltaire's *Candide* for Leibnizian Optimism.[34] Yet these continued. It was that great Victorian theologian and occasional

Prime Minister, William Gladstone, who judged that 'pain is not in its nature an evil in the proper sense, nor is it invariably attended with evil as a consequence';[35] and such views as Gladstone's serve to remind us of an enduring Christian apologetics of pain, as part of the grand mission of justifying the ways of God to man.

Broadly speaking, there were traditionally two ways to rationalize pain: it could be read as positively evil, or as mere negative deprivation, as with hunger. Dualistic creeds like Manicheism interpreted it as the Devil's work, whereas Platonists and Thomists have seen it as privation. Conventional Christians denied that pain was a design feature of Creation, having entered the world only through Sin – this Divine penalty theory being etymologically reinforced, 'pain' coming from *poena* ('punishment'). As Job's trials were meant to show, the proper response to Divine trial was to be long-suffering: being a martyr to disease was no less glorious than martyrdom by the infidel. Especially within traditional Catholicism, mortification was an induction into holiness, flagellating the flesh to liberate the spirit.[36]

Yet caution was always urged, lest pain were fetishized, making a proud cult out of *homo dolorosus*. Christian charity in any case required the relief of pain – Luke had been 'the beloved physician', Christ had performed some thirty-five healing miracles, and the promise of Heaven was not more agony but bliss. Hence apologetics required nuance: suffering was a gift of Providence, a blessing indeed; yet it was also to be alleviated by appropriate medical aid and pious offices.

Calvinist churchmen adopted tough attitudes towards physical pain, but with the age of reason, theodicies had to be refined. According to William Paley's influential *Natural Theology* (1802), pain was a 'lesser evil', designed to prevent 'greater'.[37] Today's twinge in the toes should be read as a Providential hazard-sign, directing us to cut alcohol consumption lest tomorrow we get gout. Ingenious apologists even speculated that the Divine Designer might have brought physical suffering into the world out of sheer creative superfecundity. The blind and deaf, freaks and cripples, averred Soame Jenyns in the mid-eighteenth century, enriched Creation through enhancing the dazzling heterogeneity of existence. Almost anticipating Leriche, Samuel Johnson gave Jenyns' special pleading for the omnipresence of pain the drubbing it deserved – such apologetics were tantamount to suggesting that the Almighty took sadistic 'delight in the operations of an asthma, as a human philosopher in the effects of the air pump' – the sting in Johnson's tale being that, unlike God, scientific experimenters were cruel indeed.[38]

Meanwhile the new Enlightenment sensibilities associated with the age of feeling finally rebelled against and rejected Christianity's apparent collusion with pain, and modern secularism follows suit. If the medieval mind regarded sickness and scarcity as divinely ordained, our political manifestos promise their eradication. Ancients craved the good death, Moderns, as the ex-priest Ivan Illich protested in his *Limits to Medicine*, hanker after the prolongation of painfree, if drugged-up, life.[39]

By Victorian times if not before, pain was in danger of becoming a scandal and its ubiquity an inducement to doubt and a gift for sceptics. Throughout and despite all her sufferings, the Unitarian-bred Harriet Martineau thus deplored the moral repugnance of Evangelical teachings on pain. Pieties about the beauties of suffering, claimed her *Life in the Sick-Room* (1854), glamourized morbid self-pity and sapped the will to be well. Christianity was locked into a culture of woe, was implicitly sadistic.[40] Charles Darwin regarded Scripture as no less vicious than Nature: he was not prepared to stomach the 'cruel' Christian doctrine that unbelievers would be condemned to eternal hellfire. And faced by the murderous struggle for survival, he and other sensitive souls could no longer accept that the wise man automatically looked, as Pope had recommended, 'from Nature up to Nature's God'.[41] Muscular Christian evolutionists, of course, had their unflinching riposte: God had programmed suffering into the evolutionary economy to weed out weaklings.[42]

Pain and Progress

The Enlightenment made its philosophical manifesto not the uses of adversity but the minimization of suffering, notably, of course, through the principle of utility. That great atheistic cat-lover, Jeremy Bentham, urged an end to wanton cruelty towards animals, because they too suffered.[43] This left the medical profession on the horns of a dilemma. Many doctors were prominent humanitarians, campaigning against the slave trade, child labour, and other abominations. Yet medical progress seemed to hinge upon experimental physiology, and British experimentalists increasingly came under fire for their alleged indifference to the pain they inflicted upon dumb animals. Experimenters responded with the 'lesser evil' defence; certain Continental physiologists, by contrast, upheld the Cartesian 'automaton' position on the brute creation (lesser animals could not feel) or flaunted a lofty indifference in the name of scientific research.[44]

This Enlightenment upheaval in attitudes to pain reopens that old question: has the endurance of pain changed over time? Do Moderns deplore pain not because they are less callous but because they have become too soft to bear it? Everyone knows that pain experience can be subjective: that pioneer demographer, Thomas Malthus, noted that he could block out a painful toothache, temporarily at least, by concentrating on writing. Likewise, different societies respond dissimilarly to 'painful' sensations – some 'psychologize' more while others 'somatize'. Some cultures encourage operatic wailing and stylized screaming rituals, others the stiff upper lip: dependent upon cultural conditioning, either may prove an effective coping strategy.[45]

It has often been claimed that the civilizing process has brought increased sensitivity to pain: 'the savage does not feel pain as we do', judged the nineteenth-century American, Dr Silas Weir Mitchell. This alleged phenomenon might be read positively (the evolution of humanity) or negatively – a lamentable weakening of moral fibre. 'That anybody should be in pain and not be immediately relieved – that sharp pain should ever be inflicted upon any one', grumbled the eminent Victorian jurist, James Fitzjames Stephen, 'shocks and scandalizes people in these days': such mawkishness was to be deplored.[46]

What is undeniable is that the medical profession has become more responsive to the widespread clamour for pain relief. Sedatives and narcotics had long been used to quell pain – mandragora, henbane (hyosciamine) and sedative sponges were well known to Antiquity – but painkilling was not central to the agenda of the Classical physician. Analgesics were to grow more important in prescribing practice. This was partly due to greater access to effective drugs: from the seventeenth century, opium was easily available, while the rise of the pharmaceutical industry led to major synthetic compounds: morphine (1806), codeine (1836), and, a century ago, acetylsalicylic acid, the humble aspirin.[47]

Attitudes altered alongside. There is little sign that the Renaissance physician made pain-control a high priority. Growing customer assertiveness changed that, stimulated by competition from quacks promising gentle remedies. Pain management developed. Eighteenth-century physicians began to calm the dying with generous doses of laudanum, and the nineteenth century brought the anaesthetics revolution. That idea, or its uptake, came tardily, however – retrospectively it seems remarkable that Humphry Davy could be involved in the 1790s in auto-experimentation with nitrous oxide (laughing gas) as a putative remedy for respiratory disorders, without capitalizing upon its anaesthetic properties. By the 1840s, however, ether was being used to aid dental extractions, and chloroform was employed for painless childbirth; Queen Victoria had her fourth son, Prince Leopold, delivered under chloroform in 1853. The hypodermic syringe, invented in the same year, allowed the injection of narcotics, and cocaine came into use in the 1880s, popularized not least by Freud. Hypnosis enjoyed a vogue, rather like acupuncture today (needling, we now know, has a physiological effect, stimulating endorphin release).[48]

Ivan Illich and other critics of 'medical imperialism' have deplored the modern shrinking from gladiatorial confrontations with pain.[49] Such aversion from reality, they allege, undermines integrity and autonomy: those who cannot face pain will not be able to face death. Yet, as is amply shown by the liberal policy with morphine dosages followed in British hospices, all the indications are that effective pain control can materially enhance the quality of life in the terminal and chronic sick. In times when fears are growing that health-care costs will spiral unsupportably, attention to pain and its reduction may help order our priorities.[50]

NOTES

1. Eric M. Sigsworth (ed.), *In Search of Victorian Values* (Manchester: Manchester University Press, 1988).
2. For the history of pain within medicine, see K. Keele, *Anatomies of Pain* (Oxford: Blackwell Scientific Publications, 1957). Such developments must be understood in context of wider shifts in the theory of the nature of disease. See F. Kräupl Taylor, *The Concepts of Illness, Disease and Morbus* (Cambridge: Cambridge University Press, 1979); Walther Riesse, *The Conception of Disease. Its History, Its Versions and Its Nature* (New York: Philosophical Library, 1953).

   For modern developments, especially the Pain Society, I am greatly indebted to Sarah Natas, 'The Relief of Pain: The Birth and Development of the Journal *Pain* from 1975 to 1985 and its Place within Changing Concepts of Pain' (B.Sc. Dissertation, University College,

1996). For the 'gate' theory see Ronald D. Melzack and Patrick Wall, *The Challenge of Pain* (New York: Basic Books, 1983).

3. See Dorothy Porter, 'John Ryle: Doctor of Revolution?', in Dorothy Porter and Roy Porter (eds), *Doctors, Politics and Society* (Amsterdam: Rodopi, 1993), 247–74. Competence in pain management has been, in recent years, one of the special professional claims of the nursing profession. See Sioban Nelson, 'Care of the Sick: Nursing, Holism and Pious Practice' (Ph.D. thesis, Faculty of Humanities, Griffith University, Queensland, Australia, 1996).
4. See Lester Grinspoon and James B. Bakalar, *Marihuana: The Forbidden Medicine* (New Haven: Yale University Press, 1993).
5. Jeffrey Barnard, 'Too Many Pretty Girls', *The Spectator*, cclxxv (14th October 1995), 61–2, p. 62: 'But it allowed me to air some grievances about the medical profession, particularly its meanness and slowness in giving patients relief from pain, and the stupid and exaggerated idea and fear of making people morphine addicts.'
6. Quoted in Roselyne Rey, *History of Pain*, trans. Elliott Wallace and J.W. and S.W. Cadden (Paris: Éditions la Découverte, 1993), 295.
7. For the shortcomings of the physiological theory of pain, see Ann Dally, 'The Significance of Pain in the History of British Psychiatry', in G.E. Berrios and Roy Porter (eds), *History of Clinical Psychiatry* (London: Athlone, 1993), 203–11. For nineteenth century worries, see A.D. Hodgkiss, 'Chronic Pain in Nineteenth-Century British Medical Writings', *History of Psychiatry*, ii (1991), 27–40, and *idem*, 'From Lesion to Metaphor: Chronic Pain Without Lesion in British, French and German Medical Writings 1800–1914' (University of London MD thesis, 1996).
8. Quoted in Edward Shorter, *From Paralysis to Fatigue. A History of Psychosomatic Illness in the Modern Era* (New York: Free Press, 1992), 290.
9. Roselyne Rey, *History of Pain*.
10. David B. Morris, *The Culture of Pain* (Berkeley: University of California Press, 1991); David B. Morris, 'The Languages of Pain', in Richard M. Caplan (ed.), *Exploring the Concept of Mind* (Iowa City: University of Iowa Press, 1986).
11. J. Hemlow (ed.), *The Journals and Letters of Fanny Burney (Madame D'Arblay)*, 12 vols (Oxford: Clarendon Press, 1972–84), vi, 598f.
12. Roger Cooter, 'Dichotomy and Denial: Mesmerism, Medicine and Harriet Martineau', in Marina Benjamin (ed.), *Science and Sensibility: Gender and Scientific Enquiry, 1780–1945* (Oxford: Basil Blackwell, 1991), 144–73; Roy Porter and Dorothy Porter, *In Sickness and in Health: The British Experience 1650–1850* (London: Fourth Estate, 1988), 213. For the modern clinical dimension see M. Balint, *The Doctor, His Patient, and the Illness* (London: Pitman, 1957); Ronald D. Mann (ed.), *The History of the Management of Pain: From Early Principles to Present Practice* (Carnforth: The Parthenon Publishing Group, 1988), especially ch. ix: Jennifer Beinart, '"The Snowball Effect": The Growth of the

Treatment of Intractable Pain in Postwar Britain', 179–86.

13. T. Beddoes, *Hygeia*, 3 vols (Bristol: Phillips, 1802–3), vol. 2 Essay viii p. 78; Roy Porter, '"Expressing Yourself Ill": The Language of Sickness in Georgian England', in P. Burke and R. Porter (eds), *Language, Self and Society: The Social History of Language* (Cambridge: Polity Press, 1991), 276–99.
14. For this genre see, for instance, Susan Bordo, 'Reading the Slender Body', in Mary Jacobus, Evelyn Fox Keller and Sally Shuttleworth (eds), *Body/Politics: Women and the Discourses of Science* (New York/London: Routledge, 1990), 83–112.
15. Roy Porter and Dorothy Porter, *In Sickness and in Health: The British Experience 1650–1850* (London: Fourth Estate, 1988). See also Barbara Duden, *Geschichte unter der Haut* (Stuttgart: Klett, Cotta, 1987), translated as *The Woman Beneath the Skin. A Doctor's Patients in Eighteenth-Century Germany*, trans. by Thomas Dunlap (Cambridge, Mass.: Harvard University Press, 1991); Andrew Wear, 'Historical and Cultural Aspects of Pain', *Bulletin of the Society for the Social History of Medicine*, xxxvi (1985), 7–21.
16. George Steiner, *Language and Silence* (London: Atheneum, 1970); Elaine Scarry, *The Body in Pain* (Oxford: Oxford University Press, 1985); Scarry's book is the most searching attempt to explore the Judaeo-Christian tradition of thinking about pain and suffering within philosophy and literature. Bending criticizes it: see below, ref. 35.
17. V. Nutton, 'Humoralism', in W.F. Bynum and Roy Porter (eds), *Companion Encyclopedia of the History of Medicine* (London: Routledge, 1993), 281–91.
18. M. Foucault, *Naissance de la Clinique: Une Archéologie du Regard Médical* (Paris: Presses Universitaires de France, 1963), trans. A.M. Sheridan Smith, *The Birth of the Clinic* (London: Tavistock, 1973; 1976).
19. See the essays in *The Puzzle of Pain* (East Roseville, Australia: G & B Arts International, 1994).
20. Malcolm Nicolson, 'The Art of Diagnosis: Medicine and the Five Senses', in W.F. Bynum and Roy Porter (eds), *Companion Encyclopedia of the History of Medicine* (London: Routledge, 1993), 797–821; Roy Porter, 'The Rise of Physical Examination', in W.F. Bynum and Roy Porter (eds), *Medicine and the Five Senses* (Cambridge: Cambridge University Press, 1992), 179–97.
21. For discussion see David Armstrong, *Political Anatomy of the Body: Medical Knowledge in Britain in the Twentieth Century* (Cambridge: Cambridge University Press, 1983); Colin Jones and Roy Porter (eds), *Reassessing Foucault: Power, Medicine and the Body* (London; Routledge, 1994), especially Thomas Osborne, 'On Anti-Medicine and Clinical Reason', pp. 28–47.
22. Stanley Joel Reiser, *Medicine and the Reign of Technology* (Cambridge: Cambridge University Press, 1978; 1981); *idem*, 'The Science of Diagnosis: Diagnostic Technology', in W.F. Bynum and Roy Porter (eds), *Companion Encyclopedia of the History of Medicine* (London: Routledge, 1993), 822–47.
23. For Von Frey, see Rey, *History of Pain*, 200, 302.

24. For this historical succession see Rey, *History of Pain*, chs 3–6.
25. For Utilitarianism see E. Halévy, *The Growth of Philosophic Radicalism*, new ed. (London: Faber and Faber, 1972) and Martin Wiener, *Reconstructing the Criminal. Culture, Law and Policy in England, 1830–1914* (Cambridge: Cambridge University Press, 1991)
26. Rey, *History of Pain*, 294f.
27. Oliver Sacks, *A Leg to Stand On* (London: Duckworth, 1984). Sacks' *Migraine: Evolution of a Common Disorder* (London: Pan Books, 1981) is a fascinating exploration of certain positive dimensions of pain.
28. For clarification of such questions in medical philosophy see Lester S. King, *The Philosophy of Medicine: The Early Eighteenth Century* (Cambridge, Mass.: Harvard University Press, 1978).
29. See E.M. Tansey, 'The Early Scientific Career of Sir Henry Dale FRS (1875–1968)' (University of London Ph.D. thesis, 1990).
30. For Freud and the interpretation of hysteria see Sander Gilman, Helen King, Roy Porter, George Rousseau and Elaine Showalter, *Hysteria Beyond Freud* (Berkeley: University of California Press, 1993); for Groddeck see G. Groddeck, *The Meaning of Illness: Selected Psychoanalytical Writings* (London: Hogarth Press, 1977).
31. See T. Szasz, *Pain and Pleasure. A Study of Bodily Feelings* (London: Tavistock Publications, 1957).
32. Randolph M. Nesse and George C. Williams, *Evolution and Healing. The New Science of Darwinian Medicine* (London: Weidenfeld & Nicolson, 1995).
33. Quoted and discussed in Rey, *History of Pain*, 306.
34. Henry Vyverberg, *Historical Pessimism in the French Enlightenment* (Cambridge, Mass.: Harvard University Press, 1958).
35. Quoted in Wiener, *Reconstructing the Criminal*, 111. Helpful for the late Victorian period is Lucy Bending, 'The Representation of Bodily Pain in Late Nineteenth Century English Culture' (D.Phil., University of Oxford, 1997).
36. C.S. Lewis, *The Problem of Pain* (London: Centenary Press, 1940); D. Bakan, *Disease, Pain and Sacrifice: Towards a Psychology of Suffering* (Chicago and Boston: Beacon Publications, 1971).
37. William Paley, *Natural Theology* (London: R. Faulder, 1802), ch. xxvi.
38. Mona Wilson (ed.), *Johnson. Prose and Poetry* (London: Rupert Hart Davis, 1968), 365.
39. I. Illich, *Limits to Medicine: The Expropriation of Health* (Harmondsworth: Penguin, 1977).
40. See the discussion in Roy Porter and Dorothy Porter, *In Sickness and in Health: The British Experience 1650–1850* (London: Fourth Estate, 1988). Harriet Martineau, *Life in the Sick-Room: Essays by an Invalid* (2nd edn, London: Moxon, 1854); *idem*, *Autobiography*, 2 vols (London: Virago, 1983; 1st edn, 1877).
41. On Darwin's sensibilities see Janet Browne, *Charles Darwin: Voyaging, Volume I of a Biography* (New York: Knopf, 1995; London: Jonathan Cape, 1995).
42. Richard Hofstadter, *Social Darwinism in American Thought*

(Philadelphia: University of Pennsylvania Press, 1944); Robert C. Bannister, *Social Darwinism: Science and Myth in Anglo-American Social Thought* (Philadelphia: Temple University Press, 1979).

43. D. Harwood, *Love For Animals And How It Developed In Great Britain* (New York: Ph.D. Thesis, Columbia University, 1928); Keith Thomas, *Man and the Natural World* (London: Allen Lane, 1983; Harmondsworth: Penguin, 1983).
44. Nicolaas A. Rupke (ed.), *Vivisection in Historical Context* (London: Croom Helm, 1987).
45. Catherine Gallagher, 'The Body Versus the Social Body in the Works of Thomas Malthus and Henry Mayhew', in C. Gallagher and T. Laqueur (eds), *The Making of the Modern Body: Sexuality and Society in the Nineteenth Century* (Berkeley: University of California Press, 1987), 83–106; D. De Moulin, 'A Historical-Phenomenological Study of Bodily Pain in Western Medicine', *Bulletin of the History of Medicine*, xlviii (1974), 540–70. For cross-cultural perspectives, see A. Kleinman, *Social Origins of Distress and Disease: Depression, Neurasthenia, and Pain in Modern China* (New Haven, Conn.: Yale University Press, 1986); Robert T. Anderson and Scott T. Anderson, 'Culture and Pain', in *The Puzzle of Pain* (East Roseville, Australia: G & B Arts International, 1994), 120–38.
46. Quoted in Wiener, *Reconstructing the Criminal*, 178.
47. Miles Weatherall, *In Search of a Cure: A History of the Pharmaceutical Industry* (Oxford: Oxford University Press, 1990); Martin S. Pernick, *A Culculus of Suffering. Pain, Professionalism and Suffering in Nineteenth Century America* (New York: Columbia University Press, 1985).
48. L. Gwei-Djen and J. Needham, *Celestial Lancets: A History and Rationale of Acupuncture* (Cambridge: Cambridge University Press, 1980).
49. I. Illich, *Limits to Medicine: The Expropriation of Health* (Harmondsworth: Penguin, 1977).
50. On hospices see Sandol Stoddard, *The Hospice Movement. A Better Way of Caring for the Dying* (London: Jonathan Cape, 1978); R. Lammerton, *Care of the Dying* (Harmondsworth: Penguin, 1980); E. Kubler-Ross, *On Death and Dying* (London: Tavistock, 1970). There is much wisdom in Eric J. Cassell's *The Nature of Suffering and the Goals of Medicine* (New York: Oxford University Press, 1991), but he hardly gets to grips with the specifics of medical attitudes towards pain and pain relief.

BEYOND THE FRONTIERS OF SCIENCE? RELIGIOUS ASPECTS OF ALTERNATIVE MEDICINE

Mike Saks

Introduction

This chapter focuses primarily on the growth and development of alternative medicine in Britain since the mid-nineteenth century. It starts by charting the meaning of the concept of alternative medicine in this country, which is contrasted with that of medical orthodoxy. The notion of medical orthodoxy became increasingly associated with the ideology of 'science' as it developed through the nineteenth into the twentieth century. This link with 'science' can be seen as an attempt to legitimate the biomedical approach on which orthodoxy came to be based in a situation of intense occupational interest-based rivalry between those lying within the newly established ranks of the medical profession and outsiders who challenged their position. The corollary of this is that alternative medicine was castigated for being 'unscientific' in its approach to health and suffering – a critique of unorthodox therapies that continues to be echoed in contemporary Britain by the medical establishment, comprised of leading figures in the Royal Colleges and the British Medical Association.

The charge of being 'unscientific' levelled against alternative medicine by the medical elite was further accentuated ideologically when the therapies concerned were also tainted by the profession with the labels of sorcery and superstition. Such labels were – and, to the extent to which they are employed today, still are – heavily laden with religious overtones designed to associate them with earlier, allegedly more primitive, health care practices. Judged against the touchstone of a tightly drawn concept of 'religion', it is noted that some of the therapeutic approaches encompassed within the umbrella of alternative medicine can indeed be seen to have religious connections – affinities which become even more apparent when the definition is stretched more widely. It is argued, however, that paradoxically – despite the ideological invective – even religiously based alternative therapies may not differ greatly from orthodox medicine in the degree to which they can be viewed as being scientific. The chapter begins, though, by outlining the more general development of alternative medicine in this country.

The development of alternative medicine in Britain

The notion of alternative medicine is defined here relativistically to include those health care practices employed to promote health and alleviate suffering that are not typically supported by the medical establishment – according to such indicators as the degree of incorporation into the orthodox medical curriculum and the level of orthodox medical research funding that they receive.[1] Crucial to its emergence in Britain was the professional underwriting of medicine in 1858 through the Medical Registration Act, which for the first time formally defined the parameters of both orthodox and unorthodox medicine at a national level. Thereafter, the single register that was established by the medical profession, together with its monopoly of title and preferential legal rights in terms of scope of practice and state employment, clearly distinguished the two fields – even if non-medically qualified alternative therapists were still able to treat patients under the provisions of the Common Law.[2]

In this context, the watershed that was reached signalled the transcendence of the comparatively open field that prevailed in the health care arena in the period preceding the mid-nineteenth century, in which a plurality of groups ministered to the needs of the sick on a more level playing field in an increasingly market-based system. From the sixteenth and seventeenth century onwards this included practitioners whose repertoire ranged from the use of herbs and minerals to the employment of charms and incantations in ritual healing. Religious ideas played an important part in these areas in the pre-industrial era, as highlighted by the belief in the King's touch, which was thought to cure such diseases as scrofula and linked to the powers associated with the divine nature of kingship.[3] In addition, prayer and pilgrimage were seen as antidotes to melancholy and other conditions, while diet and exercise were viewed as being important for maintaining a state of Christian wellbeing.[4] Healing, though, also had strong associations with witchcraft, in which a supernatural cause of the person's condition could be invoked in a tradition where women healers challenged the male dominance of the Church.[5]

While the role of the Church in healing declined,[6] the range of health care practices on offer in this pluralistic system expanded still further in the eighteenth and early nineteenth centuries. In this period, the emphasis began to transfer in a shifting socio-political order from increasingly discredited fields like astrology – which did not sit too comfortably with the notions of free will and the omnipotence of God in Christian belief [7] – towards an even wider span of entrepreneurial activity in the ever more competitive environment that was developing. This covered the operation of the growing band of purveyors of patent medicines, as well as bonesetters, naturopaths and hydropaths, whose activities still encompassed a significant religious element – as illustrated by the symbolism embodied in the names of Friar's Balsam and the Golden Vatican Pill, preparations which were widely on sale to the public of the day.[8] In this vein, it is important to stress that, notwithstanding the array of health practitioners involved – amongst whom numbered physicians and surgeons in addition to the so-called 'irregulars' – a heavy onus was also placed on self-help in health care without direct economic reward, not least in relation to the support provided in cases of ill health based on neighbourliness and religious duty.[9]

What was to follow from the mid-nineteenth legislation that legitimated the newly forged medical monopoly, however, was the emergence of a more secularly based and unified medical profession, largely set against the diverse cluster of alternative therapies with which its members had previously been more closely associated. These initially included practices such as homoeopathy and herbalism which have subsequently developed into an even broader span of approaches, ranging from acupuncture and chiropractic at one end of the spectrum to aromatherapy and spiritual healing at the other. Despite the escalating power of the medical profession, however, there has been an expansion of the numbers of the non-medically qualified exponents of this growing range of therapies since the 1950s – such that by the early 1980s these had reached some 30,000 practitioners[10] who are increasingly grouped into organised protoprofessional bodies in this country.[11]

This trend was fuelled by a significant rise in popular interest in alternative therapies. This was encouraged by the development of a counterculture in the West from the 1960s onwards, as growing links were made with philosophies derived from the East through the opening up of cultural boundaries. This exacerbated the attack on the safety and efficacy of orthodox 'scientific' medicine at this time, as well as serving as a platform for exploring alternative approaches in the health arena – not to mention cultivating a more egalitarian relationship between client and therapist. However, it would be mistaken to see this trend as simply representing the effects of a mass New Age conversion to a different belief system, not least because most consumers of the alternatives have by no means abandoned orthodox medicine. Whatever the explanation of the developing interest in the medical alternatives, the scale of such interest is well reflected in a recent public opinion poll indicating that approximately three-quarters of the British population want more mainstream unorthodox treatments to be delivered within the National Health Service, from which – notwithstanding the rights of practice conferred by the Common Law – they have hitherto been conspicuously excluded.[12]

Nonetheless, despite this contemporary desire for incorporation, such therapies remain counterposed in a number of respects to the biomedical orthodoxy that became established as the mainstream fount of knowledge of the British medical profession. It should be emphasised, though, that the development of unorthodox medicine has not followed a completely linear pattern. Indeed, in the decades before its recent revival in this country from the mid-twentieth century onwards, alternative medicine had generally lapsed into a period of marked decline in popularity in the wake of the establishment of the new medical orthodoxy.[13] This was undoubtedly partly related to the initial promise felt to derive from the emergence of 'scientific' medicine, in a situation where intense occupational rivalry between those inside and outside the ranks of the medical profession provided a backcloth to a succession of ideological assaults by the elite of the profession on alternative practitioners.

Alternative medicine as unscientific superstition

In this sense, a major thrust of the attack by medical orthodoxy on alternative medicine may well have originated from the economic, political and status interests of the elite of the medical profession in retaining and extending its position of monopolistic privilege won in the mid-nineteenth century.[14] Such interests seem to have formed at least a partial basis for the development of the new era of scientific medicine centred on the concept of the body as to a large extent separate from the mind and divisible into parts that can be repaired when they break down – whether through drugs, surgery or some other mechanism. As Jewson describes, this biomedical conception arose from the shift from the eighteenth-century notion of 'bedside medicine', in which affluent clients could influence the treatment provided by the practitioner in a patronage system, to the nineteenth-century rise of 'hospital medicine' where the classification of disease was central. The process of scientific transformation then moved on in the twentieth century to the stage of 'laboratory medicine', where stress was placed on intervention based on laboratory diagnosis, which was even further removed from the individual patient as the body came to be conceived in terms of the cell.[15]

Within this conception of medical science, leading figures in the British medical profession have for long considered alternative therapies – which are typically underpinned by more holistic philosophical conceptions, bringing together both physical and mental processes – to be beyond the bounds of credibility at the ideological level. To be sure, alternative practitioners from the mid-nineteenth century onwards were subject to many accusations, including that of trading on public gullibility by fleecing clients of their money while building up their own personal fortunes and threatening the very health of the population through the practice of quackery.[16] However, a major and increasingly pronounced aspect of the attack on their integrity was that they were not concerned with scientific understanding in the same way as their medical counterparts, being seen as at best involved in the 'so-called' science of healing.[17] Crucially, in this context, following the Enlightenment, alternative medicine was not just held to be non-scientific, but also labelled as irrational superstition[18] – thereby highlighting the religious basis of such therapies in an increasingly secular society.[19]

This line is also reflected in the response of the medical establishment to the resurgence of public interest in alternative therapies in Britain and other Western societies since the 1950s. While there have been many ideological strands to the contemporary medical critique of unorthodox therapies, this has been even more forcefully centred on the claim that they are non-scientific – whether through their overt association with fraud or other related methodological flaws.[20] Homoeopathy, for instance, has characteristically been seen as based on anecdotal evidence as opposed to rigorous scientific evaluation,[21] while spiritual healing has usually been dismissed by the leading medical journals as 'hocus pocus'.[22] It was but a few small steps from these accusations of scientific irrationality to tarring such therapies with the brush of witchcraft. Thus, for example, not only was acupuncture disparagingly likened by the medical establishment to snakes' blood and crocodiles' teeth in the treatment of illness,[23] but it was also felt that chiropractic 'ought to be as extinct as divination of the future by examination of bird's entrails'.[24]

Similar themes are also intriguingly expressed in the 1986 report by the British Medical Association on alternative therapy.[25] The first half of this report in fact is devoted not to alternative medicine itself, but to reviewing the history of medicine and extolling the achievements of modern scientific progress – from the introduction of vaccinations to the development of surgical anaesthesia. Only at this point do the alternatives to medicine come into the frame, when they are generally disparaged. This is largely because they are held to derive from different systems of understanding to orthodox medicine which 'are incompatible with the corpus of scientific knowledge'[26] as they do not accord with the scientific method based on systematic observation to discover the laws governing natural phenomena. Modern medicine is consequently declared to have become 'increasingly separated from doctrines embracing superstition, magic and the supernatural',[27] thereby providing a pivotal axis for distinguishing it from primitive and outmoded alternative therapies – and particularly those involving religious sects and cults directly claiming to cure disease.

Religious aspects of alternative medicine

In view of this ideological assault, it should not be too surprising that some religious aspects of alternative medicine persist today, notwithstanding arguments about increasing secularisation in the modern era. This is clear even when judged in terms of a narrow definition of religion, based on a belief in supernatural beings.[28] The classic example within this conceptual framework is that of healing, in which the largest number of alternative practitioners in Britain are currently concentrated. Such an approach is typically held to involve the use of therapeutic energy in enhancing the health of the patient. This is a diverse area with a very long history deriving from shamanism and magic – the latter of which has created a strained relationship with the Church since medieval times in Western societies. It comes closest to being classifiable as religious when it is believed that divine intervention occurs – as in the case of certain forms of faith healing based on marshalling the energy of the patient and spiritual healing involving the transmission of energy from the healer to the patient.[29] These healers tend to see the source of their healing as being God or discarnate entities who have been healers or doctors when alive – such as Harry Edwards, one of Britain's best known spiritual healers, who held that his spirit guides were Lister and Pasteur.[30]

But if this example raises the question of how 'alternative' alternative medicine really is, it is worth emphasising that even these types of healing have tended to be viewed as heresy by organised religion. Here too, however, there is something of an irony in the contemporary context when healers in this country have increasingly themselves become more systematically organised into specific bodies like the National Federation of Spiritual Healers and the Confederation of Healing Organisations, an umbrella group. In relation to organised religion, though, note should be made of the Churches' Council for Health and Healing which was established in the 1940s with the aim of encouraging the Healing Ministry and a membership including all the main church denominations, the Royal Colleges, hospital chaplaincy organisations and healing groups.[31] The founding of the Churches' Council underlines that a boundary exists between the orthodox and unorthodox in relation to both medicine and religion. This has been formalised for British pilgrimages of the sick and dying to Lourdes where a committee of doctors has traditionally decided which, if any, cures might be deemed divinely miraculous by the Church.[32]

One type of religious healing which has been influential in Britain that is certainly medically unorthodox is Christian Science, based on the nineteenth-century work of its American founder, Mary Baker Eddy. For Christian Scientists pain, disease, injury and death are illusions centred on mistaken thoughts resulting from 'malicious animal magnetism' which can be overcome with the assistance of authorised Christian Science practitioners.[33] In this sense, it contrasts with faith healing in which pain and suffering are not only believed to exist, but also regarded as fulfilling a purpose in God's plan and being incapable of correction by humankind alone, without divine intervention.[34] There are links here with the more recent development of Scientology that emerged from Dianetics, which was invented by L. Ron Hubbard in the early 1950s.[35] This philosophy is based on the dual tenets that the mind is reincarnated and that the majority of human ailments are psychosomatic. Paralleling Eddy's belief system, illness is seen to be derived from the recording of 'engrams' of painful experience which fulfil a similar role to 'malicious animal magnetism' and can be treated by trained 'auditors'.[36] It was on this basis that auditing or processing became the central method of knowing and controlling the self in Scientology, a self-proclaimed applied religious philosophy.[37]

At this point it should be stressed that not all alternative therapies with an overtly religious dimension involve trained therapists; self-help can also play a significant part. The case of Pentecostalism, where the most common type of healing is either personal or collective prayer, often with a direct plea for divine intervention, provides a classic illustration. This is highlighted by the account by Allen and Wallis of the health behaviour of members of the Assemblies of God in Scotland where many of the congregation believed that disease could be caused by the Devil and that God sometimes sends illness as a punishment. In this context, divine healing through the special gift of the Holy Spirit or faith in Christ was held to facilitate recovery, either by itself or in conjunction with medical treatment. Prayer was undertaken through the direct laying on of hands, at a distance or via a material medium taken to the patient. Interestingly, it is argued in this study that this particular 'deviant' belief system was sustained in face of the dominance of medical orthodoxy through both internal legitimations and the relative sectarian isolation of members of the Assemblies of God from the wider community in their everyday interactions.[38]

There may be parallels here between the contemporary practices of the Assemblies of God and the use of relics in healing in earlier times. As far as the modern context is concerned, though, it should be noted that much alternative medicine is not directly related to religion in the more restricted understanding of this term. However, while there seems at first sight to be very little linkage between alternative therapies like herbalism and acupuncture and religion, this is a chimera – particularly given wider debates about how the concept of 'religion' should be defined. This is very apparent when looser conceptions are employed which place less stress on the supernatural and more on deeply held convictions finding expression in moral imperatives, not least those involving reference to the human spirit.[39] This opens up the consideration of alternative approaches based on differing cultural conceptions of the human body to that conceived by orthodox biomedicine.

This is well exemplified by some forms of ethnic medicine, such as Ayurvedic medicine which is primarily used to serve the Asian community in Britain through practitioners like hakims.[40] This system derives from ancient texts covering all aspects of living that provide a complete guide to health, well-being and spiritual energy. Within this system three types of activity are held to exist – the active creation of energy (Rajas), the passive destruction of or resistance to energy (Tamas) and the unifying preservation of energy (Sattva). These interrelate with the five elements (Doshas) of the human being and the universe, which comprise earth, water, fire, air and ether. The aim of the system is to bring the internal environment into balance through appropriate diet and living habits – following diagnosis and treatment based on such practices as massage and meditation – in order to counteract adverse alterations in the external world.[41]

There are similarities here too with traditional Chinese medicine – including that of moxibustion, herbalism, shiatsu, exercise and acupuncture, the classical practice of which is centred on Taoist notions of the harmony of the universe.[42] As such, it too involves balancing forces, in this case the polar forces of Yin and Yang – particularly in relation to the energy flows along the twelve meridians located in the body. Like Ayurveda it also involves a process of diagnosis based on the total health profile of the patient, encompassing the physical, mental, emotional and spiritual – a profile to which a response is made through a combination of one or more of the treatments on offer in this medical system.[43] Acupuncture is undoubtedly the most popular of the various forms of traditional Chinese medicine in this country in terms of both patients and practitioners.[44] In this respect, it is more widely employed than Ayurvedic medicine, although admittedly not always by practitioners fully embracing its ancient philosophy.[45]

Central to the current demand for such therapies, therefore, is their characteristic philosophical tenet that they are underpinned by a holistic approach encompassing mind, body and spirit. This they share with many other related alternative therapies, including practices like homoeopathy and naturopathy. Indeed, the popularity of these alternatives to medicine in part rests on the fact that, in a society in which consumer health preferences have shifted, they typically claim to go beyond the physical reductionist approach on which orthodox biomedicine is primarily based.[46] As such, they can be regarded as reviving a discourse akin to that underlying the theory of humours that formed an important part of health care up to the mid-nineteenth century in Britain – which was equally pivoted on maintaining equilibrium between the various elements in the conceptual universe.[47] In its modern incarnation, the focus of the holistic New Age approach to health and suffering in the latter half of the twentieth century is also on balancing the flow of bodily and mental energy in treating the client in his/her broader environmental context.[48] As such, holism, which strongly embraces the concept of the spirit, could be construed as at least having more loosely cast religious overtones.

Even where they have apparently been successful, however, religiously based unorthodox therapies – whether directly or indirectly derived – have generally been decried by leading figures in the medical profession for being based on factors like spontaneous remission and the power of suggestion rather than the principles typically outlined by their practitioners.[49] This mirrors the earlier reaction of the Church to doctors who were distrusted as being potential aetheists and subjected to persecution – especially as far as anatomical dissections, which were felt to preclude resurrection, were concerned.[50] The contemporary medical response could be seen to represent a parallel attempt to assert the superiority of orthodox medical science over religiously-oriented unorthodox approaches. Does, however, alternative medicine really lie beyond the frontiers of science as defined in the context of medical orthodoxy? Or are there more continuities than first meet the eye?

Alternative medicine and orthodox medicine: two sides of the same coin?

In answering this question, much depends on how the operation of science is conceived. Traditional conceptions of science tend to be based on the notion that it is centred on rational and open-minded investigation in pursuit of the truth.[51] However, while this is the image that the medical establishment has sought to cultivate in its self-presentation as 'scientific', it has come under radical challenge over the last few decades for misrepresenting the nature of the scientific community, particularly in terms of its truth claims. In this regard, pivotal critiques have been made by Popper[52] and Kuhn[53] respectively highlighting the pitfalls of verificationism and drawing attention to the socially constructed paradigms of untestable assumptions within which 'normal science' takes place. Such work has led a number of recent contributors to deny that there is a clear division between science and non-science in terms of its impartiality and transcendental objectivity.[54] This is perhaps most clearly thrown into focus in this context by the work of Horton who has sought to underline the parallels between magic and witchcraft in traditional African religious thought and orthodox Western science.[55]

As a result of this debate, the issue can be raised as to whether there is a fundamental difference between orthodox medicine and even narrowly defined religiously based strands of alternative medicine in terms of their scientific credentials. This is accentuated by the fact that the scientific status of biomedicine has itself come under serious challenge in Britain from a variety of quarters in the modern era – not least from public disaffection with the safety of orthodox medicine in the wake of revelations from the 1960s onwards about the potentially dangerous side-effects of a number of drugs and the consequences of unnecessary surgery.[56] For all the achievements of medical orthodoxy, this challenge highlights just how few of its practices are indeed based on rigorous research. It also underlines the limitations of the randomised controlled trial which has so often been held out as the key methodological standard for the evaluation of treatments in mainstream biomedicine, yet is of debatable applicability to many aspects not only of orthodox medicine, but also of unorthodox medicine – given the focus on the individualised treatment of the person rather the condition itself that is usually involved.[57]

But if this dilutes the potency of the ideological attack by the medical establishment on alternative medicine as unscientific, this is even further accentuated by its specific response to alternative medicine which has been far from even handed. This is exemplified by the initially negative reception given to classical acupuncture in the 1960s and early 1970s despite its therapeutic promise in areas where orthodox treatment seemed relatively ineffective[58] and, more recently, by the methodologically shaky medical critique of the Bristol Cancer Help Centre – with its spiritual, psychological and emotional approach to illness – for increasing mortality rates as compared to conventional medicine.[59] Its reaction to more overtly religious aspects of alternative medicine has also often appeared to be less than impartial. Inglis argues, for instance, that medical research into healing was effectively blocked by the medical establishment up to the mid-1970s largely because of the threat to doctors of being struck off for collaborating with the medically unqualified. He amplifies this claim by describing how the *British Medical Journal* ignored reports in the 1960s of the fieldbreaking and favourable double blind trials undertaken on the effect of the laying on of hands by two biochemists, Professor Bernard Grad of McGill University and Justa Smith, a Franciscan nun.[60]

This case also indicates that alternative medicine – including religiously based unorthodox therapies – may be more positively sustained by evidence than is suggested by the link made by the medical elite with non-scientific superstition. Certainly, small-scale randomised controlled trials in fields such as chiropractic and homoeopathy lend some support to this claim.[61] This support is extended further if a more pluralistic view is taken of the most fruitful research methodologies for evaluating health care. In this respect, for instance, measurement of the relatively high levels of consumer satisfaction commonly associated with unorthodox therapies increases their currency, although it is by no means a perfect tool.[62] This is not, of course, to deny that there are substantial shortcomings in the empirical basis of unorthodox practice, nor that some of the alternatives to medicine centred heavily on religion – such as Christian Science and Pentecostalism – can be set within the self-fulfilling frame of reference of believers.[63] However, as Brooke observes, it is difficult historically to disentangle science and religion and this appears to apply no less to the epistemological threads of both orthodox medicine and unorthodox forms of therapy in Britain today.[64]

The parallel between these two areas is confirmed by the increasing appreciation by orthodox practitioners of the need to take a more holistic spiritual approach.[65] In this vein, even the critical 1986 report of the British Medical Association acknowledged that the appeal of alternative therapies was the compassion offered to patients and stressed that good doctors 'recognise the close relationship between mind and body and the importance of the patient's emotional and spiritual perceptions'.[66] Indeed, the latest report of the British Medical Association on complementary therapies in 1993 takes a strikingly more positive stance on the medically unorthodox, including healing and other religiously oriented therapies.[67] In the wake of rising public demand for unconventional therapies, it is felt that orthodox doctors should work more collaboratively with practitioners of such therapies, with greater emphasis placed on unconventional medicine in both the orthodox medical curriculum and research.

This stance has also been reflected by a growing number of doctors themselves offering alternative therapies at grass-roots level – whether this be in pain clinics or indeed in general practice contexts where such therapies are becoming increasingly commonly offered in Britain. Such shifts in the nature of practice have clearly been sustained by the support not only of members of the public, but most critically of a growing number of politicians and influential public figures. In this latter respect, it should be noted, for example, that it was Prince Charles, in his role of President of the British Medical Association, who instigated the recent consideration by this organisation of alternative therapies.[68] These developments have progressively helped to transform these therapies from being the quackery of yesterday to the more respectable complementary medicine of today.[69] In this light, there now seems to be a stronger case than ever before for seeing alternative medicine in general and the religiously based elements of unorthodox practice in particular as one of the two sides of the same medical coin.

Conclusion

Such a conclusion should not, of course, mask the very real limits on the extent to which the medical and allied health professions are taking up alternative therapies, particularly as regards faith and spiritual healers of the more narrowly defined religious kind. And even where doctors and other health professionals like nurses and physiotherapists employ therapies like acupuncture that have some quasi-religious overtones, they frequently tend to do so in transmuted form – such that the traditional holistic emphasis on the spirit is sacrificed within a biomedical frame of reference, restricting both the scope and the theoretical underpinning of the therapy concerned.[70] This trend is counterbalanced by the fact that religiously based alternative therapies are themselves not always applied in a holistic manner by unorthodox practitioners, who occasionally appear only to be making a ritualistic nod in this direction to affirm their ideological purity.[71] This reification of physical technique by some alternative therapists raises further questions about how far religious aspects of unorthodox medicine really do lie beyond the frontiers of science as understood in this context.

It may, however, be beneficial to reformulate the question at hand to consider not so much whether it is reasonable for orthodox medicine to label religious and other forms of alternative medicine as distinctively unscientific, but rather to ask why leading figures in the profession have deployed the ideology of non-science and superstition against unorthodox practitioners in the manner described. There are a number of possible explanations, the most benevolent of which views the stance taken by the medical elite as part of its altruistic desire to protect the wellbeing of the population. However, as the foregoing discussion indicates, there are sufficient cracks in the edifice of orthodox medicine to cast doubt on how far this account stands up to critical scrutiny. It seems more likely in fact from recent work that the anti-scientific ideology has been advanced against unorthodox practitioners since the mid-nineteenth century primarily to bolster professional self-interests in establishing and maintaining the medical monopoly – in order to legitimate the income, power and status of the profession in a situation of intense occupational rivalry.[72]

Having said this, the medical profession is not simply a privileged island operating in a sea of occupational competition, but can also be seen – in a perhaps not totally unconnected manner – to be carrying out a wider societal role, including that of social control. In this respect, Turner argues that many of the previous regulatory moral functions of mainstream religion have been taken on by medicine, in its policing of social deviance.[73] On this interpretation, other professionals too are becoming increasingly involved in these functions in a more secular society – including alternative practitioners as they become incorporated into mainstream medicine – with the doctor replacing the priest as the primary guardian of social values, under the guise of an ideology of scientism. This only serves to highlight the complexities of locating the boundaries of science and religion, as exponents of orthodox and alternative medicine grapple with the dilemmas of addressing health and suffering in contemporary Britain, as in many other countries in the international context.

Glossary of terms

The following basic glossary of terms used to describe some of the more popular forms of alternative medicine that figure in the text is included to assist the reader unfamiliar with such therapies.[74] It is illustrative of the range of approaches on offer, rather than comprehensive:

Acupuncture: The insertion of needles into the body for therapeutic purposes.

Aromatherapy: The use of essential oils extracted from plants, typically administered through massage.

Chiropractic: A type of manipulation of the spine and other joints based on the effects on the nervous system.

Faith Healing: The use of the energy of the subject to promote healing, relying on faith.

Herbalism: The employment of plant material to prevent and treat illness.

Homoeopathy: A therapy based on giving minute dosages of remedies and the principle that 'like cures like'.

Hydropathy: A water-based therapy such as drinking spa water or taking remedial showers/baths.

Naturopathy: An approach to prevention and treatment that is based on natural processes, including diet and exercise.

Osteopathy: A form of manipulation of the spine and other joints centred on realignment.

Spiritual Healing: A therapy based on energy being transmitted to the subject from the healer, who is at the heart of the process.

NOTES

1. Mike Saks, 'Introduction', in Mike Saks (ed.), *Alternative Medicine in Britain* (Oxford: Clarendon Press, 1992), 1–21.
2. Ivan Waddington, *The Medical Profession in the Industrial Revolution* (Goldenbridge: Gill & Macmillan, 1984).
3. Christina Larner, 'Healing in Pre-industrial Britain', in Saks (ed.), *Alternative Medicine in Britain*, 25–34.
4. Bryan Turner, *Medical Power and Social Knowledge* (London: Sage, 1987).
5. Anne Oakley, 'The Wisewoman and the Doctor', in Saks (ed.), *Alternative Medicine in Britain*, 35–42.
6. Charles Webster, 'Paracelsus Confronts the Saints: Miracles, Healing and the Secularization of Magic', *Journal of the Social History of Medicine* 8 (1995), 403–21.
7. Peter Wright, 'Astrology in Seventeenth-century England', in Saks (ed.), *Alternative Medicine in Britain*, 43–54.
8. Roy Porter, *Health for Sale: Quackery in England 1660–1850* (Manchester: Manchester University Press, 1989).
9. Roy Porter, *Disease, Medicine and Society in England 1550–1860* (London: Macmillan, 1987).

10. Stephen Fulder, *The Handbook of Alternative and Complementary Medicine*, 3rd edition (Oxford: Oxford University Press, 1996).
11. Mike Saks, 'The Wheel Turns? Professionalisation and Alternative Medicine in Britain'. Paper presented at International Sociological Association conference on Occupations and Professions: Changing Patterns, Definitions, Classifications, University of Nottingham, September 1996.
12. Mike Saks, 'The Alternatives to Medicine', in Jonathan Gabe, David Kelleher and Gareth Williams (eds), *Challenging Medicine* (London: Routledge, 1994).
13. See, for example, *Report as to the Practice of Medicine and Surgery by Unqualified Persons in the United Kingdom* (HMSO: London, 1910).
14. Mike Saks, 'From Quackery to Complementary Medicine: The Shifting Boundaries between Orthodox and Unorthodox Medical Knowledge', in Sarah Cant and Ursula Sharma (eds), *Complementary and Alternative Medicines: Knowledge in Practice* (London: Free Association Books, 1996), 27–43.
15. Nick Jewson, 'The Disappearance of the Sick Man from Medical Cosmology 1770–1870', *Sociology* 10 (1976), 225–44.
16. Paul Vaughan, *Doctors Commons: A Short History of the British Medical Association* (London: Heinemann, 1959).
17. BMJ, 'The Puff Professionals: New Cures', *British Medical Journal*, 3 October (1863), 375; Lancet, 'How Quackery Is Supported', *Lancet* 6 July (1889), 51.
18. See, for example, Lancet, 'Psychology of Quackery', *Lancet* 3 February (1934), 246.
19. Kenneth Thompson, 'Religion, Values and Ideology', in Robert Bocock and Kenneth Thompson (eds), *Social and Cultural Forms of Modernity* (Cambridge: Polity Press, 1992), 321–66.
20. Mike Saks, *Professions and the Public Interest: Medical Power, Altruism and Alternative Medicine* (London: Routledge, 1995).
21. Robert Eagle, *Alternative Medicine* (Futura: London, 1978).
22. Brian Inglis, *Natural Medicine* (Fontana: London, 1980).
23. BMJ, 'BMA Clinical Meeting, Cheltenham 24–27 October', *British Medical Journal* 2 November (1968), 320.
24. BMJ, 'The Flight from Science', *British Medical Journal* 5 January (1980), 1.
25. British Medical Assocation, *Report of the Board of Science and Education on Alternative Therapy* (London: BMA, 1986).
26. British Medical Assocation, *Report of the Board of Science and Education on Alternative Therapy*, 35.
27. British Medical Assocation, *Report of the Board of Science and Education on Alternative Therapy*, 61.
28. John Brooke, *Science and Religion: Some Historical Perspectives* (Cambridge: Cambridge University Press, 1991).
29. Fulder, *The Handbook of Alternative and Complementary Medicine*.
30. Jeremy Kingston, *Healing without Medicine* (London: Aldus Books, 1976).
31. Fulder, *The Handbook of Alternative and Complementary Medicine*.
32. Inglis, *Natural Medicine*.

33. Rennie Schoepflin, 'Christian Science Healing in America', in Norman Gevitz (ed), *Other Healers: Unorthodox Medicine in America* (Baltimore: Johns Hopkins University Press, 1988), 192–214.
34. John Lee, 'Social Change and Marginal Therapeutic Systems', in Roy Wallis and Peter Morley (eds), *Marginal Medicine* (London: Peter Owen, 1976), 23–41.
35. Roy Wallis, 'Dianetics: A Marginal Psychotherapy', in Wallis and Morley (eds), *Marginal Medicine*, 77–109.
36. Bryan Wilson, *Religious Sects: A Sociological Study* (London: Weidenfield and Nicolson, 1970).
37. Roy Wallis, 'The Sociology of the New Religions', *Social Studies Review* September (1985), 3–7.
38. Gillian Allen and Roy Wallis, 'Pentecostalists as a Medical Minority', in Wallis and Morley (eds), *Marginal Medicine* (London: Peter Owen, 1976), 110–37.
39. Brooke, *Science and Religion*.
40. Fulder, *The Handbook of Alternative and Complementary Medicine*.
41. J. Patricia Martin, 'Eastern Spirituality and Health Care', in Verna Carson (ed.), *Spiritual Dimensions of Nursing Practice* (Philadelphia: W. B. Saunders, 1989), 113–31.
42. Effie Poy Yee Chow, 'Traditional Chinese Medicine: A Holistic System', in J. Warren Salmon (ed.), *Alternative Medicines: Popular and Policy Perspectives* (London: Tavistock, 1985), 114–37.
43. Martin, 'Eastern Spirituality and Health Care', in Carson (ed.), *Spiritual Dimensions of Nursing Practice*.
44. Fulder, *The Handbook of Alternative and Complementary Medicine*.
45. Saks, *Professions and the Public Interest*.
46. Janet McKee, 'Holistic Health and the Critique of Western Medicine', *Social Science and Medicine* 26 (1988), 775–84.
47. Cecil Helman, *Culture, Health and Illness*, 2nd edition (London: Butterworth-Heinemann, 1990).
48. Kristine Alster, *The Holistic Health Movement* (Tuscaloosa: University of Alabama Press, 1989).
49. Bryan Turner, *Regulating Bodies: Essays in Medical Sociology* (London: Routledge, 1992).
50. Lee, 'Social Change and Marginal Therapeutic Systems', in Wallis and Morley (eds), *Marginal Medicine*.
51. See, for example, Robert Merton, *Social Theory and Social Structure* (New York: Free Press, 1968).
52. Karl Popper, *Conjectures and Refutations* (London: Routledge and Kegan Paul, 1963).
53. Thomas Kuhn, *The Structure of Scientific Revolutions*, 2nd edition (Chicago: Chicago University Press, 1970).
54. See, for instance, Michael Mulkay, *Sociology of Science: A Sociological Pilgrimage* (Milton Keynes: Open University Press, 1991); Andrew Webster, *Science, Technology and Society* (London: Macmillan, 1991).
55. Robin Horton, 'African Traditional Thought and Western Science', in Michael Young (ed.), *Knowledge and Control* (London: Collier-Macmillan, 1971), 208–66.

56. Donald Gould, *The Mĕdical Mafia* (London: Sphere, 1985).
57. Dennis MacEoin, 'The Myth of Clinical Trials', *Journal of Alternative and Complementary Medicine* 8 (1990), 15–18.
58. Mike Saks, 'The Paradox of Incorporation: Acupuncture and the Medical Profession in Modern Britain', in Saks (ed.), *Alternative Medicine in Britain*, 183–98.
59. Margaret Stacey, 'The Potential of Social Science for Complementary Medicine', *Complementary Medical Research* 5 (1991), 183–86.
60. Inglis, *Natural Medicine*.
61. Saks, 'The Alternatives to Medicine', in Gabe, Kelleher and Williams (eds), *Challenging Medicine*.
62. Ursula Sharma, *Complementary Medicine Today: Practitioners and Patients* (London: Routledge, 1992).
63. Arthur Nudelman, 'The Maintenance of Christian Science in a Scientific Society', in Wallis and Morley (eds), *Marginal Medicine*, 42–60; Allen and Wallis, 'Pentecostalists as a Medical Minority', in Wallis and Morley (eds), *Marginal Medicine*.
64. Brooke, *Science and Religion*.
65. See, for example, Jane Thompson, *Spiritual Considerations in the Prevention, Treatment and Cure of Disease* (Stocksfield: Oriel Press, 1984); Olly McGilloway and Freda Myco (eds), *Nursing and Spiritual Care* (London: Harper and Row, 1985).
66. British Medical Assocation, *Report of the Board of Science and Education on Alternative Therapy*, 78.
67. British Medical Assocation, *Complementary Medicine: New Approaches to Good Practice* (London: BMA, 1993).
68. Saks, 'From Quackery to Complementary Medicine', in Cant and Sharma (eds), *Complementary and Alternative Medicines*.
69. Saks, 'The Alternatives to Medicine', in Gabe, Kelleher and Williams (eds), *Challenging Medicine*.
70. Saks, 'The Paradox of Incorporation', in Saks (ed), *Alternative Medicine in Britain*.
71. Mike Saks, 'Alternative Therapies: Are They Holistic?', *Complementary Therapies in Nursing and Midwifery* 3 (1997), 4–8.
72. See, for example, Saks, *Professions and the Public Interest*.
73. Turner, *Regulating Bodies*.
74. For further information see, amongst others, Anthony Campbell, *Natural Health Handbook* (London: New Burlington Books, 1991); Andrew Stanway, *Complementary Medicine: A Guide to Natural Therapies* (Harmondsworth: Penguin Books, 1994).

AGENCY AND COMMUNITY: THE LOCATION AND DISPERSAL OF INVIDIA

Roland Littlewood

Community, as Raymond Williams[1] has reminded us, is a 'warmly persuasive' word. Who could protest against its engaging connotations of unifying common identity, of local solidarity and grounded purpose? Indeed, what location could one find better for alleviating human suffering than among one's empathetic neighbours? The word *care*, despite its earlier sense of a particular suffering or affliction which has to be endured, now has similar resonances of nurturance and support, as opposed to, say, *treatment* or *cure*. And yet in 1997, the popular connotations of those public health practices which in Britain are known as *community care*[2] are of violence, failure and fragmentation.

Over the past decade, the practice and the image of psychiatry in the British *inner-city* (like the term community, an apparently spatial designation, and one introduced from the United States for urban areas with a high concentration of poor, sick and non-white residents) has been dominated by a succession of moral panics involving black patients, generally young men diagnosed with schizophrenia, who are portrayed as the perpetrators of homicidal violence. Christopher Clunis, a black man who killed, apparently at random, a white stranger in an underground station, is one of a number of young men whose psychotic violence has led to the hasty enactment in the 1990s of legislative and administrative measures (notably the Supervision Register and Supervised Discharge Order) aimed at preventing severely mentally ill people from harming members of the public.[3] Under the new Care Programme Approach and Section 117 of the last Mental Health Act, detailed arrangements now have to be made to supervise and observe an involuntary patient's subsequent living arrangements and to ensure access to training and work:[4] a problematic undertaking when unemployment among young Afro-Britons is three times as high as for whites of the same age. There is an emphasis on the value, and on the regular administration, of injected antipsychotic medication.

British psychiatrists generally agree that whatever a schizophrenic illness may be, it cannot be easily eradicated yet it can be attenuated, or its recurrence avoided, by such *depot drugs*. When patients who have a diagnosis of schizophrenia together with case reports of socially disturbing behaviour are reluctant to take their medicine (*failure to comply*), the local *mental health team* are expected to take action to 'prevent another *Clunis*' as threatened disaster is now termed: for this particular individual has given his name to a public fear. Prescribed measures include increased medical and social work surveillance (*supervised discharge*) of the implausibly named *user* (or *consumer, client* or even *survivor*[5]), to provide early warning of danger, together with proposals to enforce compulsory treatment after discharge from hospital. Hospital staff have an increasingly custodial role, supervising users placed in *seclusion*, or sitting at the door of the now generally *open wards* to prevent their recalcitrant clients from running away. The more violent consumer will be transferred, sometimes at a distance of one hundred miles or more (in one case known to me, to Holland) into one of the new *intensive care units* provided by the private sector which parallel the closing of the old county mental hospitals in the move to *care in the community*. The actual national figures on the numbers of psychiatric patients in Britain are no longer collected,[6] and the current public debate follows personal anecdote or scandal, generally one involving the threat of extreme violence.

While progressing along this *pathway to care*, the consumer, their *carers* and the mental health professionals participate in a drama which spatially recapitulates themes of power, class, colour and locality. The carer (a rare person in the inner-city where young black men tend to live alone in one bedroom flats or not infrequently on the streets) is now well aware of the reported deaths of young black men with schizophrenia in Britain's most well-known security hospital, and frequently proposes cannabis as the cause for their relative's disturbed actions, recreational drug use being regarded by black Britons as less stigmatising and certainly less hazardous than an ascription of illness.[7] Black Britons have rates of diagnosed schizophrenia ten to fifteen times that of the white population; extrapolating from incidence rates to lifetime risk, perhaps one in ten will eventually be diagnosed as schizophrenic.[8]

Doctors and nurses are increasingly wary of the clients described in their casenotes with unctuous civility as 'this Afro-Caribbean gentleman'. Whilst the nurses, who spend their working lives on the ward, are more likely to be injured by patients than are doctors, both professions are voting with their feet, and there is a crisis of recruitment in urban psychiatric services. Whereas twenty years ago the weekly ward round might deal with psychodynamic or descriptive psychopathology, with the minutiae of diagnosis or with debate on the illness in relation to personality, environment and life experiences, ambitious nurses are now funded by their employers to take part-time degrees in business management, and just two themes now occupy the limited time available for each patient. The first is the assessment of violence to staff and others, *risk management* and *containment*, together with ways of reducing this by the deployment of medication. The second is the shortage of beds and staff and hence the continuous discharge of unwell consumers. Only the more *challenging* (dangerous) can be admitted. The staff juggle conflicting obligations: the Department of Health and the *purchasers* (not the actual users of the services but the health authority acting as the commissioning body in the new *internal market*), seeking to avoid further scandals, require all potentially dangerous patients *in the community* to be admitted, whilst at the same time no patient who is still a *potential risk*, whether to themselves or to others, should be discharged. With the diminishing number of available beds, all inner-city psychiatric units (the *providers*) are in a permanent state of *throughput* crisis, with the beds of those patients who are temporarily home on leave being occupied by newly admitted patients. Staff are warned by their *line managers* (whose salary – or at least its bonuses – are dependent on their financial acumen) when their *bed occupancy* rates fall below a local or national level agreed by the purchasers or when the *percentage overspend* rises. Uncompetitive units are closed and their staff *downsized* in a *skillmix*: that is, they lose their jobs.

It is hardly surprising that patients' advocates and support groups condemn this reliance on medication, the overcrowding of the remaining wards, the increasing use of compulsory admission and treatment procedures, the lack of psychotherapy and the regular transfer to locked wards and *secure units* specialising in *challenging behaviour*. Afro-British voluntary organisations in particular tend to perceive the mental health enterprise as white, middle class and racist, as adhering to a coercive biomedical model of containment which is too ready to mobilise the police, to have their children taken into the custody of the local authority, to interpret religion as madness, and to condemn anger as mania.[8] Yet the same organisations (which are now often publically funded), despite their commitment to a 'holistic' approach and their advocacy of less coercive non-medical therapies (aromatherapy, *shiatsu*, homeopathy, neoshamanic 'African healing'), summon the hospital psychiatric services and seek compulsory admission 'from the community' when a *survivor's* disruptive or threatening behaviour passes the limits of their own tolerance.

In this chapter I propose that the current clinical notion of the *community* is not just a physically delineated arena in which people live and work, and in which their suffering occurs and is alleviated, but as the virtual location to which suffering and misfortune are now dispersed. The current situation in British mental health policy is the positioning of humanistic and highly personalistic concepts of mental suffering within the unregulated health market of the last fifteen years, with resulting ambiguities over personal agency in sickness and health.

During the twentieth century, public policy governing the treatment of the severely mentally ill has generally not been inconsistent with professional theories which proposed a biological malfunctioning of the brain which ideally could be identified structurally or functionally (for example, Wing 1978[9]). And hence mentally ill people could not be held fully accountable for their illness nor for their actions, and treatment, aimed at reversing the malfunction, should be based in the hospital, the biomedical centre for restitution of suffering, where the isolation of the patient from the pressures and stigmas of everyday life contributed to their recovery, as well as making possible detailed clinical assessment (*the mental state interview*), trials of various medical drugs, and on eugenic grounds prevention of sexual relations.[6] Only in 1919 was a post-discharge psychiatric service contemplated outside the hospital, and out-patient clinics appeared as late as the 1930s. The county mental hospitals remained self-contained and closed institutions, often with their own farms, industrial units, staff housing and recreational facilities on the same site. Psychoanalysis, the alternative and private psychiatry, with its downplaying of biological difference in favour of interpersonal and intrapsychic processes leading to variations in individual psychological development, with its therapy of communication between the identified patient and their therapist which re-evoked earlier stages of development,[10] generally restricted itself to alleviating problems which were popularly identified as continuous with everyday circumstances – anxiety, depression, dissatisfaction with life – rather than as insanity. And psychoanalysis has been generally available to the middle classes only, as a contractual practice in private consulting rooms and outside the public health service.

In the 1950s and 1960s, a number of popular accounts of the social world of psychiatric hospitals and of the process of hospitalisation (such as Goffman 1961[11]) concluded that many of the symptoms of mental illness identified by the doctors in their patients were not brain diseases but rather the consequence of patterns of medical segregation and public stigmatisation. And these were reinforced by psychiatrists' own, similarly critical, studies of 'institutionalism'.[12] The 1959 Mental Health Act allowed compulsory treatment in hospitals without the old stigma of legal certification, following the 1954–7 Royal Commission on mental illness which had first proposed the expression *care in the community*. The location of much psychopathology was argued to be not in biology but in hospital life and in stigmatising and invalidating attitudes which promoted segregation. To some extent, this had always been professionally appreciated, and the large county asylums had provided farmwork and small-scale industrial workshops, less to speed the patient back to their home and work than to provide an environment which resembled everyday life whilst providing security and treatment: these activities, regarded as exploitative, dull and repetitive, had begun to fall out of favour in the early 1950s as the newly available antipsychotic drugs promised a cure.

The group of doctors who identified themselves in the 1960s as 'anti-psychiatrists' joined the new sociological critiques of hospitals to psychoanalytical hypotheses (derived from Winnicott) on the family origin of schizophrenia, the most common major psychiatric illness whose cultural ubiquity was then under question.[13] Mental illness was reread as the child's psychological response to the claustrophobic power of parents in the nuclear family: a family which was primarily coercive and from which any individual, particularly the putative patient, had to be liberated.[14] Parallels were repeatedly made between the then intellectually fashionable anti-colonial liberation movements and the individual's struggle against Western institutions of social control, notably the family but also public education, the criminal, law, religion and social policy.[15] Herbert Marcuse proposed our 'liberation from the affluent society',[16] and 'liberation' became a concept for public discussion: individualistic and dramatic, political, visual and medical theories and images cross-cutting in a distinct sociocultural milieu. The critical influence of the French philosopher Michel Foucault was acknowledged (even though he had himself favoured a therapeutic role for the family). Whilst not providing any socialist interpretation of mental illness,[17] anti-psychiatry's quest for individual liberation from closed institutions was subsumed into the voluntaristic rhetoric of what came to be known as the 'Counterculture'. Following the popular antiquarian anthropology which proposed the Amazonian shaman as a lunatic cured in an inspirational vision quest validated by his own society,[18] the anti-psychiatrists set up a number of communal living houses where patients could heal themselves in an 'open milieu' of empathy and supported self-healing, and which were termed *communities*. The psychotic was acclaimed less as the victim of an oppressive social order than the autonomous culture hero whose unfettered madness was a creative act of resistance.[19] Some *survivors* (of medical treatment) formed themselves into liberation groups such as the Mental Patients Union and the later Network For Alternatives to Psychiatry with the support of sympathetic doctors.[20] By the 1970s, social work students were taught to regard themselves as protectors of their patients against the medical establishment who simply sought to contain legitimate dissent.

In 1982 Peter Sedgwick questioned the equation of anti-psychiatry with political radicalism, and in a close reading of Laing denounced him as a reactionary romantic.[21] So far from being a socialist, Laing, he maintained, had simply drafted into a new theory of the family such fashionable leftist idioms as 'alienation' and 'mystification' quite independently of any specified economic and historical processes. Yet Sedgwick[21] still declared himself in favour of a holistic 'anti-positivist' and 'anti-Cartesian' affirmation of mind/body unity; and the idea that what psychiatrists read as a disease was at some more profound level meaningful was influential in a public debate which blamed society – or at least its psychiatrists – for the stigmatisation of mental illness (even if the image of the psychotic as a contemporary prophet did not prove quite so enduring). Since the eighteenth century, there had always been a popular suspicion of doctors for falsely imprisoning the sane, or which more radically proposed psychotic illness as a potentially valid communication.[18,22] The Counterculture, reframed as political libertarianism – increasingly right-wing libertarianism – allowed this view greater publicity in national debate, and certainly made it intellectually respectable. Few university students in the late sixties and early seventies (medical students always excepted) did not have a copy of Laing or Cooper on their shelves; by the late eighties, they were to hold political and administrative office. If the European anti-psychiatrists offered a superficially 'left' libertarianism, the American psychiatrist Thomas Szasz[23] had provided a rigorous 'right' market critique, less popular then in Britain than in the United States, in which he proposed that mental illnesses were never brain diseases, and therefore the individual was always responsible and coercive treatment could never be justified: if he or she wanted help for a perceived problem they could find themselves a private psychoanalyst in what he termed *contractual psychiatry*. If they didn't request advice, they were to be left alone or if guilty of a crime sent to prison in the usual way. Szasz antagonised his medical colleagues by noting parallels between their procedures of investigation and evidence and those of the Inquisition, as he denounced not only involuntary hospitalisation but all *institutional* [publically funded] *psychiatry*.[24]

In Britain, Laing had emphasised the liberatory potential he perceived in Foucault's writing on the politics of psychiatry, and after some initial reluctance the Royal College of Psychiatrists was persuaded to join the American Psychiatric Association in criticising the medical internment of Soviet dissidents. These concerns and influences came together in a shared public acceptance that psychiatric hospitalisation, whether coercive or not, was potentially dehumanising, and that hospital procedures for dealing with what was really psychological *stress* (another warmly persuasive term and one in which the cause of illness lay in actions outside the individual) were, at best, doubtful. A number of scandals in psychiatric hospitals, particularly those for the mentally handicapped in the 1960s and 1970s, strengthened the influence sought by pressure groups such as the National Association for Mental Health (now renamed MIND) which moved from providing training towards political advocacy, particularly after MIND's appointment of an American civil rights lawyer. Together with the example of the earlier hospital-based 'therapeutic communities', which had generally worked with personality difficulties and non-psychotic illness to emphasise group processes in a systems-theory model rather than attempting the cure of individual disease,[25] this led to a general agreement – shared by the Ministry of Health, liberal doctors and social workers, and by the informed public – that psychiatric facilities should be provided close to peoples' homes rather than in the distant Victorian asylums. In 1962, the government's Hospital Plan for England and Wales had already recommended that the mentally ill needed only brief hospital admissions for the administration of drugs, for after that they could be cared for primarily by the local social services.[6] Psychiatrists enthusiastically agreed that their future location would be in small 'district' general hospitals alongside their colleagues in other medical specialisms. In 1981 the Conservative Government proposed that within fifteen years all psychiatric hospitals would be finally closed.[26]

Thus so far: a move from biomedical objectification of disease processes to a liberal humanitarianism, with an optimistic assumption that popular attitudes to mental illness were not stigmatising. The notion of 'health' was changing from something (*pace* Isaiah Berlin) we might call 'negative health' (the absence of the doctor's disease) to 'positive health' as promoted by the World Health Organisation and various schools of complementary medicine – a moral and totalising ambition of complete bodily and mental fitness and personal transformation at the very highest level of functioning and life satisfaction: with a consequent shift from treatment (by others) to (self) achievement.

The passage of socialist intellectuals and professionals towards the libertarian and 'anti-welfarist' New Right in the 1970s and 1980s has been recently noted in many bracing British and American memoirs. Whilst this was perhaps a not uncommon generational phenomenon, in the 1980s British social politics as a whole moved closer to the American: from a paternalist welfare consensus with its recognition of the corporate role of trade unions and professional bodies, to an open acknowledgement of robust individual competition, a distrust of professional expertise, with settlement of differences increasingly determined by the courts, with a media-articulated appeal to the individual voter as an interested consumer rather than as a member of a political grouping. The civil service, BBC, trade unions, social workers, the medical profession and even lawyers (the emergent power in the area of health) have all had their powers of determining standards and practice curtailed. As public organisations they have been drastically reduced in influence, whilst a series of new particular interest organisations – on the quality of housing, health and manufactured goods – has grown up. Once known as *pressure groups*, since they have themselves gone into business as *service providers* they are now generally termed the *voluntary sector* as opposed to the *public* (governmental funded and publicly accountable) *sector*. Anti-psychiatry seems to have proved remarkably congenial to market capitalism. With support from biological psychiatrists, who favoured psychophysiological interpretations of insanity but whose pharmaceutical drugs still do not 'cure' but merely 'alleviate' schizophrenia, *mental health care* (as it became termed) was dispersed into the hypothetical community with increasingly shorter stays in psychiatric units now based in the local general hospitals. Mental health policy as determined by the Conservative governments has increasingly shifted from the medical profession's goal – the professional elimination of disease – to the appealing idiom of *therapy*: to individually contracted and paid expert consultation, loosely modelled on psychotherapy and recalling American human potential training for business managers in self-presentation and self-actualisation.[27]

And in all of this, the idea of illness has changed. A recent paper by David Parkin[28] argues from his fieldwork among local healers in Zanzibar that one can usefully identify two rather general ways of resolving illness and misfortune. One, which we can identify with biomedicine (but not only with biomedicine) is 'eradication' – killing the objectified cause stone dead – surgery and antibiotics, exclusion, excision and exorcism. Local therapeutic practices may rather favour a practice of 'dispersal' or restoration of harmony between a person and their social and physical environment (as in Chinese medicine: Bray this volume), in which a problem may be resolved by returning it onto its sender or displacing it out into the social world (as in sorcery and counter-sorcery), or simply placating and accommodating it in an attenuated form in what anthropologists term 'cults of affliction' (spirit possession cults, Alcoholics Anonymous).[29] Current Western idioms are, for the former, 'treatment'; for the latter, 'healing' or indeed 'care'. If the former is identified particularly with hospital medicine, the limitations of medicine in dealing with chronic disability or pain in Western societies may lead to 'folk' or 'alternative medicine' being recognised as more valuable. 'Healing the whole person' is the contemporary idiom, but neither option is necessarily individualised in practice. I would suggest that the current dispersal of patients away from the psychiatric hospital with its localised procedures but institutional public accountability is a recognition of the earlier failure of the eradication of disease by clinical psychiatry; for who would doubt that the development of new but potentially dangerous pharmaceuticals which effectively eliminated psychosis, alcoholism and everyday dysphorias would lead to a rapid return to intensive hospital-based care? But community care is also a dispersal of both patient and illness away from the medical expert back into the world of everyday decisions over employment, commodities, lifestyles, values and so on; an amoral and statistical world where a multitude of individual and self-interested choices provide the hidden hand of a liberal market economy and thence some form of natural order and predictability. If the model for the old hospital psychiatry was that of a mechanical age, then the new model, following the prominence of service industries in European economies, is perhaps one of shopping malls;[30] instead of diagnoses reflecting hypothetical biomedical entities, we have commercial relations characterised by market idioms of *choice, communication, user contract, budgetary control, consultancy, corporate plans, needs level assessments, case management, quality assurance* and *packages of care* as the new clinical discourse. For the provision of personally targeted individual care is necessarily more expensive than that of a 'production line' hospital; and the libertarian right has been concerned to reduce taxation.

The nosology is no longer one of individual dysfunction, whether biomedical or even psychodynamic, but rather of performance and negotiation, sales and managerial aptitude. The clinical currency now used by *mental health care providers* (nurses, doctors, social and housing workers) in their *mission statements* privilege issues of exact finance but of imprecise individual danger and trauma: *damaged, chaotic, dependency levels, high dependency behaviour, challenging behaviour, post-traumatic stress*: the whole emerging out of market negotiations between *purchaser* and *provider* (as represented in health service trusts with government appointed part-time directors), and *the voluntary sector*; market units whose names recall those of American human potential therapies or even small businesses (Focus, Positive Care, New Perspectives, Compass, Sunrise Care, Anglian Harbours for example); and which are publicised through standardised logos which recall both doctor-directed advertisements for antidepressants and successful output graphs in their optimistic upward and rightward movement.[31] If the changes of the last twenty years appear to have shifted responsibility for providing health care from hospitals to *the community*, local authorities were informed in 1989 that they simply 'should be arrangers and purchasers, not providers of services'.[6] It is increasingly difficult to distinguish local health trusts (which are nominally part of the remaining public health service, yet required to seek private investment under the 1992 Private Finance Initiative) from the private agencies which bargain to provide equivalent services and which are themselves increasingly controlled by United States health corporations.[32] Publically elected individuals are no longer accountable as responsibility is pushed 'downwards' to individual units whose failures of *management* or *good practice* are to be resolved in the courts, in adversarial Mental Health Review Tribunals, or simply by their bankruptcy. The mentally ill consumer is *empowered* (made responsible) to attend *mental health advice centres, workshops, drop-in centres* and *self-help projects* whose language and ambitions recapitulate those of New Age therapies or Alcoholics Anonymous and the other 12-step programmes: less the eradication of an illness than (to take a term from the anthropology of spirit possession) its uncertain accommodation.[33] As if, spread out thin among the population, it will cease to be quite so pathological. And the achievement of *health* is one of autonomy and holistic self-actualisation recalling that of the managers addressed by Dale Carnegie and Vincent Peale. It becomes increasingly difficult to differentiate a multitude of improbably named projects, trusts, enterprises, centres, groups, units and workshops from which the consumer (as self-manager) is expected to obtain their desired *package*. Many are the now commercialised interests of the mental health pressure groups themselves: MIND has moved from its 1980s critique of health policy to becoming the provider of the services it then advocated. And the very distinction between patient and professional is eroded: the *occupational stress* of the new situation for nursing staff themselves involves them in *putting in a bid* to obtain *funding* for a contracted therapist to provide staff therapy modelled on that for survivors of disasters and indeed for their own clients, a therapy which aims to avoid staff *burnout* in maximising their productivity, let alone their personal goals. Nurses who would once have taken supplementary qualifications to train in psychotherapy or psychology now seek a qualification in business administration and marketing. *Savings* are conceived of in terms of greater efficiency alone; any local suggestion that savings lead to a reduced service is deprecated and is treated as incompetent management. The doctors, gradually stripped of their authority, seek to blame matters on the *managers* who cut their budgets and *audit* their *performance*; yet, in a sense, there are no longer any managers, for every employee (doctors included) are now themselves managers, responsible to their own *line manager* for budgets and *co-ordinating services flexibly* and *creatively* (that is economising). In a further move from biomedical empiricism to marketing, the preferred language has shifted recently from *unmet needs* (the illness and its social consequences as assessed by professionals) to *unmet choices*:[6] desires articulated by the apparently not disabled patient as consumer yet only to be assessed as *fundable* (legitimate) by the manager.

Community is not simply a recourse to politically congenial and less paternalistic spatial metaphors;[34] the very location and nature of mental illness has changed. (And this involves us in the ironies which my placing here of italicised policy terms might have suggested.) Following Kant and Schopenhauer, I would propose that we can understand ourselves and the world in two fundamentally different ways: either as a consequence of cause and effect processes 'out there', generally independent of, but potentially accessible to, human awareness – the naturalistic mode of thought; or we can understand the same matters personalistically – as the motivated actions of volitional agents employing such characteristically human attributes as intention, responsibility, suffering, self-awareness, inter-subjectivity, representation and action. Whilst Euro-Americans conventionally allocate one or other area of interest to the naturalistic or the personalistic, perhaps objectifying them as separate domains (nature: culture:: symptom: choice), we can apply either mode of thought to any phenomenon. The experiencing self may be explained mechanistically, the natural world may be personified. In small scale societies, analogues of the psychiatrist's concept of 'mental illness' are often understood in a personalistic way – as the consequence of failed ambition or antisocial actions by the individual or others, of divine retribution, and so on.[18] Biomedical considerations of such psychiatric phenomena as self-harm (symptom of depressive illness? intention to die?) or myalgic encephalomyelitis (disease? malingering?), like debates on criminal responsibility (mad? bad?), continually slip between one and the other, for only one mode can be correct at any one time. The pragmatic legal categories of tort and diminished responsibility generally duck any attempt to examine their mutual relationship, nor can courts easily allocate financial compensation after accidents according to an index of 'real' versus 'public' disability; the eighteenth-century workhouse was similarly faced with the problem of distinguishing the 'impotent poor' who were unable to work from those who would not work.[6] Both libertarian and popular anti-psychiatry, like holistic and ecological medicine, proposed that the psychiatrist's understanding of schizophrenia as a brain disease was dehumanising, and that it should rather be approached as an intelligible and meaningful response by an individual to certain stressful events; and thus behind illness, the individual remained intact and inviolable as the potential agent of their own fate.

Ambiguities and ironies inevitably emerge for neither mode of thought can be demonstrated as completely true, nor false: we always live with the two options. In certain areas – anthropology, psychiatry, medical jurisprudence, economics and the sociology of knowledge – the practical problems of reconciling causation and volition become especially salient. Practicable solutions generally reduce one position to the other as prior and essential: whether in ontology, in epistemology or, usually, in both.

This is not a paper on scientific or popular rationality and I do not wish to detail current attempts to resolve the antinomy but rather to take it as an inescapable ambiguity in everyday life, and thence in public policy. There has been an apparent shift in the moral and political economy between these two modes of thought in the last twenty years in Britain, in a more personalistic and contractual direction, towards Szasz's bracing 'ethic of autonomy'.[23] If, as Margaret Thatcher put it, 'there is no such thing as society' (*the* community being merely a term for a number of individuals), debate on public policy has moved from the idea of public actions and demands as reconciling social interests (whether those of a social class, a political party or a professional body) towards an American emphasis on individual responsibility for sickness, unemployment and poverty, and on the contractual rights and responsibilities of the mentally ill, with diminished space in a natural world dominated by self-sufficient individuals for 'accidents' – which have now become violating traumata (post-traumatic stress disorder, multiple personality disorder, repetitive strain injury, environmental causes of ME) occasioned by the mischief or negligence of others, responsible agents whom legal process hold accountable for the failed *management* of our risks.

Should this not enhance public responsibility? In what is still only a 'quasi-market'[6] – for the purchases of the psychiatric consumer are generally paid out of income derived from national insurance and taxation – the attempt to achieve purely contractual goals has not been successful. The patterns we term 'mental illness' are always ironically poised between human action and disease process. Insanity is not plausibly regarded in contemporary Britain as a 'choice' nor as a consequence of the malevolence of others. The mentally ill are not taken as responsible for their experiences or actions, and the modern state is still expected to intervene on their behalf. But they are required to press for their autonomy as the achievement of health. The 1983 Mental Health Act encourages patients hospitalised involuntarily to appeal for early release to special Review Tribunals, supported by a (generally appointed) lawyer who takes their task as arguing to the Tribunal on their behalf solely for such liberty.[35] Unelected Community Health Councils and *voluntary sector* agencies, arguing that they represent through their employees the *community* or *consumer voice*, make regular complaints about *elitist* medical decisions and instead propose *support networks*. Psychiatrists and nurses, conscious of a further diminution in status and of their policing office, complain that their work has become increasingly adversarial, with patients encouraged to refuse treatment at the insistence of *voluntary sector* professionals who speak in the name of *the community*.[36] Nurses are required to issue to users details of the appeal process which necessarily equates discharge from hospital with health and normality, medical treatment with illness.[37] (Other medical decisions – on the withdrawal of life-support technologies, the environmental causes of ill health, the ownership and sale of body parts such as ova and the foetus – are increasingly made by lawyers; as Jones[6] notes, the shift from medical (naturalistically justified) power to the legal (personalistic) recalls the earlier struggle between doctor and lawyer for control over the nineteenth-century asylum.) Despite the occasional campaigns to destigmatise mental illness, the emphasis on legal rights and the avoidance of involuntary hospitalisation has the consequence of increasing the stigma of treatment; and thus a greater unwillingness on the part of anybody to be admitted. The recent rise in the proportion of involuntary admissions is, I suggest, not only the market consequence of admitting only the 'sicker' patients.

This culture of autonomy, consumerism and adversarial law, of individual choice and thence individual responsibility, is problematic at moments of psychiatric drama when accountability for actions is demanded; these particularly involve Britain's black minorities whose large number of wandering patients, passing from *high intensity care* to *secure units*, to police stations, magistrates' courts and prisons, to *homeless peoples' centres* and resettlement units, to general practices, to *cold-weather shelters*, hostels and lodging houses, and the streets – now recall the wanderings of the medieval insane once conjured up by Michel Foucault or the John O'Bedlams (the licensed beggars once released from Bethlem Hospital to seek their livelihood).[38] But now under the aegis, not of rejection by their fellows, but of their own choice.

Public accountability has systematically evaporated whilst something like a natural process – the market – have reemerged in its stead. Responsibility for alleviating mental illness lies less with elected and identifiable individuals than with commercial advantage as an essentially ultrahuman phenomenon. Elected officials have been replaced by part-time government-appointed businessmen.[39] Staff themselves are prohibited from publicly discussing their work through 'gagging clauses' in the new *locally agreed contracts* in which individual nurses and doctors negotiate as best they may for their salaries. The 'hidden hand' of the market is indeed hidden, supposedly allowing natural order and structure to develop out of a multitude of self-interested events which are no longer available as public information; as Jones[6] has observed, the quasi-market of health has led in the 1990s to the government declaiming any responsibility for the new mental health scandals; indeed, she notes there are no longer any published national statistics for the incidence of mental illness nor for bed occupancy. Public responsibility has disappeared into *the community* where in some elusive way, *needs* will be *addressed* through a multitude of negotiations between anonymous individuals translated into a natural mechanism in which attempts to understand or direct matters can only disrupt them (as in the recently fashionable Theory of Rational Expectations). Yet *needs* are hardly natural phenomena, and once a level of need is quantified by health economists, the cost of funding above a certain level may be centrally disallowed through emphasis on the *nation's health* (financial) *priorities*.

By a *community*, we refer to a group of people with a shared sense of belonging and identity, and with a common responsibility to provide assistance. Peter Wilmott has suggested that the term paradoxically came into prominence among the British after the last war with the dissolution of culturally homogeneous neighbourhoods characterised by common residence, interests, occupation and mutual assistance, with the appearance of impersonal local government officials who administered welfare and directed urban redevelopment and who, after the 1959 Mental Health Act, took on responsibilities for alleviating psychological illness.[40] In other words, when any institution one might easily recognise as a bounded and accountable collectivity was disappearing; and now accelerated as local planning power is transferred to centrally-controlled Development Corporations. *Community* recalls its own absence, a 'fictive'[41] space into which entities like illness may usefully be dissipated. The term is not applied to the middle-class suburbs (where one might indeed argue for at least some uniformity of shared interests and action), but to holes in the national fabric characterised by unemployment, higher levels of physical and psychological illness, ethnic minorities, poverty and poor housing – as if these had some shared way of life which plausibly compensated for, or caused, their poverty.[42] *Community* is no longer an identifiable political or economic structure but a state of mind, a way of thinking and acting.[43] As Benedict Anderson has argued,[44] it is increasingly imagined, not inhabited, as a social reality.

If the community through which care is provided appears to be a topos with no plausible physical location, there is one sense in which mental illness is now very specifically located among a group of real people. And in which something we might term politics has re-emerged. The image of the wandering lunatic is primarily that of a black person. I have argued elsewhere that the conflict between black and white in the modern period was initially couched as simple conquest or civilising mission; when equality threatened, European supremacy was justified to the faint-hearted through arguments of biological *race* and inherent inferiority, and then in the twentieth century through psychological and psychopathological arguments which justified black people's poverty, unemployment and failure.[45] In Europe and America they were regarded as having more psychiatric illness (and thus more of them required hospital treatment) either because their own culture was itself pathogenic or because of the stress of living up to a

European society (*ibid.*). (After the period of widespread migration to Britain, during the 1970s one solution was the ejection of the Black mentally ill back to another alien space, through repatriation under the 1959 Mental Health Act (*ibid.*).) Our current euphemism for dealing with issues of ethnicity and racism is to allocate black Britons to a particular *community* named for the origins of their parents: 'the Asian community', and so on. The psychiatry of 'race' has been replaced by that of 'culture',[8] less biological but equally essentialised. And thence we get 'problems of mental illness *of* the West Indian community': invidia initially dispersed away from public responsibility, yet in a public crisis then localised in a problematic group which becomes the occasion for increased surveillance under the paradoxical idiom of its representatives *purchasing care.*

The anthropologist Paul Heelas[46] has proposed, following locus of control experiments by psychologists, that when there is a strong personalistic emphasis on an autonomous self, we attribute undesired deviations to some discrete agency external to this self: recalling what Douglas Hofstadter has recently called America's 'paranoid political style', Michael Kenny's 'paradoxes of liberty'. (A not uncommon psychotherapist's observation is that the increasingly personalistic direction of that discipline results in increasing referral of accountability from the suffering individual onto their parents.) Enhanced competitive individualism is the bedfellow of externally directed blame, whether we understand this competition in terms of social policy or of political action.[47]

The notion of 'the community' in Britain articulates an uncertain and ironical contradiction between market choice and adversarial confrontation; and the localisation of medical problems is, if no longer in the abnormal brain, in something perilously close to 'race'. And 'the Black community' now purchases its own surveillance, the failure of the libertarian dispersal of mental illness calling up fresh demands, if not for eradication, then at least for focused incarceration.

Acknowledgements

Pages 1–3 paraphrase, with Maurice Lipsedge's kind permission, his material published in Littlewood, R. and Lipsedge, M., *Aliens and Alienists*, third edition, 1997, published by Routledge, London. I am grateful for comments from David Parkin.

NOTES

1. Williams, *R. Keywords*. (London: Fontana/Croom Helm, 1986). Italics are used here to refer to particular policy and other idioms in current British use. This continued emphasis is inevitably tiresome but it is perhaps easier on the eye than repeated 'scare quotes'.
2. Mears, R. and Smith, R. *Community Care: Policy and Practice*. (London: Macmillan, 1994). Utting, W. *et al. Creating Community Care: Report of the Mental Health Foundation into Community Care For People with Severe Mental Illness*. (London: MHF, 1994).
3. Ritchie, J., Dick, D. and Laingham, R. *The Report of the Inquiry into the Care and Treatment of Christopher Clunis*. (London: HMSO, 1994).
4. Department of Health *The Care Management Approach*, (Health Circular (90) 23/LASSL (90) 11. London: HMSO, 1990).
5. Pembroke, L. Surviving psychiatry. *Nursing Times, 87*, 1993, 29–32.
6. Jones, K. *Asylums and After*. (London: Athlone, 1993).
7. Lloyd, K. and Moodley, P. Psychiatry and ethnic groups. *British Journal of Psychiatry, 156*, 1990, 907.
8. Littlewood, R. and Lipsedge, M. *Aliens and Alienists*, (3rd rev. edit. London: Routledge, 1997).
9. Wing, J. *Reasoning About Madness*. (Oxford University Press, 1978).
10. Among the few universals one can identify historically and cross-culturally in understandings of sickness is that treatment is generally the reciprocal or resolution of the presumed aetiology (homoeopathy being a notable exception).
11. Goffman, E. *Asylums: Essays on the Social Situation of Mental Patients and Other Inmates*. (New York: Anchor/Doubleday, 1961).
12. Wing, J. and Brown, G.W. *Institutionalism and Schizophrenia*. (Cambridge University Press, 1970).
13. Laing, R.D. and Esterson, A. *Sanity, Madness and the Family*. (London: Tavistock, 1964).
14. Cooper, D. *The Death of the Family*. (London: Allen Lane, 1971).
15. Cooper, D. *The Dialectics of Liberation*. (Harmondsworth: Penguin, 1968).
16. Ibid.: 175.
17. Laing later claimed that he had never been politically on the left, and indeed denied that his writing was concerned with the origin of mental illness at all.
18. Littlewood, R. *Pathology and Identity*. (Cambridge: Cambridge University Press, 1993).
19. In practice the Counterculture failed to establish a social context in which mental illness could be perceived as meaningful. In his autobiography, Mark Vonnegut describes how the hippie commune members with whom he lived proved unwilling to cope with his episode of schizophrenia: after a certain amount of anguished debate,

they took him to the local mental hospital where he was given electroconvulsive therapy (cited in Littlewood 1993).[18] Their hesitations and guilt were identical with those of the bourgeois families so trenchantly denounced by Laing. And the anti-psychiatrists' most well-known patient, Mary Barnes, has been subsequently described as having an unusual personality rather than schizophrenia which was the classic illness for the movement.

20. As late as 1986, Madness Network 'demand[ed] the termination of psychiatry as a medical profession, including the cessation of all training programmes [and] the dismantling of the entire "mental health" system' (Madness Network News Collective working draft to abolish psychiatry. 1986 Reprinted, *Phoenix Network Mental Patients Publication*, 1995, No. 3, 17–23.)
21. Sedgwick, P. *Psychopolitics*. (London: Pluto, 1982). At a meeting of the Royal College of Psychiatrists in 1982 some months before his death, Sedgwick proposed this in an invited lecture and was greeted with rapturous applause. It was difficult to escape the conclusion that the psychiatrists (who, then and now, consider themselves as politically on the left) supposed themselves spared the opprobrium of radical critiques: for their major critics had been revealed as reactionaries.
22. Porter, R. *A Social History of Madness: Voices of the Insane*. (London: Weidenfeld & Nicholson, 1989).
23. Szasz, T. *The Myth of Mental Illness*. (New York: Harper & Row, 1961).
24. Szasz, T. *The Manufacture of Madness*. (London: Routledge & Kegan Paul, 1971).
25. Jones, M. *Social Psychiatry*. (Reprinted 1969. Harmondsworth: Penguin, 1952).
26. Psychiatric hospital bed numbers had already started falling in the 1960s; doctors attributed this to the new antipsychotic drugs.
27. Littlewood, R. *Reason and Necessity in the Specification of the Multiple Self*. (London: Royal Anthropological Institute, 1996).
28. Parkin, D. Latticed knowledge: eradication and dispersal of the unpalatable in Islam, medicine and anthropological theory. In R. Fardon (ed.), *Counterworks: Managing The Diversity of Knowledge*. (London: Routledge, 1995).
29. Janzen, J.M. Drums Anonymous: towards an understanding of structures of therapeutic maintenance. In *The Use and Abuse of Medicine*, (eds) M.W. De Vries, R.L. Berg and M. Lipkin. (New York: Praeger, 1982).
30. Indeed, by late 1996, the Ministry of Health agreed that general practices might be owned by and sited within supermarkets, offering immediate fee-for-service medical treatment.
31. On vertical movement as a representation of health and spiritual growth, see Littlewood, R. Verticality as an idiom for mood and disorder. *British Medical Anthropology Review* (n.s.), 2, No. 1, 1994, 45–63.
32. Health Policy Network *Health Care – Private Cooperations or Public Service? The Americanisation of the NHS*. (London: NHS Consultants' Association, 1996).

33. Both AA and 'peripheral' spirit possession cults do not claim to eradicate the problem (intrusive disease or spirit) which remains liable to be activated against the individual; it can only be dealt with through an ambiguous accommodation ('once an alcoholic, always an alcoholic') or dedication to or propriation of the possessing spirit (Janzen 1982, Littlewood 1996, op. cit.). Similarly, no one claims to 'cure' schizophrenia for it is rather propriated through depot neuroleptics and a change in lifestyle and goals which ensures careful dedication to the power of the illness to prevent it overcoming the individual.
34. Whether, in their conferral of responsibility on the sick, the new terms are any less stigmatising (*i.e.* objectifying the individual as a representative of a devalued category) than 'patient' or 'hospital' may be doubted: *user* is also used for addicts, *client* for customers of prostitution; *consumer* is frankly implausible. And the popular connotations of *mental health* are those of *mental* (lunatic). My perplexity is hardly original: the House of Commons Health Committee as long ago as 1983 wondered if *community care* was not on the way to becoming a 'virtually meaningless slogan': Mayo, M. *Communities and Caring: The Mixed Economy of Welfare*. (London: St. Martin's Press, 1994).
35. Perhaps not altogether paradoxically, I have overheard enthusiastic mental health lawyers, generally young women (for this is not as yet a particularly lucrative or prestigious employment) rather crossly urge their uninterested psychotic clients to 'pull themselves together' to collaborate with the lawyer 'or you will not get out of this place [the clinic]'. To agree to compulsory treatment is a sign of sickness.
36. The American Mental Hygiene Movement, from which these British groups descend, similarly had an anti-medical ethos. Critics argued that its ideal of *mental health* was highly individualised, representing health as a robust striving towards becoming a self-sufficient entrepreneur or successful manager, acquiescence in sickness as unpatriotic social dissent. Davis, K. Mental hygiene and the class structure. *Psychiatry, 1*, 1938, 55–65
37. This frequently follows patients' own explanatory models in which experienced interference with their volition and removal of their agency by some external power (a common feature of schizophrenia) may be blamed on the treatment.
38. Against this openness of 'the community' we might counterpose the physical space inside hospital wards, centres and workshops, increasingly cramped and restrictive, with no place for physical exercise (which has been mandatory since 1877[6]) except the streets. The old county asylums (once in the country, now in the suburbs) have sold off their now valuable land for commercial building. In a meeting of my local community health trust in September 1996, I was presented with a proposed plan in which the dispersed community services would, for financial reasons (duplication of night staff, etc.), be replaced by two purpose-built hospitals where a wide variety of clinical and aftercare services could be placed economically together. One justification was that our users were increasingly harassed on the city streets and they disliked the dirty and restricted space in the units in the general

hospital where they became violent because of frustration and 'lack of space', and thus would surely prefer open grounds and peaceful gardens away from these everyday stresses. Asylums? As Kathleen Jones[6] remarks, we seem to have arrived again at the early nineteenth century: *performance* (i.e. savings) *related pay* recalls the nineteenth century pattern when hospital administrators met the cost of the establishment out of their salaries (ibid.: 62); and we might cite the return to recruitment of low paid and untrained 'care assistants', the dispersal of accountability in different professions, public opinion oscillating between sympathy and fear, tolerance and a call for action. Even the personalistic idioms of self-help 'therapy' and 'positive health' are not altogether novel (cf. Christian 'moral treatment' in the early nineteenth century).

39. Marr, A. *Ruling Britannia.* (London: Michael Joseph, 1995).
40. Littlewood, R. Review of P. Willmott and D. Thomas, *Community in Social Policy (*PSI*), Bulletin of the Royal College of Psychiatrists, 9,* No. 3, 1984, 65.
41. Harbison, R. *The Built, the Unbuilt and the Unbuildable.* (London: Thames & Hudson, 1992).
42. The dispersal of illness into 'the community' has not however been followed by publicly funded attempts to examine how illness may originate in the community (the consequences of unemployment and social dislocations (Thomas, P., Romme, M. and Hamelijnck, J. 'Psychiatry and the politics of the underclass'. *British Journal of Psychiatry, 169,* 1996, 401–4): the ethnic minority communities excepted, in what is currently termed 'transcultural psychiatry'.
43. The new 'communitarians' (Lasch, McIntyre) have been criticised for an anti-Enlightenment return to Romantic topologies of shared consciousness (Etzioni, A. *The Spirit of the Community: Rights, Responsibilities and the Communitarian Agenda,* (New York: Crown, 1994)), but 'community care', although influenced by older social welfare attitudes in Britain has less to do with the communitarianism in which it cloaks itself than with liberal individualism. (On the more general relationship between them, see Sandel, M.J. *Democracy's Discontent: America in Search of a Public Philosophy,* (Cambridge MA: Harvard University Press, 1996)); compare Scruton, R. *The Conservative Idea of Community.* (London: Conservative 2000 Foundation, 1996).
44. Anderson, B. *Imagined Communities.* (London: Verso, 1991).
45. Littlewood, R. and Lipsedge, M. *Aliens and Alienists: Ethnic Minorities and Psychiatry.* (Harmondsworth: Penguin, 1982).
46. Heelas, P. The model applied: anthropology and indigenous psychologies. In P. Heelas and A. Lock (eds), *Indigenous Psychologies: The Anthropology of the Self.* (London: Academic Press, 1981).
47. This is a common interpretation by anthropologists of sorcery accusations in 'zero-sum' peasant economies. Underlying this is the phenomenologists' study of how the flux of suffering and experience becomes congealed into such hypostatised entities as diseases, individual action or money – a process surprisingly ignored by social scientists interested in cognition but which has been variously addressed by

Marxists, Kleinians and Buddhists through the idea that nominal categories are less ambiguous than experiencing, and under problematic circumstances we essentialise a fetishised world following our own objectification of ourselves as physical entities; early in life we start to perceive the world as nominalised – as composed of entities of recurrent invariance (Schutz, A. *The Phenomenology of the Social World*, (rev. edit. London: Heinemann, 1976)) whose interaction then inevitably becomes problematic (Lukács); such reification is fundamental to social categorisation, giving ontological status to the experienced world (Lakoff, G. *Women, Fire and Dangerous Things: What Categories Reveal About the Mind*, (Chicago University Press, 1987)). And in the same way, since Kant we reify our awareness and action in the world as illness, race or community, as something like an entity. Thence the fright illnesses described by Rawcliffe (this volume): something is removed from us (or implanted within Littlewood 1996, op. cit.).

A GENERAL PRACTITIONER IN THE INNER CITY – THE REALITIES AND THE DIFFICULTIES

John Cohen

Background

Interest in the religion, culture and ethnicity of our patients arose as Britain became a much more culturally mixed society in the 1960s. It hardly featured in the medical or psychological literature until a CIBA Symposium in 1965.[1] In the 1970s and 1980s there was a great interest, particularly from the psychiatrists, and this has been reviewed by Cox.[2] Major research in the field was summarised by Leff in *Psychiatry Around the Globe*[3] published in 1988, and popularised by Littlewood and Lipsedge in *Aliens and Alienists*.[4] In the area of general practice the main authors have been Helman with *Health, Culture and Illness*[5] in 1990 and Qureshi with *Transcultural Medicine*[6] in 1994.

For an inner city general practitioner the knowledge of how different cultures understand health, illness, disease, disability, handicap and death and how they react to them is very important on a day-to-day basis. The life pattern of a Hindu, Moslem, Chinese or African family and how they interpret and deal with deviations from normal activity and behaviour is vital to help an individual patient, a family or a community, to deal with illness whether it is caused by physical, psychological or social factors or a combination of all three. This applies to white families from different part of Britain and Europe as well as people from other continents.

Understanding Culture and Religion in Primary Care Medicine

Understanding the cause and likely outcome of a patient's illness will depend on the cause of the problems and the patient's reaction to it, and this is dependent on the knowledge base of that person, his or her background and origins, education, culture, religious beliefs, personality, immediate family and close relatives or friends, and their employment, housing and financial circumstances. How and why he or she chooses and presents at the time will be determined, in part, by social and cultural and religious issues.

The doctor needs to know the way in which symptoms, signs of illness, disability, handicap and disease are understood in a particular family or culture, and if he is not sure he must ask the patient or a knowledgable relative or friend.

Migration from one country, culture and accepted norms and behaviour to another which has different parameters of climate, environment, language, diet, social and cultural behaviour is a major stressor to personal identity for the migrant and also for other family members who have arrived with them. This affects the next generation in their turn, as they struggle to determine their place in two cultures, that of their parents and that in which they have grown up.

The elderly parents of the migrants may come to live with them and the family may be further confused and severely strained by the conflicts between the generations, and the old and new cultures. This was true for the Jews of the East End of London at the beginning of the twentieth century as it is in the nineteen-nineties for the Bangladeshis living there now.

The general practitioner has to be aware that patients of Afro-Caribbean origin living in Britain appear to have a higher incidence of chronic mental illness than those of Caucasian origin, when compared to the incidence in the West Indies.[7, 8] Indians living in Britain have a higher incidence of chronic mental illness than those of Pakistani origin – the causes of these differences remain unclear.[9]

The doctor may also come across 'culture-bound syndromes' which are illness or diseases which are confined to a particular culture.[10] Loss of soul (Susto) in South America, post-natal depression (Amakiro) in Uganda and possession by spirits (Sar) in Somalia are examples. Anorexia nervosa is perhaps the European equivalent, where dieting, and maintaining a slim figure are culturally encouraged, and where emphasis on adolescent individuality and separation from parents and the parental home is accepted as normal.

There are other conflicts in Western Society not seen to the same degree elsewhere. The fear of old age, of loss of, youth, vitality and dignity affects people in the West as they get older, and they have concerns and fears for the future. When they are unable to care for themselves, they may be shunned by friends, neighbours and family and placed in the care of strangers, however kindly, in a 'rest home', 'retirement home', or an even more sheltered and isolated 'nursing home'.

The time frame and aetiology of diseases and conditions in Western medicine often conflicts with the longer term and more accepting views held in other cultures, and their compliance and response to drug treatment may be biologically and socially different.

Death does not end the problem for people of cultures who may wish to bury or cremate the deceased as soon as practical, even on the day of death if that is practical. For the British it is sometimes seen as unseemly haste, not waiting a decent time to allow the body to cool and the relatives to come from a long distance. There may be a false assumption that bribery on the part of the relatives is the way to organise a quick arrangement for the disposal of the body, and this may offend funeral directors, registrars of deaths and crematoria.

There may be considerable distress in some cultures if a post mortem must be held under the auspices of Her Majesty's Coroner, as the delay in making arrangements for the disposal of the body and the resting place of the soul or spirit causes distress, often not considered or understood by officials and bureaucratic organisations.

The doctor does not come to the relationship with a patient as an 'empty vessel'. He or she has ideas, beliefs, religion and a culture which may affect or interfere with the interpretation of the causes of the problems that the patient and the patient's family may present. It may also affect the judgement as to the best treatment for the condition, if the views of the receiver are not considered. And yet the patients may be uncomfortable about expressing views to the doctor, because 'the doctor knows best'; he or she is regarded as the expert.

The patient might feel that the doctor would not wish to hear their views anyway, and we cannot express them in a form and language that he or she can understand. Unfortunately, it may be easier, and quicker, for the doctor to agree with this view and treatment may be provided which may not be in the patients' best interests.

The mental health services in Britain were not designed for a multicultural society and often have difficulty dealing with problems which occur in immigrants and ethnic minority patients. Racist attitudes are often only just below the surface, patients from these communities may not conform to the usual patterns of behaviour and may not easily accept conventional forms of treatment.

Even what constitutes mental illness varies from culture to culture and between societies. What might be perfectly well tolerated in Kingston, Jamaica may be unacceptable in London, England. Many European countries laugh mockingly at our attitudes to public morality and behaviour while we are faintly sceptical of their 'obsessions and preoccupations'.

The view of depression and schizophrenia varies widely across Europe and psychiatrists from different countries have problems in collaborative research because of uncertainties about meaning and definition. For example, attitudes to mental illness became highly politicised in Germany and in the former Soviet Union, and many kept their concerns and depressive symptoms to themselves, or sought physical solutions to psychological problems through doctors, and sometimes through alcohol and illicit drugs.

Even in Britain there are a wide variety of views about what constitutes mental illness, and while there is general agreement about the most disturbed, psychotic and deluded patients, amongst the less severely ill there is far less certainty about the causes, natural history, treatment and social consequences.

Ethnic Populations in Britain and in the Inner Cities

In Britain in the nineteen-nineties, people born abroad and belonging to ethnic minority groups constitute 5.5% of the population (3.1 million). Of these 1.5 million (2.6%) belong to the Asian cultural group and this includes Hindus, Moslems, Sikhs and others. 0.9 million (1.6%) are of Afro-Caribbean origin and 0.7 million (1.3%) are from other ethnic groups. They are concentrated in certain areas, for example in the London Borough of Brent they make up 45% of the population, in London Borough of Newham 42%, London Borough of Tower Hamlets 36%, City of Leicester 29% and City of Birmingham 22%.

Many of the ethnic minorities have more younger and fewer older people in their communities. For example, while 19% of the white population of Britain is under sixteen, 34% of the ethnic minority community is under this age. At the other end of the age spectrum, 21% of the white population is over sixty years of age, the figure for the ethnic communities is 5%.[11]

Patients seen at our Central London general practice over two weeks in September 1996 came from the following countries – Cyprus (Greek and Turkish parts), Spain, Portugal, Russian Federation (including several wealthy businessmen and their families), Poland (including several families of Polish Gypsies), Bosnia-Hertzogovina, Croatia and Serbia, Ethiopia, Somalia and Eritrea, India, Pakistan, Bangladesh and Sri Lanka, Sudan and Egypt, Israel, Iraq, Iran, Philippines, Indonesia, China, Japan, Chile, Brazil and Peru. And these do not include the postgraduate students for the School of African and Oriental Studies who have registered with the practice.

Family Structure: Single People, Families and Communities

An individual rarely lives in isolation from his or her family of origin, relatives, friends and locality (that is neighbours). The perception of the illness from which the individual may be suffering will inevitably be affected by the history of that individual and his/her relationships, and the effects that illness may have in the future will be determined by a variety of factors, including the views and ideas of the illness as seen by the family.

Communities too share ideas about what illnesses are more acceptable and which are less. For example, alcohol and drug use are less accepted by society, lung cancer due to cigarette smoking and obesity are more tolerated, even though these examples are behaviourally motivated.

To illustrate some of these issues and make them relevant to everyday life I now present six short case scenarios of patients seen in my Central London practice in the past three months.

1. *Mrs K A-T aged 58* was born in Iran, grew up and married there. She had four children; two sons and two daughters. Her husband and two sons were killed in Iran in the nineteen-eighties and she managed to escape through family connections to Germany and then to Britain. She is very intelligent and has learnt English quickly, but finds the Social Security and National Health Service very confusing.

She is amazed that she does not have to pay the doctor and bribe 'the government officials' in the Social Services and the Department of Social Security and, not surprisingly, she finds difficulty in understanding the difference between these two organisations.

She used to be a frequent attender at the surgery with a variety of somatic complaints and all investigations for physical illness were negative. She found it difficult to discuss family and emotional issues without an interpreter, but at the same time she is worried about the credentials and motives of the interpreter. She is concerned that several of her Iranian friends have 'disappeared' and turned up in Iran. She has one daughter who escaped with her who lives in Germany and another in the United States. Religion is a comfort and a source of conflict for her as she looks back at the past.

We have attempted to help her to find a role as 'comforting mother' for new arrivals and refugees who have been in Britain for some time, and her sound knowledge and common sense has helped her to develop this role. She consults less and expects less instant cures for colds, coughs and minor illness, but I suspect that I still have some meanings for her which I can only begin to comprehend.

2. *Mr M S aged 44* was born in Bangladesh and is a devout and practising Moslem. He came to Britain to work in his uncle's restaurant and really had to work long hours for a minimal salary, most of which he was expected to send to his family at home. His uncle died and he worked in a number of low paid jobs in Indian restaurants in the West End of London. He can barely read and write and his language skills are not good. He gets very confused and tongue-tied in the presence of what he perceives as 'socially superior' people, like doctors and social workers.

His wife and children were going to come to London when he had made some money and found a home for them but his financial and social circumstances and the changes in the rules on immigration has made this an impossible dream.

Unfortunately he has had four heart attacks over the past few years and the function of his heart is poor. After investigation the cardiologists have told us that the outlook without heart transplantation is extremely limited. We have explained to him with the help of a Bangladeshi support worker what the problem is and discussed the solutions that the cardiologists have suggested. He does not believe that transplantation is possible, and in any case he could not accept anyone's heart; he believes that the donor would have to be a Moslem. As he lives alone in poor circumstances, it may well be that the cardiac team will decide that he is not suitable for transplantation anyway.

We are currently trying to get permission for his wife and children to visit him in Britain; he is not well enough to fly to Bangladesh. This has involved finding a Bengali-speaking solicitor to act on his behalf as a good deed; Mr MS has no money to pay for his services. He is very appreciative of what we are trying to do and quotes to me small snatches of the Koran which he says are blessings.

3. *Ms M M aged 60* was born in St Lucia, West Indies and came to Britain with a much older husband in the 1970s. After a few years here her husband died and she was left to bring up two daughters alone. They have since grown up and established their own families on the British model. She is still lonely and homesick after all these years and goes home to St Lucia every year to see her mother and sisters. She joined a fundamental evangelical Christian church which has provided a great deal of support for her.

She has had several nervous breakdowns, necessitating admission to psychiatric care, often initially compulsorily. The nature of the mental illness is not clear, she responds to the hospital environment and medication more quickly than one would expect, but often stops the treatment as soon as she gets home and remains well for many months.

She writes beautiful and haunting poetry and prose, which she has published, about her feelings of betrayal, isolation and loneliness. She comes to see me from time to time and asks me how I am keeping and tells me to take more time to look after myself. I do not know how to respond comfortably; it is so unusual for the doctor to be asked these things.

4. *Mrs JM aged 35* came to Britain in 1988 from an African country with her husband and three children. Her husband worked as a chauffeur in the High Commission, but after only a few months he died suddenly of pneumonia at the age of 33 years. A post mortem was carried out and showed that he had died of AIDS. It was felt as her general practitioner, I would be best placed to give her this unwelcome news.

I did not look forward to seeing her and telling her the truth, but I found that she knew that he either had tuberculosis or AIDS, and she suspected the latter. This made it easier than I had imagined to convey the message. In any case she had more experience of AIDS in her community than I had at the time in London.

It was some time before she consented to an HIV test for herself which was positive, and for the children who were all thankfully negative. Confidentiality was a problem at this time; there were a lot of health, education and social busybodies, and we tried to ensure that, as far as possible, only those who really needed to know should be informed of the HIV status of Mrs JM and her children.

The next concern was that now her husband was dead she no longer had permission to remain in Britain and was nearly deported. The children's future was discussed and plans evolved. In 1995 Mrs JM had her first serious infection and the plans swung into action. She recovered and returned home and wanted to live 'as normally as I can when I know that I am dying', she said. The older children seemed to understand, the youngest did not. In October 1996 she died peacefully at home and her unmarried sister has become the children's mother; surely a logical role for all concerned, although the immigration authorities took a good deal of persuading.

5. *Mrs AG aged 88* was born in Turkey of Russian parents and came to Britain to study after the First World War and met an Englishman, fell in love and remained here ever since. Her husband died in the 1950s and her two sons immigrated to United States and Australia. She has not seen them very much in the last few years; 'they are too busy with their own lives', she says.

Over the last few years she has become restricted by failing vision and lives a reclusive life in the bedroom of her tiny flat, increasingly living, sleeping, eating, washing, using a portable toilet and entertaining her declining circle of friends in this room. This annoys some and irritates others; 'why don't you go into a home, you'd be so much better off with other people looking after you', 'we're so worried about you at night and weekends, you might fall and hurt yourself and no-one would know', they say.

Mrs AG shrugs off these worries and polite suggestions by saying 'I've lived in this house for over fifty years and I am not moving out now. If it is God's will to go tonight I am ready, if not I will wait patiently until I'm called for'. The social workers and carers provided by the local authority are worried about her failing health and tell me that something must be done.

Even the local church concedes that it is not right that she cannot receive more help. The local authority says that its budget for home carers is cash-limited and she should sell the house and go into residential care. I have to admit I admire Mrs AG, and hope I will have the strength and dignity to act as calmly in the face of bureaucratic pressure as she does.

6. The parents of *Miss AS aged 22* came to Britain from India in the 1960s to study, got married and made their home here, and later brought their parents to live with them. While the parents went out to work, the grandparents brought up the children. The older generation have never really adapted to English customs, language or values and they have never mixed at all outside the family circle.

The parents had four children and their hope was that they would all succeed and do well. The youngest daughter was going to go to medical school but in the summer holidays before she was due to take up her place she became pregnant; the father of her child was an white middle-class student at the sixth form college that Miss AS had attended. She came to see me with him one day and asked for my support in being independent of her parents, and doing what she (and Tim) wanted to do, perhaps for the first time in her life.

A few days later her father came to see me to enlist my support against his youngest daughter for challenging his authority within the family. 'Surely you will understand what we have sacrificed to give the best to our children', he told me. He wanted Miss AS to quietly have a termination of pregnancy, forget Tim and get on with her studies.

Miss AS left home, went to live with Tim and they had a baby girl. For a long time her family refused to admit her existence, but I believe that her mother has seen the baby. The grandparents have said that Miss AS 'will be punished for her misdemeanour', and 'there is nothing else to be said'. 'She is no longer our granddaughter', they told me. I am torn between the needs of the young and the fears of the old.

Diffficulties for the Primary Care Team

Doctors, nurses and other health care workers, and especially receptionists in general practice and hospitals have little formal or informal training in understanding and caring for the needs of patients from ethnic, religious and cultural minorities. If they work in an inner city they are bound to meet such patients and they may be confused by difficulties with names, dates of birth and the nature of family relationships and their beliefs related to illness and disease.

For example, one of my young Chinese patients with a simple umbilical hernia attended the outpatient department of the local hospital with twelve relatives, and all of them expected to see the doctor. The outpatient staff were not sure what to do; for the family this was a perfectly normal experience. Their main question to the surgeon was whether they could use traditional Chinese medicine before surgery was contemplated.

There may be a problem of understanding and interpretation of culturally acceptable and unacceptable behaviour, such as spitting in the street. Family and minority groups may be reluctant to tell on family or culture members who are physically or mentally ill, or just in need of help, although they will often care for them.

For the busy general practitioner faced with a stream of patients all day with a variety of physical complaints, it may be easier and simpler merely to cope with the here and now, provide a 'pill for every ill', and not get involved with the complex business of understanding the culture and needs of the patient and the family. The problem is that the patient and the family will come to believe that all doctors are like this, and will expect similar behaviour from other doctors that they come into contact with.

General practice in Britain is not organised, nor possesses the resources to deal with all the needs of all the people, and some gain and some lose. Usually the ethnic, religious and cultural minorities are amongst those who lose out. Social services and the benefits system also face difficulties at the interface between medical and social issues. When a patient is admitted to hospital there may be further difficulties because of the strange surroundings, personnel and food, and the relative exclusion of loved and trusted family members. Interpreters and advocates will solve some of the problems but understanding, sympathy and genuine concern will go along way to relieve anxiety, fear and guilt.

Ways Forward and New Research

New ways are being developed to encourage medical, nursing and other health professions to acquire communication skills, promoting positive health, preventing disease and helping them to understand the interaction of health, illness and disease taking into account the culture and beliefs of the patient and the family.

There needs to be an increasing and ongoing dialogue between people of different cultures and beliefs to look for and emphasise what brings people together, not what separates them. Talking with others, listening to their ideas and their music and poetry, sharing their food, travelling the world all broaden and stretch the mind and encourages acceptance and tolerance. There should be a positive and genuine desire to discuss the problems faced by those of different cultures and beliefs in Britain at conferences and seminars.

The government should encourage a greater proportion of the doctors, nurses and other health and social work professionals to come from ethnic minority groups, and they should inform and educate their colleagues about the origins and meanings of the concepts that underpin their beliefs. There should be an increasing dialogue between health and social care workers to acquire knowledge, share understanding and look carefully at their attitudes.

More research is needed into communication across cultures, religions and ethnic groups, looking at the needs of patients and how they can best be met. There needs to be detailed studies that will give us more information on normal and abnormal thinking, behaviour and attitudes in all communities which make up the melting pot that is Britain today.

This country, on the North-Western edge of the European continent, has been a haven for migrants, refugees and fugitives since ancient times, and in every generation a new group has enriched our culture, traditions, and our food. We should thank them for what they have brought.

REFERENCES

1. A. De Rueck and R. Porter (eds). Transcultural Psychiatry (CIBA Symposium). 1965. Boston. Little Brown & Co.
2. J. Cox. Readings about transcultural psychiatry. *British Journal of Psychiatry*. 1991. 158. 579–81.
3. J. Leff. Psychiatry Around the Globe: a Transcultural View. 1988. London. Gaskell Press.
4. R. Littlewood and M. Lipsedge. Aliens and Alienists: Ethnic Minorities and Psychiatry. 1982. London. Penguin.
5. C. Helman. Culture, Health & Illness: and Introduction for Health Professionals. 2nd ed. 1990. Bristol. J. Wright & Sons.
6. B. Qureshi. Transcultural Medicine: Dealing with Patients from Different Cultures. 2nd ed. 1994. Dordrecht. Kluwer Academic Publications.
7. L. Hemsi. Psychiatric morbidity of West Indian immigrants. Social Psychiatry. 1967. 2. 95–100.
8. R. Cochrane. Mental illness in immigrants to England and Wales: an analysis of mental hospital admissions. *Social Psychiatry*. 1977. 12. 25–35.

9. G. Dean, D. Walsh, H. Downing and Shelley. First admissions of native-born and immigrants to psychiatric hospital in 1976. *British Journal of Psychiatry*. 1981. 139. 506–12.
10. P.Yap. Mental disease peculiar to certain cultures: a survey of comparative psychiatry. *Journal of Mental Science*. 1951. 97. 313–27.
11. P. Orton and J. Fry. UK Health Care: the Facts. 1995. Dordrecht. Kluwer Academic Publishers.

Further Reading

A. Henley. Asian Patients in Hospital and at Home. 1979. London. King's Fund.
A. Kleinman. Patients and Healers in the Context of Culture. 1980. Berkeley. University of California Press.
P. Rack. Race, Culture and Mental Disorder. 1991. London. Routledge Publications.
C. Wilkinson (ed.). Ethnic Psychiatry. 1986. London. Plenum Medical Book Co.
C. Currer and M. Stacey. Concepts of Health, Illness and Disease. 1986. Leamington Spa. Berg Publishers Ltd.
J. Cox (ed.). Transcultural Psychiatry. 1986. London. Croom Helm.
J. Cox and S. Bostock. Racial Discrimination in the Health Service. 1989. London. Penrhos.
I. McWhinney. A Textbook of Family Medicine. 1989. Oxford. Oxford University Press.
J. Kumar and J. Brockington. Motherhood and Mental Illness. 1988. Bristol. J. Wright & Sons.
S. Fernado. Race and Culture in Psychiatry. 1988. London. Croom Helm.

CONCLUSION: SUFFER MANY HEALERS

David Parkin

Animated Materiality

Medical history and anthropology have traditionally viewed the body as a site of contestable assumptions regarding the relationship between sickness and society. Scheper-Hughes and Lock (1987)[1] provide a typical overview of this relationship in identifying three dimensions of the body: it exists in material form, yet is also the means by which we live and so is part of our habitus, and culminates as the locus of conscious selfhood. The materiality of the body is thus basic and yet also that which is transcended by the way an individual gets unthinkably caught up in everyday activities. During moments of personal awareness and reflexion, one does not normally dwell on the body as a coordinated ensemble of bone, muscle, artery, vein, nerve and blood systematically carrying out a task, such analysis being judged as best left to medical specialisms.

But there is a wider sense of materiality which goes beyond the idea of the body as a visceral entity charged into life by society and consciousness. Interpersonal interaction itself involves different levels of social density: the more that people interact within a sphere of overlapping activities, the more they are likely to experience this density. The pressure of office life is contrasted with the light tranquillity of unconstrained leisure in a remote, unpopulated area. Sometimes the equation is reversed as when social isolation produces stress and a yearning for the excitement of the crowd or the energizing buzz of communal work. Whatever the variations, this sense of social density as material reality is not just additional to the anatomical idea of the body as basically a material form. They are part of each other. Society is matter. Matter is never inert.

Hinnells's discussion of Zoroastrianism provides an apt, first example of how cosmic forces and human relationships are inseparably constituted. Although nowadays much reduced in number, there are different groups of Zoroastrians in North America and Europe, as well as in India and some parts of East Asia and, very few, in Iran. The Parsis from India are the most numerous. God (Ohrmazd) is pure goodness and omniscient, but not however omnipotent. The Devil (Ahriman), who is evil, must be destroyed before God can become all-powerful.

God created first the invisible, intangible world and then the visible, tangible one. The Zoroastrian view is that the latter, the material, thus embodies the spiritual but is not opposed to it. We might call this a prime instance of animated materiality (of the physical given life), which, before the Devil's destructive intervention, was regarded by believers as a 'natural' existence free of human suffering. Pain, fever, ill health and mortality are then the 'unnatural' consequences of this deployment of evil, which is thereafter locked in a battle with the forces of good. The righteous conduct of humans helps God in overcoming evil but they themselves suffer in the conflict.

The 'unnaturalness' of a corpse and any degenerative elements which have left the body are polluting. They include menstrual and childbirth blood, excreta, nail clippings, cut hair and rotting matter. These and the corpse itself become the sites on which evil appears and fights with good, resulting in human sickness. Given its propensity in its polluted or unhealthy state to act as a locus for attacks by evil on good, the body should be kept healthy and in harmony with the soul through virtuous social behaviour.

The conventional Western contrast between medicine and religion ignores this combined bodily and social materiality. The starting point for biomedicine is the laid-out body, historically the spiritless cadaver, opened up to the surgically reductionist gaze, while religion starts with the soul which leaves behind and outlives the body. The challenge, then, is to argue that religion as much as medicine are to do with materiality. Both presuppose good and evil, or health and ill health, as resulting from appropriate or inappropriate densities of interaction with humans, gods and goods. The interactions may range from gift-giving, trade, fighting, love, sex, to supplications and prayer, and the densities are to do with frequency, range and intensity. These vary culturally as well as individually but are in all cases underwritten by expectations, rights, duties and obligations, non-fulfilment of which brings misfortune and affliction. The materiality of social density is, then, this combined sense and practice of social obligatariness and charity, according to which people measure their own well-being or lack of it, and so are constituted by it.

Complementary or alternative medical systems are generally regarded as going further than biomedicine in locating the body in social, emotional and cosmological contexts, such that cure of the soul is also that of the body, or that venal and mortal sins are corporally marked as death, disease and infertility. While this is broadly valid, we must not forget that the non-religious moralising that takes place in biomedicine over alleged abuse of the body (too much smoking, eating and drinking) may sometimes become recast as religious (AIDS as God's punishment for humanity's sins).

It is when we venture into the variety of the world's religions that we see how inadequate the separation of soul and body is. The alleged absence of non-Cartesian dualisms in Africa and Asia does not mean that medical problems of the mind/soul are not indigenously distinguished from those of the body (madness, for instance, everywhere being differentiated from stomach ulcers), but rather that problems in the one almost inevitably entail some diagnosis of the other, to the extent indeed that they appear implicated in each other.

There is a more general paradigm here. Marriott argued long ago (1976)[2] that in much Hindu theology a Brahmin is polluted (has acted in a polluting manner) in a combined bodily and moral manner if he accepts food from a member of a lower caste without realising the latter's lowly status. He has to be purified as must his co-resident fellow Brahmins who are equally polluted by the act, for they are interlinked by particles which are as much physical as moral. Food transactions, intercommunal and communal pollution and purification make up the materiality that we otherwise call socio-religious rules and their consequences if broken.

Intentionality on the part of the offender is then irrelevant to the initial, accidental act of pollution but pertains to the restorative act of purification. 'Sin' is an inappropriately translated concept in this instance but, insofar as it might have meaning, would refer to a refusal to purify and redress the unknowingly committed wrong rather than to its commission in the first place. In other words, while ill consequences flow from even unwitting transgressions, there is still room for individuals to exercise choice in their conduct.

A parallel is found in this volume in the various discussions of *karma*, in which persons' misdemeanours in past lives are not normally held against them, in contrast to their present life when they have the chance to engage in good works and so overcome present suffering and improve their future incarnation.

There are here three broad antinomies: of human against *karma* or equivalent cosmic influence, of human against God, and of good against evil. Each is used both to explain and to repair problems of human suffering. Yet each raises questions concerning humankind's capacity to challenge extra-human powers of determination.

First, then, the various strands making up what we clumsily call Hinduism, Jainism, Sikhism and Buddhism turn on the predetermination of suffering through *karmic* or *karmic*-like cyclical rebirths which individuals can strive to overcome (Leslie, Samuel, Singh and Skorupski).

Second, the theodicies of the so-called Semitic religions, including Judaism, Christianity and Islam, ask why a powerful, knowledgeable and merciful God should allow, and even inflict, human suffering (Melling, Sachedina, Solomon, Conrad and see also Wujastyk on the Hindu god, Siva's, punishment through demons).

Third, Manichaeism, partly evident in Zoroastrianism (Hinnells) and the religion of the Cathars, and parallelled in African spirit beliefs (Honwana), stands alone in admitting no definite, eventual triumph of good over evil, or of God over Satan, and may allow humankind a role in this contest between the two co-eternal cosmic principles. As Conrad notes, the dualism of Manichaeism was a challenge to the idea of monotheistic omnipotence in Judaism, Christianity and Islam, with the latter, however, eventually driving it out of Iran, its place of origin.

Structurally inverse, though of indeterminate or variable historical relationship, is the quest not for dominance of one element over another in an eternal struggle between opposing forces, but for their harmonious balance, as in Chinese medicine and Confucian philosophy (Bray) and in most non-biomedical humoural systems, including those already mentioned.

In practice elements of all three presuppositional possibilities (reincarnation, theodicy and balance/imbalance) may be present in religious explanation and activity, including those that embrace problems of human well-being and ill health.

Human Agents and Divine Omnipotence

A theme of many chapters in this volume, however, is that ordinary people are often more directly concerned with questions of personal bodily and mental health than with religious or theological issues of the kind outlined above. And yet, at the same time, these often textually based religious matters may inform the indigenous health facilities available to them, usually by way of the healer or healing agent. How does the individual human agent fit into these two overarching voices of authority, the healer and divinity?

There are in fact two kinds of relationship. First is that between healer and patient, on which so much has been written, which is both collaborative and competitive, as each draws on their respective explanatory viewpoints, which converge on some points but diverge on others. Second is the relationship of worshipper to a god, gods, demons or extra-human forces. The relationship between healer and patient may be mediated by divine inspiration, effect or substance (as in the possession of *baraka* by Sayyids in Islam or of spirits in African animism (Honwana)). Conversely, that between individual and divinity may be mediated by humans in the role of priests, clerics or shamans.

This alterity, now of human but now of divinity as mediator, inevitably throws up the problem of the relative status of human agent to divinity or divine force. It is on this status that so much discussion concerning religion and healing turns, for what is at issue is how much control over their health and well-being humans may be permitted within their religion independently of divinity.

We might at first think that this question of how much humans determine their own fate in the face of divine power is a peculiarly Christian concern, given the post-Enlightenment rejection of theories of human predestination. In fact, in different forms the question pervades the practice, if not always the texts, of many religions, especially regarding this-worldly matters of health and well-being.

As regards the religious theodicies of Christianity, Judaism and Islam, a major distinguishing feature is a concern on the part of religious authorities to suppress beliefs and practices which appeal to forces (godly or demonic) other than those of the One God, and to quash the worship of idols and craven images. There is here an interesting individualisation of three agents in the drama, which achieves fullest expression in Christianity in the Protestant ethic as classically described by Max Weber. God is one and complete in Itself, but so is Satan. Each is accompanied by smaller and much less powerful angelic and demonic entities, but these are set apart and not normally held to be refractions of the One. However, the individualism of the human agent is normally characterised as unique responsibility for his/her own divine destiny, via their sins and virtues, quite the opposite of the shared, inter-individual (dividual) Brahmanic essence described by Marriott above.

This three-part individualisation (God, Satan and Human), while distinct from the more rigidly Manichaean principles (humankind relating to two equal forces of good and evil), is not unique to the so-called Semitic religions but is a kind of underlying model in them. There are of course deviations from the model. For instance, certain Sufi Muslims hold that man and God, and good and evil as aspects of man and God, are inseparably part of each other and so not individualised in any marked way (Bousfield 1985).[3] But such exceptions are conspicuous by their unorthodoxy.

In this volume there are a number of descriptions of health, sickness and misfortune showing God, Satan and humanity meeting as distinct entities. Melling cites Cyprian, Bishop of Carthage at the time of a plague in the year 252 CE, as saying that while a Christian had to accept that his faith was no guarantee of protection against disease, he could nevertheless benefit from his suffering, both of ill health and at the hands of the devil, for it is in this way that he could be spiritually purified and know that his faith was being tested and hence confirmed. Yet, while this might be regarded as a Christian's privileged suffering, God was not above sending sickness as punishment for an individual's sin. Breaking out, so to speak, from such divine interventionism, medical advisers within the Christian tradition have sometimes also diagnosed individual sickness as due, not to God's punishment, but to a disordered and self-indulgent life: a clear indication of a theme of responsibility by and for the human individual alone.

This idea of individual autonomy before God will not of course be allowed to extend to an abuse of God's authority. Under circumstances where this may seem to be developing, ecclesiastical authorities are likely to respond by invoking faithlessness as a cause of current sickness and misery. Nevertheless, the fact that the Judaeo-Christian tradition does allow some individual human self-determination lays the ground for the development of ideas of individual responsibility in biomedicine which are not dependent on divine intercession or sanction.

Solomon distinguishes, for instance, three attitudes to healing in the Jewish tradition, one of which is what he calls the scienitific and which has always prevailed in some circles in Judaism. He notes that, even with regard to the use of medically protective amulets, the Talmud 'scientifically' distinguished between those whose validity could be tested under controlled conditions of empirical experiment and observation, and those that could not. Contrasted with this are the popular and theological healing attitudes, which, dealing with the power of demons and God respectively, portray humanity as essentially at the prey of externally imposed expectations and caprice.

Demonic caprice is confronted, but God's expectations are binding. When we surgically replace a defective kidney, do we thwart God's will? The Jewish sect, the Karaites, are not alone in rejecting the use of biomedicine for this kind of reason, it being held that a sick individual should turn not to doctors but to God in repentance. And yet the divinely revealed Torah allows that doctors may heal, with at least one major code of Jewish law obliging them to do so. A compromise is sometimes to permit the use of alternative therapies which, being "natural" in the use of God's herbs as listed in holy texts, do not offend against God's design, while man-made biomedicine does.

Sachedina notes that Islam lacks a centralised theological body such as the Vatican Council in Catholicism. There are consequently different views within and between Islamic schools of thought. There is however agreement that God is not only omnipotent and omniscient but also the ultimate healer, just as the Quran, also divinely revealed, contains all past, present and future medical and other knowledge. This does not preclude debate concerning free will and predetermination with regard to human suffering, although God's will is always absolute and hence an ultimate limit on that of the individual. Much of this debate echoes that in the Juadaeo-Christian tradition. There are a number of textually derived claims. The Umayyad rulers (660–748 CE) cited specific verses of the Quran to justify their view that human suffering was God's punishment to which mortals should unquestionably submit. On the other hand, humans bring suffering upon themselves and need to remove it through righteous works.

There is also Quranic recognition of the inexplicability of much evil suffered by people and of their need to trust to God's mercy and to his plan. The Prophet is moreover reported to have said in one tradition that suffering and sickness were means by which a true believer could expiate his sins, and in another that he could thereby purify himself, so much so that in one thanksgiving prayer, God is praised for having sent 'good' affliction. And yet afflictions can also be regarded as evils in the world against which medical and other action should be taken. Taken out of context and compared with each other, such claims might seem inconsistent and even contradictory. But they can be seen as elements in a scaffolding of reason. Islam embodies the will of God; suffering in the world is a necessary condition of knowing it and others' suffering and thence a means of knowing the beneficence of God (who is in turn the embodiment of the world); this unavoidable suffering needs no further explanation, for it is created by an unquestionably good God and can be dealt with by humans through the education and self-discipline which an understanding of the Quran and Traditions (*Hadith*) provides, an understanding which renders suffering variously as punishment, expiation, purification, a test of faith and the revelation of God's complete virtue.

There are of course alternative ways in which the reasoning can be arranged and it is such differences which have occasioned disputes within Islam and its schools. Sachedina describes one such conflict from the first half of the eighth century. The Mu'tazili emphasised a theodicy of free will and responsibility framed by God's justice, which was drawn from Hellenic and Judaeo-Christian influences. By contrast, the Ash'arites denied that such a view could be reconciled with God's tanscendent and all-powerful determination of all actions. According to Sachedina, Ash'arite predestination doctrine shaped Sunni medical theory, which saw sickness as just and inevitable, to which people could react with treatment subject to God's will. These views of humanity as either creatively pro-active or merely reactive make up the poles of the debate, with humanity and demonic forces having variable amounts of latitude permitted by God.

Again, as an exception to this pattern, we have to remind ourselves of the special case of Zoroastranism, with its dualism of good and evil as co-eternal forces, in which God does not exclusively dictate the terms of the cosmic battle and in which the human individual is of pivotal significance. For it to be possible that humans triumph over evil and so help God become omnipotent, humans become its victims and suffer affliction. They are principal agents but also at greatest existential risk.

Those religions in which individuals can better themselves through cyclical rebirths and interpret their current suffering as the *karma* of past actions place even greater emphasis on human agency and responsibility. Increasing personal merit is a route to a better rebirth, while another is through ascetic practices of self-transcendence and the elimination of desire. As Melling notes, the Christian view of suffering as enabling the afflicted individual to grow morally and spiritually is a kind of self-sacrifice or ascesis, though more in terms of helping Christ save humanity. It is at a crossroads between moral self-betterment (so preserving enhanced selfhood in an afterlife) and self-transcendence (in which selfhood is ideally rendered irrelevant). The *karmic*-related religions incline more towards the latter.

Leslie recognises that the term 'Hinduism' (to which we may add Buddhism, Jainism, Sikhism and Zoroastrianism) essentialises what are in effect different, overlapping and changing practices and beliefs. She nevertheless draws out a number of general characteristics, of which two, individual responsibility for one's own past and future *karma*, and the absence therefore of a concept of innocent victim, are especially interesting to the present discussion. The lack of emphasis in *karmic* religions on an all-powerful, all-knowing, all-merciful one God as in the Islamic and Judaeo-Christian tradition, precludes humans having to be accountable to It. They are directed instead to an existential metaphysics in which, ideally, the achievement is to be permanently released from the cycle of rebirths.

Pashaura Singh discusses the effects on contemporary life of the sacred scriptures of the Sikh Gurus, and in particular the important fifteenth and sixteenth century Guru Nanak. Singh portrays the Sikh religious perspective on *karam* (*karma*) as having undergone a radical change from the general position of *karma* in Indian thought. *Karam* as a principle of cause and effect is in fact subject to a single higher Divine Order (*Hukam*), which is ultimately the source of suffering but also that which can break the chain of bad *karam*. Guru Nanak explicity sees this balancing of opposed tendencies, which avoids rigid predestination theories and yet enables persons to see their own 'free' will as that of God (Akal Purkakh), as allowing Sikhs the opportunity to 'carve out their own destinies', a feature stereotypically associated with Sikh enterprise throughout the world.

Suffering is not sent by God but is an inevitable part of the human condition, caused by human self-centredness or desire (*haumai*) separating humanity from God. Suffering can therefore be confronted without the assumption that God is responsible for it.

There is little concern as in other theodicies with the problem of reconciling the idea of an omnipotent and kindly God with his allowing evil to occur in the world.

Buddhism shares the basic doctrine of *karma* with Hinduism and Jainism and, in its modified version, Sikhism. Popular ideas notwithstanding, none enjoin theories of human fatalism: humans may alter their destinies through their own actions. Nevertheless, according to Skorupski, Buddhism has its own distinctive understanding of *karma*. The Buddha himself defined *karma* as mental volition and as driven by the 'cravings' of desire, hatred and delusion. Such cravings can however be suppressed and open the way to freedom from the cycle of rebirths, a possibility seemingly not dissimilar in broad outline from that described by Leslie and for Hindu ascetics. Distinctive, however, is the final stage of detachment, or "snuffing out" of the unsatisfactory nature of existence, called *nirvana* which, as well as removing all desire and future rebirths, offers peace, tranquillity and deathlessness, a particularly full expression of self-transcendence or, better, of selfhood-made-irrelevant.

We have, of course, to acknowledge the different historical phases and regional versions of Buddhism (Theravada, Mahayana, Vajrayana, Japanese Shingon, Tibetan, and others found in East Asia, including Korea, Vietnam and China), a variability common to all so-called world religions. For present purposes, the focus is on one or two features that not only characterise Buddhism in general but extend also into other *karma*-related religions.

In Buddhism, *karma* is the most prevalently cited cause of suffering. Nevertheless, bodily and mental afflictions acquired at birth and therefore clearly attributable to past actions, are not regarded as grounds for discrimination or condemnation in the current life. Thus, while on the one hand a person is born with a specific personality, s/he can choose to override the behaviour that ensues from such inborn dispositions and improve their future existence.

Skorupski cites texts giving seven other causes of suffering than *karma*, including the three bodily humours (*tridosa*, comprising wind, phlegm and bile) and their imbalance, seasonal change, stress and externally induced changes. He also divides causes of specific diseases into two main categories: *karma* on the one hand, and, on the other, demons, environment, intake of poisonous substances, inappropriate conduct and humoral disorder. As general causes, these are of course shared in comparable form by most of the other "Asian" systems.

Solomon's research into refugees in the context of Tibetan Buddhism gives flesh to this abstract picture. In Dalhousie, in northern India, it is questionable as to how significant formal Buddhism is in the healing resources available to the Tibetan refugees. Few have a sophisticated knowledge of Buddhist texts and teaching, and most can be said to be engaged at best in a practical Buddhism, in which amulets, family shrines, offerings and prayers to deities and lamas, divinations, tantric rituals combine with the use of biomedicine (ironically known as 'Indian medicine').

Solomon's chapter, like some others in this volume, provides specific case histories of patients, reflecting intensive fieldwork carried out in the town. His account emphasises the intellectual distance of most people from textually based religious debates although they are indirectly affected by them. Solomon suggests, for instance, that their rudimentary and practical knowledge of Buddhism has taught the refugees that life's achievements were always likely to be hedged around with great uncertainty, such impermanence and dissatisfaction being the way of the world. This religiously derived existential uncertainty makes them wary of attaining worldly success while seeking it. It makes them equally wary and pragmatic with regard to the use and combination of whatever therapies are available.

This study shows that religions do not necessarily provide reassurance. Cults of the millennial kind try to, but are conspicuous for their short-lived nature and failed promises. Normally, given the inevitable debates within any religion over the causes, consequences and remedies of human suffering, as outlined above, the textual bases of religions provide only rough-hewn templates of possible action against ill health and misfortune.

The Spirit of Bodily Thinking

There has developed a tendency in much writing in medical anthropology and history to sharply divide western and non-Western ideas on the body-mind dichotomy. Apart from being an absolute presupposition in biomedicine, the so-called Cartesian separation of mind as the seat of reason and the body as governed by its own physicalist laws recurs in other domains. In his literary work, Emile Zola portrayed the passions as animalistically springing from bodily needs and in constant conflict with the rational and moral thinking of the soul. By contrast, African and Asian epistemologies are deemed in Western scholarship to be premised on the broad idea that thought presupposes emotional involvement, with emotional responses in turn informing intentions, and with mental and bodily ailments part of each other and neither consistently dominant. This distinction between operational knowledges starts from a Western viewpoint and can be so exaggerated as to imply that non-Western peoples, and Europeans before Descartes, hardly bother to distinguish between the head and the body as separable starting-points in diagnosis and explanation.

Numerous examples show this not to be the case and that there are interesting cross-cultural variations in the extent to which either the mind/soul/head or body are used to initiate medical judgement, however much they are then brought together within a holistic approach.

In the pre-Cartesian climate of the medieval English hospital described by Rawcliffe, prior attention to the soul is the precondition of bodily health. Although body and soul were regarded as inextricably linked, the chief concern was to promote spiritual health. The condition of the soul would then determine what could be done with the sick body: heal the spiritual state first and then supply the body with medicine. The logic of the prevalent view that physical suffering was the punishment for sin, and that confession was incumbent on the sick or dying, was to confer upon the priest the idea that he was a 'physician of the soul'.

As in much of Africa, where afflicted persons sometimes confessed to initiatory witchcraft in order to have the effects of an opponent's counter-witchcraft removed, medieval English patients might own to delicts before a surgical operation, with medical practitioners being obliged to extract confessions by a ruling of the Lateran Council of 1215.

The priority is reversed in the case described by Park for thirteenth and fourteenth century Italy, in which an idiom of the revelatory body rather than the soul is the investigatory starting-point for discovering divine as well as medical truths. Here religious dissection of the human body occurred historically at about the same time as medical autopsies were carried out to determine the cause of death or sickness.

The religious starting-point was the celebration of Christ's own suffering body as an exemplar of saintly bodies, from which could be extracted organs, objects and holy inscriptions which became sacred relics with the power to heal.

Medical dissection arose out of a revival of interest in Galen's argument that external bodily signs indicated little of the body's interior. While clerics (often nuns) and physicians sometimes helped each other interpret what they found in a body, male sceptics challenged the growing movement of penitential women clerics who were foremost in the religious dissections of other women, the potential saints. The men turned women's private religious dissections into autopsies subject to the gaze of male medical expertise, so precluding women's access to the power of sacred bodily relics and bringing them under male control. The bodily idiom here was fundamental in defining the routes to spiritual authority and knowledge.

In indigenous Japanese psychotherapy, also, as instanced by the theories of the Naikan and Morita schools (Chikako Ozawa 1997),[4] the body is the route to mental refinement and spiritual well-being. Here, bodily discipline and order have to be perfected in order to settle and restore mental disorder. Indeed, bodily balance ensures that of the mind and emotions. The two go together, but it is to bodily posture and coordination that attention must be first be given.

Bray shows that Confucian-based medical theories and practice in China do not depend on belief in a god or divinity, nor have they historically contained contestable views of the mind as the locus of either religious soul or secular rationality. Nor are such theories pervaded by debates concerning the mind-body dichotomy. However, the life-energy, *ch'i* (*qi*), is a bodily phenomenon whose proper distribution accounts for the body's overall well-being including what we would translate as the person's mental state. To that extent it presupposes the working of the human body in a combined body-mind sense and does not need even to start with such a dichotomy. Indeed, throughout her chapter, Bray does not feel it necessary to invoke reference to it.

Ch'i is responsive to seasonal and astral cyles, and should maintain a balance within bodily organs, that is, between *yin* and *yang*. The five main *yin* organs are not understood in isolation from each other but as functionally interrelating with other *yang* organs, and in terms of what are known as the five phases (not elements) of wood, fire, earth, metal and water, disorders of which may create emotional as well as physiological disturbance. Chinese medical science, whether in its Buddhist, Taoist or directly Confucian manifestations, is the least Cartesian of all. Even in medieval Taoism, there is a distinction not between soul and body but between mortal body and immortal body which eventually discards the former in order to soar free and unite with the Tao. In other words, even that which we might translate as soul is spoken of in the idiom of body.

Buddhism operates through this idiom. It both rejects the body as a repository of suffering, disease and unacceptable sensuality, and yet, through its rejection and perfection, sees it as the best means of attaining Buddhahood. Skorupski cites texts encouraging meditation on the impurities and decomposition of the body, and other texts providing instruction on how to remove bodily, emotional and mental obstructions to accomplishing this ideal. In seeking the perfection of the Buddha's body, tantric meditational exercises aim at achieving the bodily suppleness and subtlety that transcend normal bodily constraints.

We may note here Melling's reference in early Christianity to Clement of Alexandria's opposition to Gnostic contempt for the body and his insistence on physical health leading to a virtuous nature. This linking of bodily perfection with virtue, of an 'outer' with an 'inner' state, is echoed in Leslie's reference taken from Sanskrit literature to the idea that personal physical appearance denotes moral character. A good man is thus recognised by his good looks. A woman may be also, although her beauty may sometimes mask manipulative cunning. For both men and women ugliness or physical disability indicate that the person is untrustworthy. But this latter view seems to contradict the claim that one's deformity in this life is derived from past deeds and is no reason for moral discrimination in the current life.

Confronting a Cartesian dilemma, unexpected in the South Asian context, Leslie refers to a conundrum expressed in modern drama: if the head is the person's inner mental and emotional nature (their personality), and if the body, through the physical effects of *karma*, determine that inner state, then how does a bodily or facially disfigured person acquire the good personality to improve their next rebirth? Perhaps this is indeed a very recently expressed dilemma, possibly influenced by Western ideas, for the texts make clear, as with Budhhist ones, that no blame should attach to anyone for their past deeds. Or perhaps, it is again at the level of practical religion, and in defiance or ignorance of the texts, that people do in fact judge others on the basis of their bodily visible *karma*. Such questions presuppose a language of judgement, whose main terms define suffering.

The Language of Pain and Suffering

Although it is often difficult in other languages to find a translatable equivalent of the English word, suffering, words within a semantic domain connoted by the term often reflect the body's ambivalent role either as indicating a person's inner state or as the site of physically degenerative disease. The Arabic *musiba* means misfortune generally but can include bodily and mental ill health, and, as Conrad points out, there are also separate terms for pain, torment, affliction, calamity, distress and evil. Pope John Paul II regarded suffering as evil, although the translated Greek New and Old Testament term was *pascho*, for which the Latin *patior* and its English derivative 'passion' produced the ambivalence of suffering which is passively inflicted but also suffering which is actively, even ecstatically, embraced.

This ambivalent sense of suffering, and by extension pain, distinguishes its religious from its biomedical usage. Biomedically, pain is almost always negatively regarded, while in religion, within which most alternative therapies are inscribed, pain is the metaphysical space in which moral reasoning may sometimes be reconciled with bodily and mental loss and impairment. People seek relief from pain but, under certain circumstances, seek pain.

Horden provides a citation from Virginia Woolf which expresses admirably how people may be drawn to the pain of love and speak of it with great eloquence and nuanced vocabulary, while physical pain reduces the sufferer to virtual inarticulacy. Certainly, the lexicons in different languages for differentiating types of pain seem surprisingly impoverished given its overall importance as an indicator of ill health. I suggest that this is because physical pain incapacitates the whole body-mind, detracts from its cognitive as well as physical completeness, and so takes from speech the total consciousness needed to articulate subtle distinctions.

The Sanskrit term, *duhkham*, denotes suffering and misery of all mental and bodily kinds, including what we conventially understand as pain, and stands in contrast to *sukha*, happiness. According to Alexis Sanderson (personal communication), other principal Sanskrit words for pain and suffering are *pida, vedana, vyatha* and *artih* (diacritical marks are omitted). They are remarkably unspecialised in their reference, those referring to physical pain being used also for mental pain, the source or locus being differentiated by qualification, usually in a tatpurusha compound. Sanderson identifies only one word for a particular kind of pain, namely *sulam*, meaning sharp or piercing pain as experienced by a colic or gout sufferer and a metaphorical extension of its literal meaning, spike, impaling stake. There are of course terms dealing with other kinds of negative experience such as *adih* and *tapah*, connoting the mental distress of hardship, pain and loss. *Krcchram, kastam* and *klesah* refer to difficulty, trouble and distress, with *khedah* meaning fatigue and distress. Of these Old Indo-Aryan words, a few survived into Middle and New Indo-Aryan languages, of which *duhkham* is the most wide-ranging, as mentioned above.

Various elaborations of the term, *duhkham*, pervade Buddhism as well as Hinduism and related religions. The Punjabi term, *dukkh*, has broadly a comparable meaning for Sikhs, but, as Singh shows, ranges over numerous connotations in its actual textual usage, extending, as in Buddhism, to a sense of frustration and dissatisfaction with a life made heavy by previous bad ones. It is moreover contrasted with the Persian-derived term, *dard*, which means the emotional pain of, say, separation from a loved one. *Dard* is thus contrasted as emotional suffering from that experienced by the body in its purely visceral sense. A *Malar* hymn summarises powerfully this distinction and interrelationship of heart-mind-soul (*man*) and body (*sarir*): 'If there is anguish (*dard*) in the heart, there will be continued suffering in the body.'

The chapters by Horden and Porter provide the historical, social and semantic contexts in which Western ideas of pain and its treatment have developed. Porter refers to two related features. First, the legacy of certain Christian teachings is to emphasise the worthwhileness of suffering, including its most visible expression, physical pain. Pain should thus often be endured and even relished for the benefits to the soul and character it can bring. A further development of this line of thinking was to suggest that pain was evolutionarily adaptive and therefore physiologically 'healthy'. Second, Cartesian-influenced biomedicine has treated sickness as a problem of the body, of pathological anatomy, rather than of the whole body-mind-person, and so has regarded physical rather than psychological pain as the only truly authentic kind. The result is that only recently has it become less questioningly acceptable to clinicians to see the elimination of bodily pain as itself a worthy pursuit.

Is indeed the eradication of pain to be regarded as in some cases the 'cure' and not just the removal of it as pathogenic symptom? East Asian therapies based on the flow of *ch'i* (*qi*)or *ki* clearly would not accept this, for the diagnosis of pain as signifying an imbalance of life-energy is fundamental (Bray). On the other hand, as Porter concludes, effective pain control in modern biomedicine does enhance the quality of life among the terminal and chronically sick, who may be an increasing proportion of patients in wealthier, ageing regions of the world. Horden concurs that, increasingly since the 1960s, pain is indeed given due reverence.

While Cartesian dominance of French and thence European hospital medicine may from about 1800 have encouraged people to distinguish physical from psychological pain, Porter argues that earlier teachings from Hippocrates to the Renaissance 'regarded maladies holistically, and viewed the "physical" and the "spiritual" as a continuum mediated through such concepts as the humours and temperaments'.

Does this continuum, refusing to distinguish sharply between what we nowadays identify as physical and emotional pain, thus have its roots in early Hippocratic ideas? This is indeed the received wisdom. Horden argues against this and suggests that the Hippocratics, including Galen himself, revealed in their treatises a concern with pain which places them more in company with the non-holistic, laboratory-focused, rationalists of early modern medicine, in which pain generally is regarded as peripheral, and non-somatic pain as unreal. The Hippocratics were, after all, themselves concerned with scientific rationality and with the authority over patients' conduct that is associated with such specialist expertise.

Focusing on the Old Masters of medicine, mainly the writers of the *Corpus Hippocraticum* and also Rufus of Ephesus and Galen, Horden discusses the lexicon of Greek terms which we translate broadly as pain. However, against other scholarly claims, he finds that the great work does not make out of them a rich semantic field on the subject of pain. Despite referring to pain some 2,000 times, it is denoted by synonyms which, while numbering some nine basic terms, are generally unqualified by adjectives and adverbs. The

Hippocratic language of pain (as distinct from that of literature) is therefore relatively undifferentiated, like that of Sanskrit discussed above, (emotional pain being subsumed within the somatic, for instance, but with psychological trauma not treated as a matter of pain but of other symptoms and causes). Pain is not metaphysically significant for the Hippocratic doctors, who, if we follow Horden's line of argument, would be unsympathetic to the modern idea of setting up pain clinics for chronic sufferers.

In his discussion of suffering and divine justice in early Islamic society, Conrad notes the absence of Arabic words easily translatable as suffering, and that suffering has to be seen as victims' emotional response to adversity and not the adversity itself. Texts advise on the relief of suffering and less on the nature of suffering itself. The shaping of ideas of suffering through the language we use and the effect on language of the actual experience of suffering are so mutually involved that it is difficult to separate them. A challenging claim is that the use of terms, whether by religious clergy and/or makers of health policy, actually creates the stereotypes, prejudices and assumptions by which sick people are judged.

Thus, Littlewood's paper on the recent history of treatment of schizophrenics in Britain traces the development of official and clinical vocabulary. This reflects changes in health policy and moulds views of patients by the public and by the patients themselves. For instance, taken separately the terms 'community' and 'care' each connote notions of support, nurture, local solidarity, and a common purpose aimed at providing cure or long-term relief. How is it, then, that by 1997, the expression "community care" had come to be associated with violence, failure and fragmentation?

The answer lies in a major shift in government thinking. The Conservative government had proposed in 1981 that, by 1996, all psychiatric hospitals in Britain would be closed. This went hand in hand with the government's view that the new enterprise culture would allow more autonomy to the individual who would thereby be encouraged to rely less on state support. Up to that time, also, there had been a move within liberal medical circles to the view that mental illness could not consistently be objectified in terms of the normal diagnostic disease criteria, and that 'mad' patients were in fact often heroically engaged in a creative act of resistance against an oppressive social order and deserved to be allowed to live their own lives rather than be subject, as objects, to the authoritarian care of others. Persons diagnosed as mentally sick were thereafter given less care in psychiatric clinics and were sent back to the community of their families.

The staff of inner-city psychiatric clinics are expected to learn management as well as medical skills in order to make the most financally efficient use of clinics' limited bed availabilty. Given that many patients sent out into the community either lack or cannot easily be helped by their families, the result of this change in policy is to disperse them throughout society. There, however, they merge with other jobless, homeless and mendicant. Regarded as largely responsible for their own personal destiny according to the terms of the entreprise culture, they are more likely to transfer blame for their isolation onto external agencies, including society as a whole.

Since an improportionate number of diagnosed schizophrenics are young Black men, who already include many who are unemployed and without homes, a further result is the continued racial marginalisation of significant numbers of people, who often come to be regarded more as individualistic anti-social criminals than sick patients for whom society is answerable. Again, a whole new vocabulary has been evolved which reflects the official ideology of the receiving community but hides the reality that dispersal of sick people aggravates their and society's problems rather than solving them. As Littlewood puts it, 'the current (1996) dispersal of patients away from the psychiatric hospital with its localised procedures but institutional public accountability is a recognition of the earlier failure of the eradication of disease by clinical psychiatry'.

A question raised in Littlewood's work is the extent to which cross-culturally we can identify a malady such as schizophrenia. Varying socio-cultural ways of expressing emotional and psychic problems may not be acceptable to biomedical specialists working to set criteria of what constitutes schizophrenia, or customarily normal means of coping with stress in a society (e.g. beliefs in and action against witchcraft) may become wrongly diagnosed as symptomatic of schizophrenia. Moreover, within different societies, distinctively named ailments may, so to speak, serve as central, semantic and emblematic foci of a group's concerns.

Speaking from his experience as a physician in a London inner-city general practice, Cohen here draws to our attention the existence of what he calls culture-bound syndromes, citing loss of soul (*susto*) in South America, post-natal depression (*amakiro*) in Uganda and possession by spirits (*zar*) in Somalia, each of which he sees as equivalent, in terms of their indigenous nosological predominance, to the focus in Europe on anorexia nervosa. While parallels between such semantic clusters need to be compared intensively before generalisations can be made about them, the point is well made that different medical and religious rationalities inform each other in a number of culturally distinctive combinations.

Shared Templates in Religious and Medical Explanation

Pursuing the idea of Hippocratic medical diagnoses as guided by the quest for scientific rationality, King suggests why patients might for certain purposes prefer to seek cure in religion rather than in medicine. Referring to fifth and fourth century BC Greece, she contrasts the relationship at the time between Hippocratic and temple medicine, principally of the god Asklepios.

These offer alternative means of dealing with specific problems. In the case of the Asklepios temple, treatment through an understanding of an individual's dreams and narratives in the context of a wider web of family ties enables that person to make sense of their problem as one of wider human relationships and not as due to a failing on their own part. Hippocratic use of illness narrative, by contrast, subjects the patient to reflection on his/her habits as possible reasons for their malady, and so in effect lays blame on the individual.

We may here ask whether the current interest in Euro-American societies in mainly Asian and African religio-therapeutic systems (as described for Britain by Saks) is an indication of persons' assumption that these provide opportunities unavailable in biomedicine to locate their illness narratives in extended discussion of their social and emotional contexts. If so, it is only partially valid, for the increasing professionalisation of complementary medicine may well lead to a narrowing of specialist concerns which lessen, even if they do not obviate, the distinction in this respect between biomedical and non-biomedical healer-patient relations.

It would be ironic if, at the same time, the practice of biomedicine develops a more holistic perspective, as appears to be the case in limited instances. Indeed, Saks argues that, despite the biomedical characterisation in Britain through the nineteenth and twentieth centuries of alternative medicine as being unscientific and superstitious, in fact religiously based complementary therapies are not significantly different in this regard from biomedicine. He suggests that we take as our definition of religion not simply belief in the supernatural but the expression of moral imperatives sustained by reference to an idea of human spirit. By this definition, most if not all forms of alternative medicine link human well-being with holistic notions of spiritual energy and hence are religious.

Recasting this, I would say that alternative therapies generally presuppose the transformative and hence curative existence of forces which are not, however, empirically verifiable by the measures of Western science. Such forces are 'religious' insofar as they are identified in the literature as either gods, demons or spirits, or cosmic phenomena (including such notions as *ch'i* and other life-energies). Included under this definition, then, are the Chinese and Buddhist therapies (none of which are dependent on ideas of significant or high gods) as well as those of, say, Ayurveda, Yunani, African animism and of course the humoral equilibrium and herbal theories of pre-modern European medicine. The Eurocentric definers of religion would, paradoxically, regard many of these complementary medical systems as non-religious for failing to refer to a high god as ultimate source of power, knowledge and virtue.

Saks's point is that, while alternative medicines have been criticised for their scientific unverifiability, biomedicine itself has been under attack also for the way in which, following Kuhn (1970),[5] its paradigms are themselves socially constructed and based not on scientifically neutral, value-free, absolute truths but on untestable socio-cultural assumptions about what is health, disease and sickness, and how, why and what should be treated, and for whom. Whether or not we define alternative therapies as religious, they then share with biomedicine this absence of impartiality and transcendental objectivity regarding the uses to which they are put. Both forms of medicine are to that extent highly subjective, though not necessarily ineffective as a consequence, for both do make use of factual evidence based on observation in their treatments.

This is not to say that the two areas are epistemologically the same. The research procedures and results of, for example, genetic engineering, whatever their socio-cultural motivation, have a different impact on the world than the sometimes implicit attempts by alternative healers to, say, link sickness and misfortune to social and environmental disorder, as Honwana describes in her discussion of healing in post-war southern Mozambique. There is overlap rather than rigid separation in assumption, operational procedure, and results.

Regarding the latter, Honwana shows that Euro-American psychotherapy shares with African indigenous spirit beliefs a capacity to heal victims of war violence. We could, if we wished, say that African divination and remedy through the use of ancestral spirits is a form of African psychotherapy. But this privileges Western epistemology and hides the socio-cultural appropriateness and advantages of an African one. It also confuses method with aim. Both have a common goal, namely to restore the patient to their pre-traumatic state, and in both cases can be judged observationally to have some success, but their methods appear to be different. While one relies on an appeal to spirits of the dead to possess and so cure the victim, the other invokes the patient's memory and sense of an unfragmented past selfhood as a means of recovering it.

That said, such methods can always be related analogically: we might claim that the idea of past spirit (i.e. of the dead) 'stands for' the idea of past self-consciousness. We might also claim that the pantheon of named, personified and historically situated spirits in the Mozambiquan case is as complex operationally, conceptually and semantically as the vocabulary of psychotherapeutic concepts, and requires a long and demanding apprenticeship in order to understand and make use of it. That we can make such claims is no guarantee of their validity but is part of the heuristic attempt to see similarity and not just difference in the conditions under which complementary therapies are set up and practised.

From Durkheim to Lévi-Strauss, religious thought, including totemism and the classification of the cosmic, biological and spirit world, has often been analysed as analogically expressive of science, a kind of proto-science. While such parallels have their often severe limitations, it is nevertheless interesting to note the intercalary role played by spirits, demons, jinns and other comparable phenomena in religion and medicine. In addition to the Mozambiquan spirit pantheon serving psychotherapeutic ends described by Honwana, we have Conrad's and Wujastyk's portrayals of Islamic jinns and Indian demons respectively.

The ancient Indian texts analysed by Wujastyk refer to a widespread phenomenon found in many different parts of the world, namely the tendency to blame a mother for the illness of her young offspring, or its death or miscarriage. A mother or mother-to-be is enjoined to protect herself and her children from others' envy and evil, and against the demons who will punish her if they regard her as uncaring of the child or foetus. The focus in the myths discussed by Wujastyk is on child miscarriage. The demons responsible for it are listed, named and graphically illustrated in Sanskrit medical literature on care during pregnancy and child nurture. Demons commonly 'seize' the child or foetus, early symptoms of which are sometimes visible and require either medicine, better behaviour or worship on the part of the mother.

There is an amalgam here of practical and moral issues, for the mother's conduct as well as her devotion to the child's well-being is subject to judgement through the idiom of demonic scrutiny and punishment. In many African societies, similar problems of foetal and child health are ascribed to women's adultery or to their breast-feeding a young child after becoming pregnant again, but not normally through demomic attack, despite the prevalence in other contexts of possession by demons or spirits, as Honwana has described.

This onus of responsibility placed on women, in both the African and Indian cases, clearly distracts attention away from men's behaviour, and may be regarded as one of many recorded instances of male control. The more general classificatory use of demons or spirits, however, is part of an evolving explanatory structure accounting for bodily, mental and other misfortunes. It lays the ground for the possible, though not inevitable, development of empirically testable assertions. These are likely in due course to remove or lessen blame laid on women for miscarriages and the death and sickness of children, and instead mark out the special vulnerabilities of motherhood and child development. Regarded as the elements of an explanatory framework, the Indian demons contributed to an indigenous theory of mother and child care, extending into ethno-gynaecology.

Looked at also from a developmental viewpoint, Conrad discusses the challenges facing early Islam's insistence on the worship of the One, All-Powerful God. A major threat to this insistence on monotheism was the legacy of a pre-Islamic belief in fate and the machinations of demons and spirits, and in the prophylactics and medicines used against them. Destructive spirits, including those called jinns, constitute a pantheon of named forces and remain a major source of explanation of sickness and misfortune throughout the Islamic world. Belief and use of them is decried by many clerics, but, since they are described as real entities in the Quran and cannot be dismissed as fantasy and even include some which are helpful, they cannot be eliminated from popular epidemiology. As Conrad points out, the methods for avoiding or using jinns have their own internal logic. Indeed jinns and other spirits have become part of recent and modern explanations of contemporary afflictions, such as the plague and certain epidemics.

A key feature in the relationship between demons, spirits, spirit forces and gods on the one hand and humans on the other, is the way in which the former are to a greater or lesser extent personified, especially in having human-like emotions. The high gods of the Judaeo-Christian and Islamic traditions are generally held to be above such feelings, although the Old Testament Lord God was occasionally a wrathful or 'jealous God', as more often were the pantheistic deities of European antiquity, South Asia and Hinduism (see Wujastyk's descriptions and illustrations). Personifying deities or demons makes them more amenable to human ideas and possibilities of negotiation.

As Wear points out, an emotion like fear was worshipped as a god by the Lacedaemonians, just as, according to Conrad, disease contagion was regarded in Islam as a malevolent living willing being which had to be combated. Opulence is described in early Sanskrit myths as an ambivalent demoness-goddess (Wujastyk), while in Zoroastrianism demons included Violence, Fury, Greed, Wrath, Sloth and the essence of all evil, the Lie (Hinnells). In other words, demons/gods may be identified by their effects and their emotional and personality characteristics. Or such effects and emotions may personify and so constitute the being, the nominal here co-substantive with the consequence of being.

In early modern England, Wear describes the dilemma produced by the two Christian principles of self-preservation, permitting flight from the plague, and charity, requiring the fleeing rich to make provision for the urban poor obliged to stay in the city. Fear propelled flight from the city, but also gripped country residents who feared the contagion of the newly arrived Londonders, whatever their condition and status, extending to objects associated with them. With country people spurning even distant communication with Londoners, some commentators at the time condemned the exaggerated fears as causing lack of Christian charity to urban refugees.

Medically, however, exaggerated fear was seen not just as uncharitable but as itself pathological and likely to make the fear-gripped individual vulnerable to the plague. People were therefore encouraged to control their fears, the better to protect themselves, advice whose consequence might also maintain or restore social order. We are reminded here that a number of ethnographic accounts from Africa and Asia also describe how strong emotions of anger and fear make people vulnerable to sickness. Again, like destructive demons and spirits which must be thwarted, appeased or expunged, emotions can become agents in the propagation of affliction.

Conclusion

Western popular theories of disease causation often begin ontologically with an autonomous physical agent (person, virus, bacteria) acting contagiously upon other insufficiently resistant agents. Although a nod in the direction of emotional vulnerability is made, e.g. being 'run-down', this is still framed in terms of the militaristic metaphor of invader and invaded. Sometimes, beliefs in demons and other spirit forces (Western and non-Western) employ this same metaphor, and the cross-cultural similarity in folk systems may sometimes be greater than is commonly acknowledged.

What may perhaps be distinctive of the (mainly) non-Western medico-religious complexes described in this volume, however, is a readier acceptance of the idea that beings and their actions are mutually constituted. This is the idea, introduced at the beginning of this chapter, that materiality can be thought of not just as physical objects but as people's interactional densities and their socio-cultural understanding of these interactions, including the way they do or do not verbalise them.

Demons, gods and other spirit forces may cause or send sickness and misfortunes, but they are often inscribed within a wider cosmos of creation and becoming, with actions and traits conceptualised as entities, and, conversely, named beings identified by such behavioural features. But, in the end, it is humans who interpret. Thus, the spirits who destroy and harm humanity may sometimes be understood by indigenous religious specialists as co-substantive with humans who have abused other humans and their divine representatives, and so in effect are punishing themselves for their transgression.

In the case of *karmic* rebirth cycles, blame is always generationally deferred, so to speak, and the transformation of lives is normally from creature into creature. But there is even here the idea that one is made up in the present life of the actions and emotions of one's past which are prior to current agency and autonomous of it, even though their future course can be altered and present effects mitigated.

The many subtle variations in such cosmic materiality defy banal generalisation. Overall, however, they may be contrasted with bio-medical assumptions of physical agents acting upon each other independently of the human judgements, beliefs and objects that partly constitute them.

NOTES

1. Scheper-Hughes, N. and M. Lock. (1987). The mindful body: a prolegomena to future work in medical anthropology. *Medical Anthropology Quarterly*. 1: 6–41.
2. Marriott, M. (1987). Hindu transactions: diversity without dualism. In B. Kapferer. (ed.). *Transaction and meaning*. Philadelphia: Institute for the Study of Human Issues.
3. Bousfield, J. (1985). Good, evil and spiritual power: reflections of Sufi teachings. In D. Parkin. (ed.). *The anthropology of evil*. Oxford: Blackwell.
4. Ozawa, Chikako. (1997) (June). Naikan and Morita: Japanese indigenous psychotherapies. Research Paper. Institute of Social and Cultural Anthropology. University of Oxford.
5. Kuhn, T. S. 1970. *The structure of scientific revolution*. Chicago: University of Chicago Press.

INDEX

C

D

H

INDEX

I

J

K

L

U

V

W

CONTRIBUTORS

Dr Francesca Bray,
Dept of Anthropology, University of California,
Santa Barbara, CA 93106, USA

Dr John Cohen,
31 Fitzroy Square, London W1P 5HH

Lawrence I. Conrad
Wellcome Institute, 183 Euston Road, London NW1 2BE

Professor John Hinnells,
Dept of Study of Religions, SOAS, University of London,
Thornhaugh St., Russell Square, London WC1H 0XG

Dr Alcinda Honwana,
Dept of Anthropology, University of Cape Town,
Private Bag, RONDEBOSCH 7700, South Africa

Mr Peregrine Horden
Dept. of History, Royal Holloway,
University of London, Egham, TW20 0EX

Dr Helen King,
Dept of Classics, University of Reading, Whiteknights, POB 218,
Reading RG6 6AA

Dr Julia Leslie,
SOAS, University of London, Thornhaugh St., Russell Square,
London WC1H 0XG

CONTRIBUTORS

Professor Roland Littlewood,
Dept of Anthropology, University College London, Gower St.,
London WC1E 6BT

Mr David Melling,
Directorate, the Manchester Metropolitan University,
All Saints, Manchester M15 6BM

Professor David Parkin,
Institute of Social and Cultural Anthropolgy and
All Souls College, Oxford OX1 4AL

Professor Roy Porter,
Wellcome Institute for the History of Medicine, 183 Euston Road,
London NW1 2BE

Dr Carole Rawcliffe
Wellcome Unit for History of Medicine,
University of East Anglia, Norwich NR4 7TJ

Professor Abdulaziz Sachedina,
Dept of Religions Studies, Cocke Hall, University of Virginia,
Charlottsville, Va 22903, USA

Professor Mike Saks,
Faculty of Health & Community Studies, De Montfort University,
Scraptoft, Leicester LE7 9SU

Professor Geoffrey Samuel,
Dept of Religious Studies, University of Lancaster, Bailrigg,
Lancaster LA1 4YG

Dr Pashaura Singh,
Dept of Asian Languages & Cultures,
3070 Frieze Bldg, University of Michigan,
Ann Arbor, Mi 48109-1285, USA

Dr Tadeusz Skorupski,
SOAS, University of London,
Thornhaugh St., Russell Square,
London WC1H 0XG

Dr Norman Solomon,
Centre for Jewish & Hebrew Studies, Oxford Teaching Centre,
45 St Giles, Oxford OX1 3LP

Dr Andrew Wear,
Wellcome Institute for the History of Medicine, 183 Euston Road,
London NW1 2BE

Dr Dominik Wujastyk,
Wellcome Institute for the History of Medicine, 183 Euston Road,
London NW1 2BE